Dictionary of Medical Laboratory Sciences

Dictionary of
Medical Laboratory
Sciences

Edited by

A. D. FARR
BA PhD MBIM FIMLS

Published in association with the
Institute of Medical Laboratory Sciences

BLACKWELL
SCIENTIFIC PUBLICATIONS
OXFORD LONDON EDINBURGH
BOSTON PALO ALTO MELBOURNE

© 1988 by
Blackwell Scientific Publications
Editorial offices:
Osney Mead, Oxford OX2 0EL
(*Orders:* Tel. 0865 240201)
8 John Street, London WC1N 2ES
23 Ainslie Place, Edinburgh EH3 6AJ
52 Beacon Street, Boston
  Massachusetts 02108, USA
667 Lytton Avenue, Palo Alto
  California 94301, USA
107 Barry Street, Carlton
  Victoria 3053, Australia

First published 1988

Set by Setrite Typesetters Ltd., HK
Printed and bound in Great Britain by
  Mackays of Chatham PLC,
  Chatham, Kent

British Library
Cataloguing in Publication Data

Dictionary of medical laboratory sciences.
  1. Medical technology—Dictionaries
  I. Farr, A.D.
  610′.28   RB37
ISBN 0-632-01762-7

DISTRIBUTORS

USA
  Year Book Medical Publishers
  35 East Wacker Drive
  Chicago, Illinois 60601
  (*Orders:* Tel. 312 726-9733)

Canada
  The C.V. Mosby Company
  5240 Finch Avenue East,
  Scarborough, Ontario
  (*Orders:* Tel. 416-298-1588)

Australia
  Blackwell Scientific Publications
  (Australia) Pty Ltd
  107 Barry Street
  Carlton, Victoria 3053
  (*Orders:* Tel. (03) 347 0300)

Library of Congress
Cataloging in Publication Data

Dictionary of medical laboratory sciences.

  "Published in association with the
Institute of Medical Laboratory Sciences."
  1. Diagnosis, Laboratory—Dictionaries.
  2. Medical laboratory technology—
Dictionaries. I. Farr, A.D. (Alfred
Derek) II. Institute of Medical
Laboratory Sciences (Great Britain)
  [DNLM: 1. Laboratories—dictionaries.
  2. Technology, Medical—dictionaries,
  QY 13 D554]
  RB37.D525 1988   616.07′5   87−35785

ISBN 0-632-01762-7

Contributors

R.T. Allison MSc FIMLS

P. J. Avery BSc DPhil

R. Bayston MMedSci MSc PhD MIBiol FIMLS

C. H. N. Bennett JP ATh FIMLS

J. Bertrand FIMLS

D. M. Browning FIMLS

J. Cloke JP MBIM CMLM FIMLS

A. D. Farr BA PhD MBIM FIMLS

J. L. Francis PhD MIBiol FIMLS

R. Griffin MPhil MIBiol FIMLS

D. J. Rogers BA PhD MIBiol FIMLS

P. G. Sargeaunt AIMLS

Introduction

The term 'medical laboratory sciences' covers an ever-widening range of scientific work. A century ago, workers in the early medical laboratories practised only the well-recognised disciplines of (histo)-pathology and bacteriology, but during the course of the twentieth century many other 'disciplines' have appeared and, as a number of reasonably well-defined specialist subjects came to be recognised, laboratories also became specialised. In recent years, however, there has been an increasing tendency for the specialist subjects to overlap and today's entrant to this work – be (s)he scientifically or medically qualified – has the increasingly difficult task of talking the specialist language of many such 'disciplines' as laboratory practice expands into new areas.

Very broadly, the worker in today's medical laboratory requires, in addition to a good general education in biochemistry and the biological sciences, a familiarity with the language of biotechnology, bacteriology, cellular pathology, clinical chemistry, computing, cytology, haematology, immunology, microscopy (both light and electron), parasitology, statistics, transfusion science and virology. This **Dictionary** is an attempt to provide a guide to this specialised spectrum of scientific activity.

The **Dictionary of Medical Laboratory Sciences** contains approximately 3500 entries, mostly defining terms in use particularly in the medical laboratory. Definitions from the basic sciences – especially of well-understood terms – have been avoided unless they are commonly subject to misunderstanding, seem particularly apposite, or are frequently referred to in the other definitions in such a manner that a clear understanding of them is critical to the sense. Where it has been necessary to use a trade name as an entry, this is indicated by the comment℠.

A very small number of names of individuals who are of particularly great importance in the history of medical science have been included. Entries in these cases are restricted to the dates of birth and death and one or two sentences giving the salient details of that individual's nationality and major achievement(s) in medical science. Disease states have been included only where their investigation is a major part of clinical laboratory work.

Dictionaries are not generally regarded as literature to be read as continuous prose. However, the editor and the contributors hope that all medical scientists who use it will benefit by browsing through the definitions, as well as looking up particular words of whose meaning they may be unsure.

Arrangement of entries

Alphabeticisation Entries are in strict letter-by-letter alphabetical order, disregarding spaces between individual words, hyphenation, etc. Terms which begin with a numeric digit have that number included but are alphabeticised as though the number was not present (e.g. **2-mercaptoethanol** is entered as though it were **Mercaptoethanol**). Similarly, Greek characters are given in transliteration into English but are disregarded in alphabeticisation of the term (e.g. **(gamma) Globulin** will be found entered as though it were **Globulin**).

The common order of words is used rather than reversing them to place the noun before the adjective; for example, there is an entry for **Cuboidal cell**, *not* for **Cell, cuboidal**. Similarly, where a specific technique or test is referred to this is done directly and the words are not reversed to put (e.g.) 'Test' first. For example, there is an entry for **Compatibility test**, and *not* for **Test, compatibility**. (An exception to this rule is in the case of the few entries for eponyms, where the surname comes before the given name, e.g. **Landsteiner, Karl**).

Abbreviations These are cross-referenced to the full expression, which is where the definition will be be found. Exceptions to this are the abbreviated names of scientific bodies (e.g. **IMLS**), where the title spelled out in full is sufficient definition.

Spelling This conforms to the standard of the *Shorter Oxford English Dictionary*, and English usage is preferred to American (e.g. **Haemoglobin**, not Hemoglobin; endings in -ise and not -ize). The English diphthong is used (e.g. **Oestrogen**, not Estrogen). However, where this results in the American spelling appearing far removed alphabetically from the English version (as in the example above) a cross reference is made from the American spelling to the full entry under the English spelling. A particular exception to the common rule is **Fetus**, where this older English (not native American) spelling is preferred to Foetus.

Grammar The noun is generally preferred to the verb or any other form, and the singular to the plural (e.g. entries will refer to **Elution**, not Elute, and **Bacillus**, not Bacilli).

Alternatives When a word has two or more possible meanings these are indicated by separate numbers within the definition, the more common usage being given first. When a word has both a literal and a specialised meaning, both may be given.

General Words within a definition, which themselves appear as definitions elsewhere, are printed in bold type.

The Editor is well aware of the risk of errors, omissions and ambiguities occurring in any work of this type, and would regard it as a kindness if any reader detecting any of these faults, or wishing to suggest possible additions or alterations for the next edition, would write to him at the address below, bringing the matter to his attention.

Dr A. D. Farr
Tullochvenus House
Lumphanan
Aberdeenshire AB3 4RN
Scotland

A

Ab Abbreviation for **antibody**.

Abbe condenser In microscopy, a lens system (originally designed by Ernst Abbe) which controls the light reaching the object. The system suffers badly from **spherical aberration** and **chromatic aberration**.

Aberration 1. A deviation from normal. 2. Applied to optics, referring to defects in a lens or mirror, resulting in a distorted image. 3. In microscopy, a lens defect causing the non-convergence of light rays or electrons. See **Chromatic Aberration** and **Spherical Aberration**.

ABO blood group The first **blood group system** to be discovered and the most important in clinical practice. Everyone has on their red cells one or the other, or both or neither, of two **antigens** called A and B; those who possess neither are called group O. The **plasma** contains an **antibody** against whichever of the A or B antigens is lacking from the red cells. **Transfusion** of ABO **incompatible** blood leads to severe, often fatal, **haemolytic** reactions.

Abortion The non-living product of pregnancy delivered before the period of fetal viability. In Britain this is legally set at 28 weeks gestation.

Abrasive Particulate material used in **histology** for knife sharpening. Particle size may be denoted by a two-figure system, the first figure indicating <5% of particles exceeding that figure in **microns**; the second indicates the percentage of particles present finer than one micron. Hardness also varies.

Abscess A collection of **pus** and **oedema** fluid in a space bounded by dead tissue and coagulated **exudate**. Generally this results in local swelling, heat, pain and erythema, but cold abscesses − typically caused by *Mycobacterium tuberculosis* − do not.

Absolute values The mathematical expression of **erythrocyte** volume and **haemoglobin** content calculated from the results of the red cell count, haemoglobin concentration and **packed cell volume**:

$$\text{Mean Cell Volume (MCV)} = \frac{\text{PCV} \times 1000}{\text{RBC } (\times 10^6/\text{l})}$$

$$\text{Mean Cell Haemoglobin (MCH)} = \frac{\text{Haemoglobin (g/l)}}{\text{RBC } (\times 10^6/\text{l})}$$

$$\text{Mean Cell Haemoglobin Concentration (MCHC)} = \frac{\text{Hb (g/dl)}}{\text{PCV}}$$

Absorbance The amount of incident light absorbed within a medium, as in a **spectrophotometer**. It is related to the number of absorbing particles in the medium.

Absorption The removal or assimilation of a substance from a solution. In serology, the removal from a serum of an **antibody** by permitting it to come into contact with the **antigen** for which it is specific, generally carried on red cells which also lack the antigens for which any other antibodies in the serum are specific. (From the Latin *ab* = from). See also **Adsorption**.

Acanthamoeba A free-living amoeba found in soil and water. It may cause a necrotic **encephalitis** in animals, and **granulomas** and corneal ulceration in man. Occasionally, disseminated fatal disease is seen in the **immunocompromised** patient. It is susceptible to **Miconazole**, Pentamidine and **Polymyxin** B, but not to **Amphotericin**. See also **Naegleria**.

Acanthrocyte A type of **erythrocyte** showing coarse **crenation** and varying numbers of spiky projections. These cells may occur as an inherited abnormality in association with abnormal phospholipid metabolism. Similar cells may also be observed following splenectomy, and in patients with liver cirrhosis.

ACB Association of Clinical Biochemists. Founded 1953.

Accelerating voltage The high voltage used to accelerate electrons from an **electron gun**.

Accentuator A substance which increases the **selectivity** or the staining power of a **dye** which is already capable of staining. They do not act as **mordants**, nor form **lakes** with the dye, neither do they take part in any obvious chemical union (e.g. phenol in carbol fuchsin).

Accuracy The extent of the relationship of a set of values to the true value. In clinical chemistry this true value is not always known, although concensus values will often give an indication of accuracy.

ACD See **Acid Citrate Dextrose**.

Acetylation A method of blocking 1:2 glycol groups, usually by treatment with acetic anhydride, so that they cannot be oxidised by periodic acid, thus giving a negative **PAS** reaction. Acetylation is reversible by treatment with potassium hydroxide (**saponification**).

Acetyl cholinesterase (EC 3.1.1.7) A red cell enzyme sometimes known as 'specific' or 'true' cholinesterase, which acts on esters of choline to give choline and acetic acid. Acetyl cholinesterase plays an important role in the physiology of the nervous system and is found in high concentrations at the **motor end plates**. It is directed against acetyl beta-methyl choline but almost ineffective against benzoylcholine, and is often reduced in patients with **paroxysmal nocturnal haemoglobinuria** (PNH).

Acetyl methyl carbinol Also known as Acetoin, this is the neutral precursor of 2,3-butamediol, an end product of glucose fermentation. The precursor is detected in the **Voges-Proskauer test**, which is used in the identification of **Enterobacteriaceae** and some other organisms.

n-Acetyl neuraminic acid A sialic acid found in all mammalian sera. It is an inhibitor of the **haemagglutinin** of **orthomyxovirus** and some **paramyxoviruses**, being removed from **serum** by treatment with **neuraminidase**.

Acetylphenylhydrazine An oxidant chemical capable of producing **Heinz bodies** in red cells. The greater susceptibility of red cells deficient in **glucose 6-phosphate dehydrogenase** to the action of this chemical forms the basis of the Heinz body provocation test.

Acholeplasma A **micro-organism** which is a member of the class **Mollicutes** and which, unlike its fellow member **Mycoplasma**, does not need sterol for growth. These organisms do not possess a cell wall and will pass through bacterial filters. The species responsible for human infections is *A. laidlawii*, which is resistant to **penicillins** and **cephalosporins**, but susceptible to other **anti-microbial** substances, including **Erythromycin**.

Achromat Describes a lens system constructed to correct for the principal **chromatic aberration** (i.e. when blue and red rays fail to come to a common focus). Applicable to both condensing and objective lenses.

Achromobacter An obsolete term for organisms now placed variously in the genera **Alcaligenes**, **Acinetobacter** and **Pseudomonas**.

Acid A compound which dissociates to produce available hydrogen ions when in solution, and acts as a proton donor.

Acid Citrate Dextrose An **anticoagulant**/preservative solution used for collection of blood intended for **transfusion** and consisting of 20 g/l disodium citrate and 25 g/l dextrose.

Acid dye A **dye** which carries a negative charge ($^-$): a coloured acid radicle which attaches to a basic tissue component. For example, the acid dye eosin stains the basic **protein** of **cytoplasm**.

Acid fastness The property of a substance (or, more usually, an organism) of failing to be decolourised when **stained** with hot carbol fuchsin and then exposed to a mixture of ethanol and an aqueous dilution of a mineral **acid** such as sulphuric acid. The **Ziehl-Neelsen stain** is used to determine this property. No practical distinction can be made between fastness to acid-alcohol and to acid alone. *Mycobacterium tuberculosis* is strongly acid fast, and **Nocardia** weakly so, with most other organisms being non-acid-fast.

Acid formaldehyde haematin See **Formalin pigment**.

Acid mucopolysaccharide A definition in **histochemistry** of carboxylated and sulphated polysaccharides which are **PAS** negative and found in connective tissue. Carboxylated glycoproteins are excluded.

Acidophilia The property of tissues which, by **salt linkage** and ionic binding, stain with **acid dyes**.

Acidosis An increase in the **hydrogen ion concentration** in blood. In uncompensated states acidosis will result in a change in the **pH** value. It can occur as a result of respiratory or metabolic disturbance.

Acid phosphatase A non-specific phosphatase representing a phosphomonoesterase which is active at a low **pH** value. It hydrolyses para-nitrophenyl phosphate and, although found widely in body tissues (e.g. liver, kidney, **erythrocytes**, phosphate, etc.), acid phosphatase levels are used to diagnose and monitor **carcinoma** of the prostate. Non-prostatic acid phosphatases are easily inactivated.

Acid serum test A diagnostic test for **paroxysmal nocturnal haemoglobinuria** (PNH) in which the patient's red cells are suspended in normal plasma which has been acidified to a **pH** of $6.5-7.0$. Red blood cells from patients with PNH **haemolyse** under these conditions, whereas normal red cells do not.

Acid stability test A procedure involving the **incubation** of **virus** suspensions of known concentration in media of various **pH** for fixed periods of time. Acid-labile viruses survive poorly at pH 5.0 or lower, as indicated by a 100-fold or greater loss of activity compared with suspensions incubated at neutral pH. Classically, the method is used to distinguish between acid-labile **rhinoviruses** and acid-stable **enteroviruses**.

Acinetobacter A **bacterium** of the family **Neisseria**, differing from the other members in being **oxidase** negative. While exhibiting **pleomorphism** it is usually rod-shaped. It does not exhibit **motility** and is a strict **aerobe**. Some strains oxidise glucose, but generally carbohydrates are not oxidised or fermented. Occasionally, serious infections are caused in **immunocompromised** patients. The organism is resistant to **beta-lactams** but usually susceptible to **aminoglycosides**.

Acinus See **Alveolus**.

Acoustic coupler A device which converts audible tones from a telephone into digital signals which can be read by a **microcomputer**.

ACP Association of Clinical Pathologists. Founded 1927.

Acquired antigen In **transfusion science**, a **blood group** antigen which is not the result of genetic determination but which appears on cell surfaces as a result of a disease process. (e.g. A B-like antigen sometimes appears on the red cells of group A individuals suffering from carcinoma of the rectum).

4

Acquired Immune Deficiency Syndrome A disease in which the body's **immune response** is rendered ineffective by infection with a **retrovirus** known as **HIV**. The patient has (1) a reliably diagnosed disease that is at least moderately indicative of an underlying cellular **immunodeficiency**, (2) no known underlying cause of cellular immune deficiency, nor any other cause of reduced resistance reported to be associated with that disease, and (3) an **antibody** directed against HIV.

Acquired immunity An **immune** state which develops in response to exposure to foreign materials such as **vaccines, micro-organisms** or tissues.

Acridine orange A **dye**, a **fluorochrome** derivative of acridine which binds to nucleic acids. Under **ultraviolet light**, double-stranded nucleic acids appear green and single-stranded molecules orange. The dye is useful for revealing aberrant distribution of nucleic acids in cells.

Acromegaly A **chronic** disease resulting from hyperfunction of the pituitary and secretion of growth **hormone**. Classically, patients present with an increase in size of the viscera, the soft parts and some bones − particularly the short and flat bones − without an increase in height. The hands, feet and face show the most change.

ACTH Abbreviation of adrenocorticotropic **hormone**. See **Corticotrophin**.

Actinobacillus. A group of bacteria which are negative by **Gram's stain**, fermentative, **oxidase** positive, do not exhibit **motility**, and are facultative **anaerobes**. Very sticky colonies are produced on some **culture media**. Diseases such as joint-ill are produced in animals and the organism is sometimes found associated with **Actinomyces** in lesions in man.

Actinomyces Rod-shaped bacteria, staining positive with **Gram's stain** and usually branched, not forming **spores** nor exhibiting **motility**, and not **acid fast**. They are usually **anaerobic** on first cultivation, becoming **microaerophilic**. Products of carbohydrate fermentation do not include propionic acid. These organisms are widespread in animals and man, predominantly as normal flora but *Actinomyces bovis* causes disease in cattle and *A. israeli* and others cause disease in man. Generally, **abscesses** are produced in bone and soft tissue, with **chronic** draining sinuses to the exterior. Sulphur granules are found in the **exudate**. Treatment consists of surgical drainage or excision, together with large doses of **penicillin** for several weeks or months.

Actinomyces bovis Probably the most common of six species in the genus Actinomyces. The morphology in disease tissue is of a long branching mycelium with attached 'sulphur granules'. It is found colonising the oral cavity, tonsillar crypts, and dental plaque. It is now known to be linked with pelvic actinomycosis in females using intrauterine devices.

Activated lymphocyte A **lymphocyte** in mitosis, a state of **differentiation** or proliferation in response to exposure to an **antigen** or **mitogen**. Such cells may produce **antibody**, take part in **cell-mediated immunity**, or produce **lymphokines**.

Activated macrophage A **macrophage** in a heightened state of activity following exposure to **antigen, adjuvant**, or soluble substances such as **macrophage activating factor** released by **T lymphocytes**.

Activated Partial Thromboplastin Time Test (APTT) A screening test for the **intrinsic coagulation** system in which **plasma** is incubated with a **platelet substitute** and an appropriate activator (e.g. kaolin) to promote **contact activation**. The test is also known as the **kaolin cephalin clotting time**.

Activator An inorganic co-factor which enhances the activity of a particular **enzyme** to its maximum.

Active immunity An **immunity** arising as a result of exposure to **antigen**, e.g. by vaccination or **infection**.

Acute 1. Sharp. 2. (Of a disease state), having a short and severe course.

Acute leukaemia A malignant proliferation of leucocytes, which may be of myeloid (**myeloblastic**), lymphoid (**lymphoblastic**) or monocytoid (**monoblastic**) origin. The disease is characterised by the presence of relatively large numbers of **blast cells** in the peripheral blood and/or bone marrow, and an acute − often fatal − course.

Acute phase protein A protein which is non-**immunoglobulin** in nature and which appears, or increases in concentration, in the **plasma** following **infection** or tissue damage, e.g. **C-reactive protein** or **fibrinogen**.

Acyclovir An **anti-viral drug**, more properly called acycloguanisine, and active against **Herpes simplex virus** and **Varicella/zoster virus**. Its anti-viral activity is promoted by the action of viral **thymidine kinase**.

ADCC See **Antibody Dependent Cell-mediated Cytotoxicity**.

Addison's disease This is caused by primary adrenocortical hypofunction. It is characterised by several biochemical changes which include hypoglycaemia, **acidosis**, hyponatraemia, high levels of **serum** urea and low levels of **cortisol**.

Address In computing, a number which identifies the position of an item of data in the computer's **memory**.

Adenine 6-Aminopurine, a purine base constituent of both **DNA**

and **RNA**. Used as an additive to some **anticoagulant**/preservative solutions for the collection of blood for **transfusion**, to retard **glycolysis**.

Adenoacanthoma A **malignant tumour** developing from glandular **epithelium** and showing a **benign** form of **squamous metaplasia** in addition to the architecture of **adenocarcinoma**.

Adenocarcinoma A **carcinoma** developed from glandular **epithelium**.

Adenoma A **benign neoplasm** with a gland-like structure.

Adenomatosis A condition characterised by diffuse overgrowth of glandular **epithelium**.

Adenosine diphosphate In **haematology** the main use of this adenine nucleotide is as a **platelet aggregation** reagent. See **Platelet aggregation**.

Adenosine triphosphate The major source of energy for blood cells produced, via the **Embden-Mayerhof pathway**, from glucose.

Adenosis A **hyperplasia** of ducts and acini of the breast.

Adenoviridae A large family of icosahedral non-**enveloped** DNA viruses 70—90 nm in diameter, with 252 **capsomeres**. The vertices of the **icosahedron** carry type-specific fibre **antigens**. There are two genera, one of which (mastadenovirus) affects man. They are asociated with both **endemic** and **epidemic** upper respiratory tract infections, **conjunctivitis** and **gastroenteritis**. Most of the numerous **serotypes** grow readily in a variety of **cell cultures**. The recently identified enteric serotypes are difficult to grow *in vitro*, but are readily seen by **electron microscopy**. Serological diagnosis utilises a group-specific antigen in a **complement-fixation test**.

Adenyl cyclase In **platelets**, this membrane-bound enzyme catalases the conversion of **adenosine triphosphate** to **cyclic AMP** (adenosine monophosphate), which inhibits **platelet aggregation**.

Adhesin A substance or structure borne by an organism, which facilitates its **adhesion** to surfaces. Examples of structural adhesins are p-**pili** of uropathogenic *Escherichia coli*. Slime is considered to promote adhesion of **coagulase**-negative **staphylococci** to catheters.

Adhesion The reversible or irreversible attachment of **microorganisms** to surfaces. Gonococci adhere to urethral **epithelium** by means of **pili**, which have a high affinity for glycolipids on the cell surface. **Coagulase**-negative **staphylococci** adhere to catheters, primarily as a result of electrostatic and other physicochemical forces mediated by cell surface **proteins** and carbohydrates.

Adhesive In **histology**, a substance used to improve the union between tissue section and slide. Particularly valuable in **ammoniacal silver** staining and **immunocytochemistry**. Examples are egg albumin, **chrome gelatin**, and poly-lysine.

Adipose tissue A layer of tissue in which fat is stored or deposited.

Adjuvant A substance which delays dispersal of immunogenic material injected into a living body, so that continuous slow exposure to the **immunogen** causes a maximal **antibody** response in relation to minimal doses of immunogen.

ADP See **Adenosine di-phosphate**.

Adrenal chromaffin Dark brown granular material derived from adrenalin and noradrenalin and found in cells of the adrenal medulla following **fixation** in chrome salts – the **chromaffin reaction**. A tumour of these cells is termed a phaeochromocytoma.

Adrenaline See **Epinephrine**.

Adrenogenital syndrome A series of inherited diseases in which there is a block in the formation of adrenal **corticosteroids**. There is thus no feedback to the pituitary and hypothalamus glands.

Adsorption Taking up and retention. In serology, the taking up of an **antibody** onto the surface of (e.g.) red cells. (From the Latin *ad* = towards). See also **Absorption**.

Adventitious virus A contaminant **virus**, present by chance in a **cell culture** or virus preparation. Live animals, fertile eggs and cultures of animal cells may become contaminated, interfering with laboratory procedures.

Advisory Committee on Dangerous Pathogens An expert committee set up by the United Kingdom government to advise the Health and Safety Executive and all scientists on matters concerning **infectious** diseases. The committee is responsible for the classification of known and newly-discovered agents into categories according to risk, and for recommending levels of containment for each **risk group of pathogens**. The committee is also available to give advice in the event of an outbreak of serious disease.

Aerobe A **micro-organism** which grows optimally in air. Aerobic growth involves the production of energy by transfer of electrons to molecular oxygen. Most aerobic organisms produce **catalase**. The majority, which utilise **cytochrome oxidase**, are inhibited by potassium cyanide. Facultative aerobes are those **anaerobes** which can also grow in the presence of oxygen.

Aerococcus A **bacterium**, a member of the family Streptococcaceae. The organism is **microaerophilic** and **catalase** negative, although some strains appear to be weakly positive. Tetrads of cocci are produced in liquid **culture media**, and greening **haemolysis** is produced on blood **agar**. *Aerococcus viridans*, the only species, is occasionally responsible for human infections, including **endocarditis**.

Aeromonas A bacterium, a member of the family Vibrionaceae. This rod-shaped organism is **oxidase** positive, exhibits **motility**, is **catalase** negative, ferments sugars, is negative with **Gram's stain**

and occurs widely in watery habitats. Some species are responsible for disease in fish. A hydrophiloa is associated with human cases of **diarrhoea** and may produce **enterotoxin**.

Aerosol A spray of minute fluid particles generated naturally by coughs and sneezes. In the laboratory, aerosols are generated particularly by **centrifugation** and use of **pipettes** with aqueous suspensions. Whole blood, **plasma** and **serum** are too viscous to generate good aerosols.

Aetiology The underlying pathology of a disease, especially the cause.

Affinitin Originally a synonym for **lectin**. In **histochemistry** it may now be applied to agents for visualising certain **immunocyto-chemical** reactions (e.g. **biotin-avidin**; **protein A**-immunoglobulin G).

Affinity The strength of binding between an **antibody** and an **antigen**. It can be measured by techniques such as fluorescence quenching or equilibrium dialysis, and reflected by the equilibrium constant for the reaction.

Affinity chromatography A preparative technique in which a specific substance (e.g. **antigen**) is first immobilised on a gel, resin or plastic surface. This prepared material is then exposed to a heterogenous mixture of molecules (e.g. **immunoglobulins** in **serum**). Specific molecules in the heterogenous mixture will bind to the immobilised substance and can subsequently be recovered in purified form.

Affinity labelling A technique for identifying specific amino acids in the **Fab** region of the **immunoglobulin** molecule, which bind to a particular **hapten**. **Antibody** is exposed to chemically-modified radioactive hapten, which binds to the Fab region of the immunoglobulin and subsequently forms covalent bonds with specific amino acids. Hydrolysis of the complex enables identification of the peptide responsible for hapten binding.

Afibrinogenaemia The total absence of **fibrinogen** in the **plasma**. It may be either congenital or acquired.

Ag Abbreviation for **Antigen**.

Agammaglobulinaemia Literally, a condition in which there is a complete absence of circulating **gamma globulins**. Almost always there are some traces of gamma globulins, however, and the term **hypogammaglobulinaemia** is more appropriate.

Agar A complex sulphonated polysaccharide made from certain seaweeds. Agar is not metabolised by **bacteria** and is used as a constituent of **culture media** to confer the characteristics of a gel. It melts at about 100°C and gels at temperatures below about 45°C. Various grades are available, giving different gel strengths, and media can be made stiff or semi-solid by varying the agar concentration. See also **Agarose**.

Agarose The neutral fraction of **agar**, which causes gelling and which is used in **electrophoresis** and **immunodiffusion**.

Agglutination A reaction in which cells are clumped together by the action of an **antibody** active against an **antigen** carried on the cell surface.

Agglutinin An **antibody** which reacts with cells carrying a particular **antigen** to cause **agglutination**.

Agglutinogen An **antigen** (in **blood group** serology, usually carried on red cells) which will react with a specific **agglutinin** to form **agglutinates**.

Aggregometer An instrument for measuring **platelet aggregation** by either optical or electrical impedance techniques.

AHG Anti-human globulin. An **antibody** directed against human **globulins**.

AIDS See **Acquired Immune Deficiency Syndrome**.

AIHA See **Autoimmune haemolytic anaemia**.

AIMLS Associate of the Institute of Medical Laboratory Sciences. See **IMLS**.

AIPS Acronym for 'AIDS-induced panic syndrome', a term coined by a Sunday newspaper to describe widespread irrational fear of the **Acquired Immune Deficiency Syndrome** (AIDS), arising from ignorance of the very restricted mode of spread of the disease and the relatively low infectivity of the **virus**.

Airy disc In microscopy, describes the diffraction pattern of a series of light and dark concentric rings when viewing an illuminated hole in an opaque film. The hole is not imaged as a single bright spot due to the waveform nature of the light.

Alanine aminotransferase Aminotransferases are **enzymes** which catalyse reactions in which an amino group is transferred from an amino acid to an alpha-oxo acid. Alanine aminotransferase in the liver catalyses alanine and alpha-oxoglutarate to pyruvate and glutamate. The enzyme is widely spread in tissue with the highest concentration being found in the liver.

Albumin A readily soluble group of **proteins** found abundantly in many animal and vegetable tissues. In **blood group** serology this usually refers to Fraction V of the Cohn separation of bovine serum albumin, which is generally used in a suspension of between 20% and 30%.

Albustix™ A plastic urine test strip which has an absorbent area at one end, impregnated with tetrabromophenol blue **buffered** at **pH** 3·5. The stick is dipped into urine and the presence of **albumin** indicated by a change in the indicator to green.

Alcaligenes A group of bacteria which are **aerobic, oxidase** positive, **catalase** positive rods exhibiting **motility** and not producing acid from carbohydrates in conventional **culture media**. They often produce a strong fruity odour, and can utilise various organic acids. They are widely distributed in nature.

Alcoholic hyaline A proteinaceous amorphous eosinophilic type of aggregate found in liver cells in alcoholic **hepatitis**, and which stains positively with luxol fast blue. Also known as a **Mallory body**.

Aldosterone Aldosterone is formed from **progesterone** in the adrenal cortex and has the effect of regulating the transport of ions across cellular **membranes**, particularly in the renal tubule. Increases in concentration cause the kidney to retain sodium and excrete potassium and hydrogen ions.

Aleukaemia The term given to the finding that there are no leukaemic cells in the peripheral blood of a patient with acute **leukaemia**.

Alexin Obsolete term originally used to describe thermolabile substances in **serum** which are now called **Complement**.

Algorithm A series of well-defined instructions or operations which comprise a procedure for solving a mathematical problem.

Aliquot One of a number of equally sized portions into which a substance (usually a liquid) may be divided. (Note: aliquot is a noun, i.e. a thing; there is no verb 'to aliquot').

Alkaline denaturation test A test used for the demonstration and measurement of **fetal haemoglobin** (HbF), utilising the fact that HbF is more resistant to denaturation by alkali than is normal haemoglobin (HbA). See **Kleihauer test**.

Alkaline haematin method A method of measuring **haemoglobin** in which blood is added to sodium hydroxide and heated in a boiling water bath. The colour is compared with that of the **Gibson and Harrison standard**.

Alkaline phosphatase A non-specific phosphatase representing phosphomonoesterase, and which is active at high **pH** values. It hydrolyses para-nitrophenyl phosphate and is found widely in body tissues. It is used particularly to diagnose and monitor the treatment of liver and bone disease.

Alkalosis A decrease in **hydrogen ion concentration** in blood. When uncompensated it results in a rise in the **pH** value. It usually occurs as a result of a metabolic disturbance.

Alkaptonuria The **excretion** in urine of homogentisic acid. This is due to an **inborn error of metabolism** and a lack of the **enzyme** homogentisate oxidase. This results in a failure to convert homogentisic acid to 4-maleyacetoacetic acid.

11

Alkylating agent   One of a group of chemotherapeutic drugs useful in anti-tumour therapy. The most commonly used compounds are nitrogen mustard, chlorambucil, cyclophosphamide, busulphan and melphalan.

Allele   One of a number of alternative **genes** which may occupy a given position on a **chromosome**. Alleles occupy the same relative positions on each of a pair of **homologous** chromosomes.

Allelomorph   See **Allele**.

Allergen   An **antigen** capable of producing a **hypersensitivity** (allergy), stimulating and reacting with an **antibody** of the **IgE** class.

Allergy   A **hypersensitivity** to particular **antigens**. The term is most usually applied to **immediate hypersensitivity**.

Allo-   A prefix word. Pertaining to another of the same type, within the same species.

Allo-antibody   An **antibody** produced in response to an **antigen** from the same species of animal.

Allogenic   Genetically different, but of the same species.

Allograft   A graft from one individual to another of the same species. The two individuals involved are genetically dissimilar. See **Transplantation**.

Allotype   Genetically determined **antigens** which vary in different individuals of the same species. The antigens are located on **proteins** (e.g. **Gm** groups on human **IgG**).

Alpha chain   The **heavy chain** of IgA.

Alpha fetoprotein   An **oncofetal antigen** which may be present in the blood of individuals with hepatic **carcinoma**.

Alphanumeric   A series of characters comprising both letters and numbers.

Alpha virus   A genus of the **virus** family of **Togaviridae**, which includes some important **pathogens**. None occur naturally in Britain. They are transmitted to man and animals by **mosquitoes** (**Anophiline** or Culicine) and are **zoonotic** in man.

ALT   See **Alanine aminotransferase**.

Alternative pathway   A pathway for the activation of **complement** components C3 to C9, without the involvement of components C1, C4 or C2. It is occasionally called the **properdin** pathway, since this **protein** is an integral part of it.

Alum haematoxylin   A complex formed between aluminium salts and **haematein**, the coloured oxidation product of **haematoxylin**, and the most common nuclear oversight method in **histology**. The aluminium salt, which acts as a **mordant**, may be replaced by other metallic salts for special purposes.

Aluminium hydroxide   Widely used in **blood coagulation** studies to absorb **coagulation factors** II, VII, IX and X selectively from **plasma**.

Alveolar cell carcinoma Terminal bronchial **carcinoma**. A localised malignant **tumour** of the lung affecting the cells lining the **alveoli**.

Alveolus A general term used to designate a small sac-like dilatation, particularly one found in various glands. (Plural = alveoli.)

Amastigote Also known as a Leishman-Donovan body. A small, conspicuous, rounded intracellular organism which is the definitive organism of both visceral and cutaneous **Leishmaniasis**. Amastigotes also occur as part of the life cycle of the **Trypanosomatidae**. See **Kala-azar**.

Amato body See **Dohle body**.

Amboceptor An obsolete term for an **antibody** used in a sub-agglutinating dose to sensitise sheep **erythrocytes** for use in a **complement fixation test**.

Ameloblast Specialist secretory cell which produces the ground substance of **enamel**. Derived from odontogenic **epithelium**.

Amenorrhoea Absence, or normal cessation, of menstruation. In primary amenorrhoea the woman has never menstruated; secondary amenorrhoea is cessation of menstruation in a woman who has formerly menstruated.

Amidolytic assay An assay based on cleavage of an amide bond. See **Chromogenic substrate**.

Amikacin An **aminoglycoside** related to **Kanamycin A**. It is more stable to inactivating **enzymes** than most other aminoglycosides because of its side chain.

Amino acid A type of organic molecule which contains at least one carboxyl group (COOH) and at least one amino group (NH_2). They are **amphoteric**. Commonly referred to as the building blocks of **proteins**, they are essential constituents of animal tissues.

Aminoglycoside A group of **anti-microbial** substances consisting of over twenty members and produced naturally by **actinomycetes** – with the exception of **Amikacin** and **Netilmicin**, which are semi-synthetic. They are **bactericidal** due to irreversible binding to the **ribosome**. Resistant organisms usually produce **enzymes** which acetylate, phosphorylate or adenylylate the drugs, and such resistance is **plasmid**-mediated. Aminoglycosides are generally active against bacteria which are positive by **Gram's stain**, with the exception of **enterococci** and **aerobic** Gram-negative rods. **Anaerobic** bacteria are usually resistant. Aminoglycosides are all (to varying extents) toxic to the kidney and to the hair cells of the ear.

Aminoglycoside-modifying enzymes These consist of acetyl-transferases (AAC), phospho-transferases (APH) and nucleotidyl-transferases (ANT). There are several **enzymes** in each class: three in AAC (2', 6', 3); five in APH (3', 2″, 3″, 6, 5″); and four in ANT (2″, 4', 3″{a}, 9). **Aminoglycosides** vary in their susceptibi-

13

lity, so that **streptomycin** is susceptible to APH 3″ and 6, and ANT 3″{a}; and tobramycin is susceptible to AAC 2′, 6′ and 3, APH 2″, and ANT 2″ and 4′. These enzymes are **plasmid**-mediated.

5-Aminolaevulinic acid (ALA) A precursor of **porphobilinogen**, which is converted by the **enzyme** ALA-dehydrase to form porphobilinogen.

p-Aminosalicylic acid This derivative of salicylic acid was discovered as a result of a systematic search for anti-**tuberculosis** drugs. It is known to inhibit folate synthesis by functioning as a competitive analogue, thus blocking purine synthesis; though it might also inhibit the synthesis of **mycobactin**. *Mycobacterium tuberculosis* is susceptible, but other mycobacteria are not. Resistance is due to inactivation by the organism and to alteration of the target **enzyme** system.

Ammoniacal silver Silver solutions of varied composition, but usually containing silver nitrate precipitated with sodium hydroxide and redissolved by the critical addition of ammonia. Used in **histopathology** in metallic **impregnation** methods, especially for demonstration of nerves and **reticulin** fibres, and in clinical chemistry in a colorimetric test for melanogens in urine. Ammoniacal silver solutions should always be freshly prepared, as storage or exposure to light may lead to the formation of readily explosive compounds within the solution.

Ammonium molybdate A heavy metal **negative stain** used in **electron microscopy** to visualise **viruses** in suspension.

Amniocentesis A procedure in which amniotic fluid is aspirated from a pregnant uterus for subsequent laboratory examination. Mostly used for diagnosis of chromosomal abnormalities, inborn errors of metabolism, and assessment of severity of **haemolytic disease of the newborn**.

Amniotic fluid The albuminous fluid that surrounds, and helps to protect, the fetus in the amniotic sac. The volume varies from 500 to 1500 ml. Early in gestation the fluid is clear and sightly alkaline, becoming cloudy during the pregnancy. The fetus excretes urine into the fluid, which can be tapped using the procedure of **amniocentesis** to enable laboratory investigation to aid pre-term diagnosis and monitoring of conditions affecting the fetus (e.g. **haemolytic disease of the newborn**).

Amoebiasis Infection with *Entamoeba histolytica*, causing dysentry with excess mucus and some blood; liver involvement may occur. Haematophagus **trophozoites** can be demonstrated in the exudate.

Amoeboid Describes elastic movement and production of pseudopodia by living amoebae.

Amorphous Without form or shape, and showing no visible differentiation in structure.

Amoxycillin A **beta-lactam antibiotic** similar to **Ampicillin**, but with the advantage of improved intestinal absorption.

Amphophilic Exhibiting **cyanophilia** and **eosinophilia** in staining of the **cytoplasm** of the same cell.

Amphoteric Describes a compound which can serve as acid (proton donor) or base (proton acceptor) depending on the **hydrogen ion concentration** of the solution. **Proteins** and **amino acids** are examples.

Amphotericin B A **polyene** anti-fungal substance produced by *Streptomyces nodosus*. It acts on **fungi** by forming complexes with ergosterol in the **membrane** of cells, so causing increased permeability to electrolytes. Most fungi (with the exception of the **Dermatophytes**) are susceptible, and resistance to it develops only rarely. Some **protozoa** are also susceptible. The drug is extremely toxic, producing a variety of effects such as vomiting, hyperthermia, anaemia, impaired renal function, Parkinsonism and cardiac arrest.

Ampicillin A semi-synthetic **penicillin**, similar to **Amoxycillin**. It is active against both Gram-positive and Gram-negative non-**beta lactamase** producing organisms, including most strains of **enterococci**.

Amylase (EC 3.2.1.1) A group of **enzymes** that hydrolyse alpha-1,4-glucosidic links in polysaccharides such as starch. Amylase is secreted by the pancreas and salivary glands and levels are greatly raised in acute pancreatitis. In **histopathology** it is used to remove glycogen from tissue sections, and as a negative control in **PAS** and Best's carmine stains. See **Diastase**.

Amyloid Amorphous extracellular material consisting of **beta-pleated sheet** protein fibrils and a globular glycoprotein-p-component. Occurs most commonly as a result of chronic inflammatory disease (type AA) but may also be primary (AL), familial (AF), senile (AS) or endocrine (AE) in origin. Shows characteristic discrete fibrils by **electron microscopy**.

Anaemia A condition in which the amount of haemoglobin, or the number of red cells, in the circulation is reduced significantly below that which is normal.

Anaerobe An organism which produces optimal growth in the absence of oxygen. Oxidation of **substrates** uses inorganic nitrates, sulphates and others as final electron acceptors. Facultative anaerobes are those **aerobes** which can also grow in the absence of oxygen.

Anaerobic jar A container constructed of metal or polypropylene, in such a way that its walls can withstand both positive and negative pressures, and with an air-tight closure. One or more valves enable a vacuum to be drawn and the air to be replaced by

15

an inert gas such as nitrogen or nitrogen-hydrogen-carbon dioxide mixtures. A platinised catalyst is incorporated within the jar so that any residual oxygen can be converted to water by combining with the hydrogen in the replacement gas. Alternatively, a commercially available sachet can be used to generate the gaseous atmosphere inside the jar. It is used for the isolation of **anaerobes**.

Analogue 1. Something which corresponds to another thing in structure and function, but is of a different origin, for example a chemical compound that closely resembles another in structure (e.g. many **anti-viral** agents are **nucleotide** analogues). 2. Continuously variable. An analogue signal is a continuously variable signal, such as an electrical quantity. See **Digital**.

Analysis of variance In statistics, a method used mainly to compare the **means** of several groups of observations, (e.g. treatment groups and **blocks**). It is also used in the calculation of **regression**. It assumes approximately **normally distributed** observations, and approximately equals **variance** within groups.

Anamnestic response Heightened **antibody** response produced as a result of a second or subsequent exposure of an individual to the same (or a similar) **antigen**. Sometimes, colloquially, called the memory response.

Anaphase The stage in **mitosis** following **metaphase**. The halves of the divided **chromosomes** move apart toward the opposite poles of the spindle, each towards one of the asters.

Anaphylactic shock A profound state of generalised shock following injection of an allergen by any route which causes it to be disseminated widely in the body. See **Anaphylaxis**.

Anaphylatoxin A peptide released during the activation of **complement**, which is a powerful mediator of inflammation. Vascular permeability is increased and **mast cells** degranulate, liberating vaso-active amines (e.g. histamine). Examples of anaphylatoxins are C3a and C5a.

Anaphylaxis An **immediate hypersensitivity** reaction which may be seen in an individual receiving second or subsequent exposure to a particular **antigen**. The response may take the form of an **anaphylactic shock** reaction, which is a generalised form of anaphylaxis. The reaction is caused by **antigen** binding to pre-formed **IgE** bound to the surface of **mast cells**. This may lead to the liberation of vaso-active amines, and the other mediators of **anaphylaxis**, from the **mast cells**.

Anaplasia A condition in **tumour** cells which have lost the morphological characteristics of the parent tissue, i.e. there is loss of **differentiation**, organisation and specific function.

Anaplastic Term used to describe a **tumour** that has **differentiation**. Amongst **carcinomas** these tumours have the worst prognosis.

Ancrod   The venom from the Malayan pit viper (*Agkistrodon rhodostoma*), used for therapeutic **defibrination**.

Androgen   Any substance which acts as a male sex hormone. Some androgenic substances are produced by the ovary, testes and adrenal cortex.

Aneuploidy   The state of having more or less than the normal **diploid** number of **chromosomes**.

Angle of incidence   The angle at which light travelling obliquely strikes an optically dense medium. See **Refractive index**.

Angle of refraction   The angle at which light passing through, and leaving an optically dense medium is bent or refracted. See **Angle of incidence** and **Refractive index**.

Anion   See **Ion**.

Anionic dye   A **dye** with a negative electrostatic charge. Such dyes are attracted to tissue carrying a positive charge (**acidophilia**). See **Ion**.

Anisochromasia   Variation in the staining intensity of **erythrocytes** in blood films stained with **Romanowsky** dyes.

Anisocytosis   Marked variation in the size of cells within a group of cells of the same type.

Anisotropic   A term used in **polarising microscopy** to describe the interference colours produced by certain crystalline substances (e.g. quartz).

Annulus   An opaque diaphragm, usually in the form of a pair of concentric circles, placed in the focal plane of a condensing lens and used in **phase contrast microscopy** to illuminate the object with a hollow cone of light.

Antagonism   The combined action of two or more **anti-microbial** substances on a micro-organism, resulting in a decrease in the activity of one or all of them. This might be due to a chemical interaction between the antimicrobials or, more usually, to the interference by one agent with the target site of another.

Antenatal   The period of gestation between conception and birth.

Anthrax   A fulminating, usually fatal, **septicaemia** of animals caused by *Bacillus anthracis*. Humans are also affected, usually by contact with infected animals or animal products such as hides, bone meal or wool. The disease can take either a cutaneous or a pulmonary form depending upon the mode of infection. *Bacillus anthracis* is a rod-shaped **aerobic** organism which forms **spores** and gives a positive reaction with **Gram's stain**. It is identifiable by its characteristic cultural morphology and by the use of a specific **bacteriophage**. It is the only species in the genus **Bacillus** (apart from variants) which does not exhibit **motility**. It produces a thick polyglutamate capsule and potent **toxins** which cause **oedema** and **necrosis**. In humans the disease is rarely fulminating but is fatal in

about a quarter of cases if not treated. The treatment of choice is
Penicillin G or **Erythromycin**.

Antibiogram An expression of the susceptibility of an organism to
a range of **anti-microbial** substances. The term usually (but not
always) denotes the use of the data for comparative purposes, as
in **epidemiological** studies.

Antibiotic A substance produced by a **micro-organism**, and which
exerts an inhibitory or lethal effect on micro-organisms − but not
the producing strain − and is active in concentrations measured in
mg/l. Many such substances are produced in natural environments, but only a minority are sufficiently safe or effective to be
used therapeutically.

Antibody An **immunoglobulin** found in the serum of animals,
generally in response to the stimulus of a **parenteral** introduction
of an **antigen** into the tissues of an animal, and which will react
with that antigen, generally in an observable manner. (Plural =
antibodies.)

7S Antibody A term used to describe the characteristics of an **IgG**
type of **antibody** when subjected to **ultracentrifugation**. The 'S'
refers to **Svedberg units**.

19S Antibody A term used to describe the characteristics of an
IgM type of **antibody** when subjected to **ultracentrifugation**. The
'S' refers to **Svedberg units**.

Antibody dependent cell-mediated cytotoxicity A reaction in which
target cells (**lymphocytes**, etc.) are killed by an **antibody** (or an
antigen/antibody complex) bound to **macrophages**.

Anticoagulant A substance which prevents **coagulation**, usually of
blood. Those in most common use include **heparin** and the salts of
ethylenediaminetetraacetic acid (**EDTA**) and of citric and oxalic
acids.

Anticomplementary Term used to describe substances present in
serum or reagents which inhibit the **complement** cascade, or activate it non-specifically without interaction between an **antigen** and
an **antibody**. The presence of anticomplementary substances seri-
ously impairs the interpretation of *in vitro* serological tests involving **complement**.

Anti-contaminator A cold baffle surrounding the specimen in an
electron microscope, to prevent the deposition of **contamination**
on the sample. See **Scanning electron microscope** and **Transmission electron microscope**.

Anti-diuretic hormone A hormone secreted by the posterior of the
pituitary gland. It contributes to the control of blood pressure by
regulating renal tubular reabsorption of water and acting as a

vasoconstrictor. Lack of the hormone leads to **polyuria** and **diabetes** insipidus. See also **Diuretic**.

Antigen   Any substance which, when introduced **parenterally** into an animal body, is capable of stimulating the production in the serum of that animal of an **antibody** with which it will react specifically, generally in an observable manner. See also **Immunogen**.

Antigenic drift   A process of **antigenic** change exhibited by some **viruses**, enabling them to re-infect apparently **immune** individuals. It is presumed to result from selection of mutants resistant to the **immune response** in the majority of the population.

Antigenicity   The power of an **antigen** to stimulate an **immune response**.

Antigenic shift   A major **antigenic** change exhibited by **Orthomyxoviridae**, resulting in an essentially new **virus** capable of infecting large populations. This potential exists in all viruses having segmented **genomes**.

Antiglobulin   An **antibody** which reacts with serum proteins, specifically with the globulin fraction.

Antiglobulin test   A test between an **antigen** and an **antibody**, in which **sensitized cells** are washed to remove free protein and then exposed to an **antiglobulin** antibody, which will attach itself to any **IgG** antibody which has combined with antigen sites on the cells, so causing **agglutination**. The indirect antiglobulin test is performed as the second stage of a procedure in which antigen and antibody are brought together *in vitro*, while the direct antiglobulin test is performed on cells which have been coated with antibody *in vivo*.

Anti-haemophilic factor   A synonym for blood **coagulation factor** VIII, which is deficient in individuals with **haemophilia A**. See also **Coagulation factors**.

Anti-lymphocyte serum   An **antiserum** raised in one species against the lymphocytes of another species. This antiserum can then be used as an agent for **immunosuppression**.

Anti-microbial   A substance which exerts an inhibitory or lethal effect on **micro-organisms** at low concentrations measured in mg/l. Naturally-occurring, semi-synthetic and synthetic substances are included in the term.

Anti-mitotic   Refers to reagents which prevent cell division without causing cell death. Their effect is often dose-dependant, too large a dose being potentially lethal.

Anti-nuclear factor   An **auto-antibody** demonstrable by **immunofluorescence** in the **serum** of individuals with systemic **lupus erythrematosus** and, more rarely, **rheumatoid arthritis**. The auto-antibody is directed against components of cell nuclei, e.g. double stranded (native) **DNA** and single stranded (denatured) DNA.

Antiplasmin　An inhibitor of the fibrinolytic enzyme **plasmin**. The major physiological antiplasmins are **alpha$_2$-antiplasmin** and **alpha$_2$-macroglobulin**.

Anti-roll plate　In **histology**, an adjustable device held close to the face of a **microtome** knife to prevent sections curling or rolling as they are cut in a **cryostat**.

Antiseptic　A chemical substance which exerts an inhibitory or lethal effect on micro-organisms at concentrations measured usually in g/l. Antiseptics are non-corrosive and suitable for topical use, but not for systemic administration. An example is **Chlorhexidine**.

Antiserum　A general term used to describe any **serum** which contains **antibody** directed against a stated **antigen** or antigens.

Antithetical antigens　Two corresponding **antigens** directly opposite to each other, i.e. produced by **allelomorphic** genes on the corresponding loci of each of a pair of **chromosomes**.

Antithrombin III　The major physiological inhibitor of those activated blood **coagulation factors** which are **serine proteases** (thrombin, IXa, Xa, XIa and XIIa).

Antithrombotic therapy　Treatment which is given to prevent the occurrence or the extension of a **thrombus**.

Antitoxin　An **antiserum** directed against a **toxin**. This usually means a bacterial **exotoxin**, but could refer to any **antigen**ic toxin.

(alpha 1) Antitrypsin　The major component of the alpha 1-globulins. It inhibits trypsin and other proteolytic **enzymes** and may be assayed immunologically or enzymatically by measuring the inhibition of trypsin activity.

Anti-viral drugs　A heterogeneous group of chemicals having antiviral activity *in vivo*. Many of them are **analogues** of **nucleotides**, and some are quite toxic. A number of these drugs are prophylactic, and do not improve resolution of established disease.

Anucleated squame　A large flat **squamous cell** without a nucleus, reflecting the ultimate level of **keratinisation** of the squamous **epithelium**.

Apathy's medium　Largely obsolete gum or sugar mixture used as an aqueous **mountant** in **histopathology**. It is non-**fluorescent**.

Aperture　1. An opening. 2. In microscopy, a small hole placed in the light or electron beam to limit the diameter (e.g. condenser aperture) or introduce contrast into the image (e.g. objective aperture).

Apheresis　A procedure in which specific components of the circulating blood of a **blood donor** or patient are removed selectively, the remaining components being returned to the circulation. See **Leucopheresis**, **Plasmapheresis** and **Plateletpheresis**.

Aplanat A term used to describe lens systems which are fully corrected for **spherical aberration** and possess good colour correction.

Aplasia Lack of development of an organ. Frequently used to describe complete suppression or failure of development of a structure from the **embryonic** stage.

Aplastic anaemia A type of **anaemia** in which there is **pancytopenia** and evidence of decreased production of all the formed elements of the blood in the **bone marrow**.

Apochromat In microscopy a term, usually confined to objective lenses, indicating total freedom from **chromatic aberration**, with the reservation that such objective lenses are used in combination with **compensating eyepieces**. Well-corrected for **spherical aberration**, such lenses are of the highest quality.

Apoferritin The protein portion of the **ferritin** molecule, comprising a number of polypeptide sub-units.

Apolipoprotein Found in various **lipoproteins**, the apolipoproteins assist in the transportation of lipid and the stabilisation of the lipid structures. They can be **immunochemically** defined.

Apoptosis A controlled method of cell deletion which ensures that normal cell turnover does not result in total cell increase, and thus tissue or organ enlargement.

Aposiderin Granular brown pigment in tissue sections which, although iron negative, is probably formed by the action of acid **fixation** on **haemosiderin**. May be confused with **lipofuscin**.

Aprotinin A polypeptide prepared from bovine lung, and which is capable of inhibiting many types of **serine protease** enzymes. It is primarily used as an anti-fibrinolytic agent.

APTT See **Activated Partial Thromboplastin Time**.

APUD Literally, Amine and amine Precursor Uptake and Decarboxylation. A diffuse system of polypeptide secreting **endocrine** cells now classified with similar cells in the central and peripheral nervous systems into the Diffuse NeuroEndocrine System (**DNES**).

Arachadonic acid A 20-carbon fatty acid which is the principal component of cellular phospholipids and precursor of the **prostaglandins**. Increasingly used for **platelet aggregation** studies.

Arachnia A **bacterium** which is a member of the Actinomycetales. A facultative **anaerobe** which is positive by **Gram's stain** and **catalase** negative, has a branched rod shape and is part of the normal bacterial flora of the mouth. Occasionally lesions similar to those caused by **Actinomyces** species are produced. Treatment normally includes surgical drainage or excision, and administration of **penicillin** or **erythromycin**, but not **metronidazole**.

Arbovirus A term applied to **viruses** which replicate in both arthropods and vertebrates. Many virus familes are represented.

Arenaviridae A family of enveloped **RNA** viruses 100—300 nm in

21

diameter and exhibiting **pleomorphism**. They occur naturally in rodents and include **viruses** causing severe **haemorrhagic fever** with high mortality but low infectivity in man (e.g. the virus of **Lassa fever** − a **risk group 4 pathogen**).

Argentaffin The reaction whereby metallic silver is deposited from solution onto tissue components without the necessity for an external reducer. See **Argyrophil**.

Argyrophil A reaction in which silver is deposited from solution onto tissue components but requires the action of an external reducer. See **Argentaffin**.

Arneth count The differentiation of **neutrophils** into sub-groups according to the number of nuclear lobes.

Arrhenoblastoma A **malignant tumour** of the ovary, consisting of immature gonadal elements with male hormone secretion, producing masculinising secondary sex characteristics.

Artefact (alternative spelling, **Artifact**) A feature not naturally present. In laboratory practice, something most commonly introduced during investigation or preparation of a specimen.

Arthritis Inflammation of a joint, which may be associated with both infective and non-infective disease and which is a feature of many **pathological** syndromes. Arthritis caused by **bacteria** can be due to **immune complex** deposition on the synovial **membrane**, or to bacterial invasion of the joint, in which case there is usually suppuration. Arthritis developing after systemic or gastro-intestinal **infection** with certain rod-shaped **bacteria** which are negative by **Gram's stain** − and in particular **Yersinia** − is often associated with the **histocompatibility antigen** HLA-B27. Arthritis is also a common feature of the **spirochaetal** infection known as **Lyme disease**.

Arthus reaction Classically seen as an inflammatory reaction following administration of an **antigen** to an individual with existing **antibody** to that antigen. The antigen precipitates with the antibody at the injection site causing **complement** activation, the accumulation of **fibrin**, **platelets** and **neutrophils**. May also be applied to type III **hypersensitivity** states, e.g. **farmer's lung**.

Arvin™ See **Ancrod**.

Asbestos body A magnesium silicate fibre coated with an iron-containing protein. Beaded and golden brown in appearance, giving a positive **Perl's Prussion Blue** reaction.

Ascaris A lumbricoides − an intestinal round worm − which is a human **parasite** responsible for an estimated 1 000 000 000 infestations in many countries. The worms are between 15 and 30 cm long and live for 1−2 years. Ova are ingested and the hatched worms migrate through blood vessels and tissues to the lungs.

They are expectorated, swallowed, and live as adults in the small intestine. Infections are usually asymptomatic.

ASCII Abbreviation for American Standard Code for Information Interchange. In computing, this is the internationally accepted code which represents **alphanumeric** characters with unique **binary** code values which are recognised by a computer.

Ascites Accumulation of serous fluid in the peritoneal cavity.

Aseptic meningitis Inflammation of the meninges, characterised by a raised **lymphocyte** count in **cerebrospinal fluid** and moderately raised levels of **protein**. A number of **viruses** and **bacteria** are known causes of this condition, including *Mycobacterium tuberculosis*, *Treponema pallidum*, **Brucella** and **mumps** virus. Rapid diagnosis is essential.

Aspartate aminotransferase (EC 2.6.1.1) Aminotransferases are **enzymes** which catalyse reactions in which an amino group is transferred from an amino acid to an alpha-oxo acid. Aspartate aminotransferase catalyses aspartate and alpha-oxoglutarate to oxalacetate and glutamate. The enzyme is widely spread in tissues, with the highest concentration found in heart muscle.

Aspartate transaminase See **Aspartate aminotransferase**.

Aspergillus A filamentous **fungus** producing characteristic **conidiophores** and a colonial appearance. *A. fumigatus*, *A. flavus* and *A. niger* are the commonest causes of disease, which can range from the superficial (e.g. otitis externa) to invasive lesions affecting all tissues, including the brain. Invasive **infections** usually affect the **immunosuppressed** individual. Secondary **infection** of tuberculous cavities may occur. Treatment involves surgical drainage or excision, and administration of **amphotericin** B.

Aspirin tolerance test A method for the assessment of primary haemostasis in which the **bleeding time** is measured before and after ingestion of aspirin. An abnormal increase in the post-aspirin time is often seen in patients with **von Willebrand's disease**.

Assay Measurement of the quantity, activity or potency of a substance or of one of its constituents.

Assay, anti-microbial The determination of the concentration of an **anti-microbial** substance in stock solutions or in body fluids. Depending on the method employed, total drug concentration or only that of biologically-active forms can be determined. Assays help to establish whether the dosage of a particular drug is giving rise to safe or toxic, effective or insufficient, concentrations in the patient.

Assembler A computer **program** which translates instructions written in a **high level language** into **machine code** which the computer can recognise.

Assembly language In computing, a **low level language** which utilises mnemonics rather than ordinary words to give instructions to the computer. These mnemonics are translated directly into **binary** code for recognition by the computer and occupy less **memory** than instructions written in a **high level language**.

AST See **Aspartate aminotransferase**.

Astigmatism 1. A form of optical aberration producing a distorted image of the object (e.g. a spherical object may be rendered elliptical in the image plane). 2. In ophthalmology, a condition affecting the human eye.

Astrocyte A large connective tissue cell of the central nervous system. Protoplasmic astrocytes have no cellular fibres but long protoplasmic processes, and are most abundant in grey matter. The fibrous types have thick fibres which may form fine branches outside the cell and are most abundant in white matter.

Astrovirus Small (20–30 nm) **viruses** associated with **gastroenteritis** and characterised morphologically by a star-like appearance in **electron micrographs**.

ATIII See **Antithrombin III**.

Atelectasis Incomplete expansion, or collapse, of the air sacs of the lung.

Atheroma A thickening of the subintima layer of the arterial wall caused by invasion of smooth muscle cells. **Cholesterol** and **platelets** may then be deposited in this subintimal plaque, leading to alterations in blood flow, and ultimately in **thrombosis**.

Atomic absorption spectroscopy The amount of light absorbed by ground atoms. Light is passed from a hollow cathode lamp, containing the element being estimated, through a flame in which the atoms are dispersed. Most atoms remain in the ground state and are capable of absorbing light at the appropriate wavelength. The decrease in the amount of incident light absorbed is measured.

Atopic 1. Used to describe individuals with **immediate hypersensitivity** states (e.g. allergic asthma and hay fever), or the states themselves (e.g. **atopic allergy**). 2. Out of place. See **Ectopic**.

Atopy A predisposition to development of reactions of **hypersensitivity** to common **antigens**, usually mediated by **IgE** immunoglobulins. See **Atopic**.

Atransferrinaemia Congenital absence of the iron-binding protein **transferrin**.

Atrophic smear pattern An appearance characterised by a predominance of immature cells of the **epithelium**.

Atrophy A regressive change or diminution in the size of a cell, tissue or organ, as a manifestation of a defect or failure of nutrition.

Attenuate To cause a reduction in **virulence** by repeated culture or prolonged storage in the laboratory. The phenomenon is exploited in order to produce live **vaccines**, which generally have a more prolonged effect than killed vaccines yet do not cause the serious disease for which the parent strain is responsible. An example is immunisation against **tuberculosis** by **BCG**.

Attenuated vaccine A **vaccine** made from live **bacteria** or **viruses** which have been cultured or treated to reduce their **virulence**, but which retain their **immunogenicity**.

Atypia Literally, a state of being not typical. In cells, any deviation from the normal morphology.

Auer rods Rod-shaped inclusion bodies which appear in the cytoplasm of **myeloblasts** and **monoblasts** − but not in **lymphoblasts** − in some cases of **acute leukaemia**.

Australia antigen Obsolete term for **hepatitis B surface antigen** (HBsAg).

Auto- A prefix word. Pertaining to self (e.g. **Auto-antibody**).

Autoagglutination **Agglutination** of cells, usually **erythrocytes**, by an **antibody** present in the **serum** of the same individual. May sometimes refer to spontaneous **agglutination** of red cells carrying a particular **antigen** and suspended in saline.

Autoanalyser™ The brand name of the original automated **continuous flow analyser**, marketed by the Technicon Corp. Ltd.

Autoantibody An **antibody** which reacts with **antigens** present in the tissues or on the cells of the individual in whom the **antibody** is found.

Autoclave A device for rendering material **sterile** by the application of steam under increased pressure, and hence temperature. Under pressure, pure steam (with no admixture of air) has a temperature of 109°C at 5 lb per square inch (psi) above atmospheric pressure, 115°C at 10 psi, 121°C at 15 psi, 126°C at 20 psi, 130°C at 25 psi and 135°C at 30 psi. Autoclaves are generally of two types. In downward displacement instruments, air is removed from the chamber by downwards displacement through an outlet valve by the admission or generation of the less dense steam; in high pre-vaccuum autoclaves the chamber is evacuated of air by a vacuum pump before admission of pure steam. (Note: sterilisation is effected by exposure to increased temperature, not to increased pressure *per se*, and references to conditions used for sterilising should indicate the temperature achieved, not the pressure applied).

Autofluorescence The property of material to absorb light of short (invisible) wavelength and emit light of longer (visible) wavelength.

Autogenous vaccine A **vaccine** prepared from the actual organisms

25

(usually bacteria) causing **infection** in an individual. The use of such vaccines is now largely obsolete, but they were used formerly to treat recurrent **infection** of the skin due to *Staphylococcus aureus*.

Autograft A graft of tissue (e.g. skin) from one area of the body to another, in the same individual.

Autohaemolysis test Determination of the amount of spontaneous haemolysis developing in blood incubated at 37°C for 48 h. By comparing the autohaemolysis with and without added glucose or **ATP** it is possible to distinguish between various red cell **enzyme** deficiencies.

Autoimmune haemolytic anaemia An **anaemia** resulting from destruction of circulating red cells by an **antibody** in the patient's **plasma**, directed against an **antigen** carried on his own red cells.

Autoimmunity A condition in which an **immune response** (either **antibody** or **cell-mediated**) occurs against the body's own tissues. If the immune response is sufficient, autoimmune disease may occur in the individual.

Autologous Related, or belonging, to self.

Autologous transfusion Re-**transfusion** of a patient's own **blood product**, either with or without prior storage.

Autolysin In **bacteria**, an **enzyme** which hydrolyses sites in the **peptidoglycan** of the cell wall during **cell wall** synthesis. In the presence of autolysins, interference with peptidoglycan synthesis by **beta Lactams** results in cell lysis. See **Autolysis**.

Autolysis Spontaneous disintegration of cells by the action of their own **enzymes**, following cell death. See **Autolysin**.

Autoradiography Delineation of the image of an object using **radioactivity** emitted by the object itself to expose a photographic emulsion.

Autosome Any ordinary paired **chromosome**, as distinguished from a **sex chromosome**.

Autotrophy The ability of an organism to use carbon dioxide as a carbon source. Such organisms derive energy from oxidation of inorganic substances such as nitrates.

Auxochrome An ionising group which gives coloured compounds (**chromogens**) the property of a **stain**. They are salts which carry an electrostatic charge opposite to that of the **chromogen**.

Auxotrophy The ability of an organism to utilise simple inorganic or organic substances, while requiring in addition one complex organic substance for growth.

Auxotype The characterisitic of a strain as denoted by its requirement for a range of organic or inorganic substrates for growth on defined media.

Average See **Mean** and **Median**.

Avidin A glycoprotein with an extremely high affinity for **biotin**. As one biotin molecule binds to one molecule of avidin, while avidin has four biotin binding sites, it is a useful 'bridge' between biotin-labelled **antibodies**, **lectins**, etc., and biotin-labelled markers (e.g. peroxidase). It is also a useful label of nucleic acid probes.

Avidity In **serology**, the relative speed with which an **antibody** will react with cells carrying its specific **antigen**.

Axenic A culture containing a single species of organism (e.g. growth of **parasites** in culture, completely free of bacteria, which are restrained by antibiotics).

Axon A nerve fibre which may be surrounded by flattened Schwann cells, coated in a **lipid (myelin)** sheath or naked. They conduct impulses from nerve cells and form motor or effector endings.

Axoneme Core of a **flagellum** or **cilium**, composed of microtubules. Originates in the **blepharoplast**.

Axostyle An elongate tube-like **organelle** running lengthwise through some flagellated organisms, such as the **Trichomonads**, and often projecting posteriorly.

Azlocillin A ureido-substituted **penicillin** similar to **mezlocillin**. It has a broad spectrum of activity, particularly against Gram-negative rod-shaped **bacteria**, but is susceptible to **beta lactamases**. Most strains of *Pseudomonas aeruginosa* are 10 times more susceptible to azlocillin than to **carbenicillin**.

Azo dye A **dye** in which the **chromophore** group $-N-N-$ joins two benzene or naphthalene rings. The product of **simultaneous couplings**, where an **enzyme** liberates alpha-naphthol from **substrate**, and this reacts with a diazonium salt to produce an insoluble azo dye at the site of enzyme activity.

Azthreonam A **monobactam** active against **bacteria** which are negative by **Gram's stain**, but having no useful activity against Gram-positive organisms.

B

Babesia A **protozoa** found within **erythrocytes**, causing **zoonosis** in cattle, domestic animals and rodents. It is tick-borne and sometimes causes a disease superficially resembling **malaria** in humans, particularly if they are **immuno-suppressed** or asplenic. Many species exist but *B. divergens* and *B. microti* are those usually implicated in human disease.

Bacillus A **bacterium**, a rod-shaped member of the family **Bacillaceae** which is positive by **Gram's stain**, forms **spores**, is an **aerobe** and is usually **catalase** positive and exhibits **motility**. The main exception is *B. anthracis*, the causative organism of **anthrax**, but non-motile variants of other species occur. *B. cereus*, *B. subtilis* and others occasionally cause disease in man. The organisms are widespread in nature, some causing **epidemic** infections in insects — a property which is sometimes exploited as a control measure.

Bacitracin A polypeptide **antibiotic** isolated from *Bacillus licheniformis*. It acts by inhibiting the removal of phosphate from **bactoprenol** during cell wall synthesis, and therefore has a different action from the **penicillins**, being active at the level of the **cytoplasmic** membrane. Its action is exclusively against Gram-positive organisms and **Neisseria**, but **Streptococci** of **Lancefield groups** B, C and G are resistant, and it is used in the laboratory in a presumptive test for *Streptococcus pyogenes*. The drug is highly nephrotoxic but is safe for use topically and in irrigating fluids.

Back titration The determination of **anti-microbial** activity in a body fluid by **incubation** of an organism in successive dilutions of the fluid. **Bacteristatic** activity is recorded after initial incubation by observation of turbidity, and **bactericidal** activity by subculturing the non-turbid dilutions. Usually the organism causing the **infection** for which treatment is being given is used, but an **indicator** organism (such as the Oxford **staphylococcus**) can be used. The method is useful for assaying **anti-microbial** drugs, specific and non-specific **antibodies**, cellular components, etc. It does not indicate anti-microbial concentration.

Bactec™ A proprietary method of culturing blood which depends on the production of radio-labelled carbon dioxide from radio-labelled **substrates** in the **culture medium**. If viable organisms are present in the **blood culture**, the gas is released into the head space and detected by **radiometry**, triggering an alarm. The system is automated and can cope with large numbers of blood cultures. Some fastidious or relatively inert organisms are not reliably detected.

Bacteraemia The presence – possibly transiently – of **bacteria** in the blood stream. The difference (if any) between bacteraemia and **septicaemia** is one of degree, the latter implying a more severe illness with probable multiplication of the bacteria in the blood.

Bactericidal Capable of killing **bacteria**. Usually applied to **anti-microbial** substances, the term is not absolute and depends on conditions of growth, and particularly on the concentration of the anti-microbial substance. See **Bacteristatic**.

Bacteriocin A **protein** produced by an organism which is lethal to other organisms, generally of the same species. Bacteriocins are much more potent than **antibiotics** and a single molecule is sufficient to kill a susceptible cell. Many exert their effect by stopping oxidative phosphorylation, or some other vital synthetic process.

Bacteriology The study of **bacteria**, including their structure, physiology, taxonomy and ecology. Specialities, such as veterinary or medical bacteriology, are recognised. Traditionally, **fungi** and some **parasites**, but not **viruses**, are often included.

Bacteriophage A type of **virus** which infects **bacteria** and **fungi**. They usually have complex structures with a head containing **DNA** or, less commonly **RNA**, and a tail with a contractile sheath. After attachment to receptors on the cell surface and **infection** of the nucleic acid, the host **micro-organism** is induced to manufacture more bacteriophage components. The bacteria may be disrupted, as in a **lytic infection**, or immature prophages may replicate with the host cell without causing it to disrupt. Because of the specific **susceptibility** of micro-organisms to certain bacteriophages they can be used for the purposes of **epidemiological** typing.

Bacteristatic Capable of killing **bacteria**. **Anti-microbial** substances which are **bactericidal** are also usually bacteristatic at low concentrations, and bacteristatic substances are often bactericidal at high concentrations, although in many cases these cannot be achieved in clinical use.

Bacterium A type of unicellular prokaryote in which the cytoplasmic **membrane** is the only membrane within the cell, all other **organelles** being in direct contact with the **cytoplasm**. Bacterial ribosomes are smaller than those in eukaryotes and their designation on the basis of **ultra-centrifuge** sedimentation characteristics is 70S. The bacterial 'nucleus' consists of a single, extremely long **DNA** molecule and **mitosis** does not occur. Most intact bacteria, with the exception of the **Mollicutes**, possess a rigid **cell wall** containing **peptidoglycan**. Multiplication is by cell division.

Bacteriuria The presence of **bacteria** in the urine. Conventionally, if greater than 10^5 organisms per ml are present in pure culture,

infection is indicated. The term is often used to imply the absence of **pyuria**. In women the infection may be asymptomatic, but is not necessarily innocuous.

Bacteroides A rod-shaped **bacterium** which is an **anaerobe**, negative by **Gram's stain**, is **catalase** negative and which may exhibit **motility**. They are found in the mouth, intestine and genital tracts of man and animals, and consequently are often associated with sepsis following surgery involving these areas. Bacteroides species are susceptible to **metronidazole** and usually to **clindamycin** and **chloramphenicol**. *B. melaninogenicus* is susceptible to **penicillin** but *B. fragilis* is not.

Bactoprenol The carrier lipid, Undecaprenol, which is responsible in **bacteria** for transfer of muramic acid pentapeptide from the hydrophilic **cytoplasm** to the hydrophobic cell **membrane** during synthesis of peptidoglycan for **cell wall** construction. The active carrier is diphosphorylated and returned to the cycle once the pentapeptide has left the cell membrane and entered the cell wall.

Baermann apparatus An apparatus used to separate nematode larvae from soil or **faeces**. Rubber tubing carrying a spring clip is attached to a funnel and warm water is used to moisten the infected material. Larvae migrate down the tubing and are released into a collecting vessel.

BALB/c mouse An inbred strain of mouse with a genetic predisposition to develop **myelomatosis**, either spontaneously or following **intraperitoneal** injection of paraffin oil or complete **Freund's adjuvant**.

Balloon cell See **Koilocyte**.

Band pass The width or range of wavelength that is allowed to pass through the exit slit of the wavelength selecting device in a **spectrophotometer**.

Band width See **Band path**.

Bar code A machine-readable pattern of vertical black and white lines of varying thickness which represents alphabetical and numerical characters. Read by a **light pen**, the code is interpreted by a computer and compared with the machine code version of the characters stored in its memory.

Barr body An ovoid mass of sex **chromatin** situated at the periphery of the nucleus of a cell and attached to the nuclear membrane. It consists of heterochromatic X **chromosome** and is present in the normal female but not in the normal male.

Barrier nursing Procedures for the care and treatment of patients which minimise the risk of spread of **infection** from that patient to others. Reverse barrier nursing is intended to protect a susceptible patient from infection from the environment, or from other patients and staff. The terms do not necessarily imply isolation or nursing in cubicles, but are components of measures to prevent the spread of infection.

Bartonella Bacteria which are negative by **Gram's stain**, rod-shaped and **aerobic**, exhibiting **motility** and **pleomorphism** and growing on **serum** and blood-enriched **agar** at 30°C. Transmitted by the sandfly, the organism adheres to **erythrocytes** and gives rise to profound **anaemia** with fever and later chronic **granuloma**tosis. *Bartonella bacilliformis*, the causative species, is susceptible to various **anti-microbial** substances, including **penicillin**.

Base A compound which accepts hydrogen ions (protons). See also **Hydrogen ion concentration**.

Basement membrane A non-cellular zone underlying the **epithelium** of mucous membranes and secretory glands.

BASIC An acronym for 'Beginners All-purpose Symbolic Instruction Code'. In computing this is the most commonly used **high level language** for writing **programs**.

Basic dye A dye which carries a positive charge $^{(+)}$. A coloured basic radicle which attaches to an acid tissue component (e.g. methyl green) which stains the phosphate groups of **deoxyribonucleic acid**.

Basophil A member of the **polymorphonuclear leucocyte** class of cells, characterised by the presence of large **basophilic** granules when stained by **Romanowsky staining** methods. This cell is normally the least frequent $(0.2-2.0\%)$ of the peripheral blood leucocytes.

Basophilia An increase in the number of circulating blood basophils, seen mainly in chronic myeloid **leukaemia** and in **polycythaemia rubra vera**.

Basophilic Tissue which, by salt linkage and ionic binding, stains with basic dyes.

Batroxobin See **Reptilase**.

Baud In computing, a unit of signalling speed indicating the number of signals per second. If each signal equals one **bit**, then one baud equals one bit per second. Common Baud rates are 110, 300, 1200, 2400, 4800 and 9600 bits per second.

BBTS British Blood Transfusion Society.

B cell A **lymphocyte** derived from the **bursa of Fabricius** in birds. In mammals, B cells are derived from the fetal liver and/or bone marrow. These cells carry surface **immunoglobulin**, which is predominantly monomeric **IgM** and **IgD**, as receptors for **antigen**. On contact with antigen, B cells transform and proliferate to form **plasma cells**, which synthesise and secrete **immunoglobulins**.

BCG Abbreviation for the *Bacillus of Calmette and Guerin*. This is a live **attenuated** strain of *Mycobacterium bovis*, used as a **vaccine** to confer a degree of **immunity** to **tuberculosis**. Vaccination does not prevent **infection** but limits dissemination so that usually it does not become clinically evident, and is naturally eradicated. It should be used only in **tuberculin**-negative people, and should be avoided in the **immuno-compromised** patient. Calmette and Guerin first attenuated the organism by sequential culture (passage) of it in a medium containing **bile salts**.

BCR See **British Corrected Ratio**.

BCSH British Committee for Standardisation in Haematology.

BDOS In computing, the abbreviation of 'Basic Disc Operating System'. The portion of an **operating system** which handles all of the **file** transactions on the **floppy discs**.

Beer-Lambert law A law applying to monochromatic light, stating that the optical density of a homogeneous layer of absorbing material is proportional to the amount of absorbing material which the light traverses. It is given by the formula A = kcl, where A = optical density, k = absorptivity of the material, c = the concentration of the material, and l = the path length of the light. (Also known as Beer's law and Lambert's law. The variation of absorbance with concentration was stated by Beer, and the variation with path length by Lambert.)

Bell and Alton Platelet Substitute See **Platelet substitute**.

Bence Jones protein A **protein** of the **light chain**, excreted in the urine of some patients with **multiple myeloma**. Traditionally it has been characterised by its ability to precipitate on heating at 40°C to 60°C. Modern methods characterise it using **electrophoresis** and immunological techniques.

Benign Mild. Offering a favourable chance of recovery. The opposite of **malignant**.

Benzyl penicillin Otherwise known as **penicillin G**, this is a **beta lactam** type of **antibiotic** produced by the *Penicillium* species. It inhibits **peptidoglycan** synthesis by preventing removal of the terminal D-alanine from the pentapeptide chain, thus preventing incorporation of the latter in the cell wall. Benzyl penicillin is susceptible to **beta lactamase**, and this is the main mechanism by which organisms exert resistance. Gram-negative rods and **mollicutes** are not susceptible, neither are most staphylococci.

Bertrand lens An additional lens fitted to the optical train in the body of a microscope, and having the effect of converting the eyepiece into a telescope for viewing the back focal plane of the objective lens. It is of particular value in **phase contrast** microscopy.

Bethesda unit A means of expressing **factor VIII** inhibitor levels, based upon the ability of a test plasma to inhibit a known amount of added factor VIII.

BHK 21 A **clone** of baby hamster kidney cells, capable of indefinite laboratory passage. Some **viruses**, particularly **rubella** and **herpes simplex**, can be grown to high **titre** in these cells. They are particularly useful in studies of **transformation** by viruses.

Bias A systematic under- or overestimation of a quantity, caused by not allowing for a certain effect (e.g. maladjustment of a recording device).

Bichromasia The property of taking up both acidic and basic dyes.

Bichromatic A system of measuring light absorption at two different wavelengths simultaneously. The system enables the effect of interfering absorption to be eliminated or reduced.

Bifidobacterium Bacteria which are **anaerobes**, do not form **spores**, are **catalase**-negative, positive by **Gram's stain** and are rod-shaped organisms which branch to form Y-shaped pairs. They are found in the alimentary tract and the vagina and rarely cause disease, although occasional cases of **endocarditis** have been reported.

Bile A generic term used to describe the fluid in the gall bladder which contains the bile pigments.

Bile pigment See **Haematoidin**.

Bile salts Conjugates of bile acids with glycine or taurine, known as glycholate or taurocholate (respectively). The conjugates are formed in the liver and secreted in the bile. In **bacteriology** they are used in **culture media** to enhance the growth of some intestinal **pathogens**. In **cellular pathology** they are used empirically for the selective removal of **ribonucleic acid** from tissue sections.

Bile solubility A test to distinguish *Streptococcus pneumoniae* from other streptococci exhibiting alpha-**haemolysis**. Bile salts stimulate the **autolysis** of *Streptococcus pneumoniae*. The test can be carried out on suspected colonies on an **agar** plate.

Bilharzial pigment A consequence of protozoal infection, seen in tissue sections, where it behaves like **formalin pigment**, but from which it may be differentiated by its intracellular distribution.

Bilharziasis See **Schistosomiasis**.

Bilirubin An orange-yellow pigment, insoluble in water but soluble in organic solvents, which is the main constituent of bile. It is a breakdown product of **haemoglobin** and is found in the **plasma** of individuals who have suffered *in vivo* **haemolysis**. See **Kernicterus**.

Biliverdin The precursor of **bilirubin**, which is formed from the **porphyrin** part of the **haemoglobin** molecule.

Binary 1. An arithmetical system which utilises only two alternative values, '0' and '1', each symbol representing a decimal power of two. 2. Any system that has only two possible states, such as 'On' or 'Off'.

Binary fission The division of a single organism into two offspring.

Bio-assay A method of determining the concentration of an **anti-**

microbial substance in a solution of body fluid by measuring its ability to inhibit the growth of a susceptible organism under controlled conditions in the laboratory. Both the pure drug and any active metabolites are detected. The method is technically undemanding but is slow and inaccurate compared to chemical **assay** methods.

Biochip Biological and chemically synthesised molecules which act as conductors in the same manner as circuits etched on a silicon **chip**, thus allowing electrical circuits of molecular size. Biochips avoid the problems of tunnelling losses and heat dissipation associated with silicon chips, and it may prove possible to interface them with living systems to provide (e.g.) brain and cardiac implants, and implants to control artificial limbs.

Biogenic amine A term reserved for naturally occuring amines which may be induced to fluoresce (for example, by formaldehyde). Although other methods may be used to demonstrate these substances, over 20 amines and precursors have been identified by **FIF**.

Biological activity A term often applied to the blood **coagulation factors** and referring to the amount of the factor measured by a technique which utilises its normal biological (i.e. enzymatic) function. This should be contrasted with 'total' protein, usually measured by immunological or chemical techniques. A discrepancy between 'biological' and 'total' activity may be indicative of a qualitatively abnormal protein molecule (e.g. **dysfibrinogenaemia** or **disprothrombinaemia**).

Biological safety cabinet An enclosed cabinet with a ducted air supply for the safe handling of **high risk samples**. Three classes of cabinet are available with differing levels of containment and protection for the operator. See **Class I exhaust protective cabinet**, **Class II cabinet** and **Class III exhaust protective cabinet**.

Bioluminescence The emission of light by some **micro-organisms**, usually of marine origin, as the result of cellular oxidation of a substrate (Luciferin) by the **enzyme** Luciferase.

Biopsy 1. A surgical procedure in which tissue is removed from the living body for subsequent examination in the laboratory. The biopsy may be (i) incisional, to determine the nature of the lesion, or (ii) excisional, when it is hoped to remove the lesion completely. 2. A piece of tissue removed from a living body for laboratory investigation.

BIOS In computing, the abbreviation of 'Basic Input/Output System'. The portion of the **operating system** used to handle all machine-dependent transactions.

Biosensor A device used in patient monitoring as a **transducer** to convert biological phenomena into electrical data which can be processed and displayed in a form intelligible to the operator. Biosensors may be of three types: (i) *in vivo*, the sensor being implanted or introduced percutaneously into the subject; (ii) on-line, the sensor being connected in a non-invasive manner to the subject (e.g. as with an electrocardiogram); or (iii) *in vitro*, the sensor being used in an analytical laboratory instrument without any direct connection to the subject.

Biotechnology A generic term for the (usually industrial) application of scientific and engineering principles to the processing of materials by biological agents, to provide goods and services.

Biotin A vitamin (H) for which the glycoprotein **avidin** has an exceptionally high affinity. It is used as a label for the detection of many affinity procedures (e.g. **antibody/antigen** reactions, **lectin** binding, nucleic acid probes). A particular property is that it possesses only a single ligand binding site.

Biotype A variety or strain within a species which, while possessing the essential characteristics of the species, displays variation in biochemical tests which might enable sub-division of the species for purposes of **epidemiology**.

Bird fancier's lung A respiratory condition caused by inhalation of **antigens** derived from the **plasma** of birds (usually parrots). The antigens may be present in the skin, feathers and faeces of the birds. The condition is due to a **hypersensitivity** reaction of the **Arthus** type.

Bird's eye cell A description applied to a **malignant** squamous cell that possesses a second **squamous cell** as an **inclusion** in the **cytoplasm**.

Birefringence Applicable to **polarising microscopy**, and indicating differences in **refractive indices** within a mineral.

Bisalbuminaemia A genetical variant condition in which the albumin fraction is divided on conventional **electrophoresis** into two distinct bands which behave similarly on immunological examination. However, it has been shown that the variant has a change in one amino acid. The condition apparently has no clinical significance.

Bis-chloro-methyl ether (BCME) A potent carcinogen formed by the vapour phases – but not solutions – of **formaldehyde** and hydrochloric acid.

Bit In computing, a **binary** digit; either '0' or '1'.

BK virus A polyoma **virus** of man, normally causing prolonged asymptomatic **infection**. In patients who have undergone renal **transplantation** it is associated with ureteric damage. Infection can persist for long periods.

Blast cell A general term indicating the earliest recognisable types of blood cell precursors. See also **Erythroblast, Lymphoblast, Myeloblast** and **Normoblast**.

Blast cell crisis The transformation of a **chronic** form of **leukaemia** to an **acute** form, with a greater proportion of **blast cells** and a more acute clinical course.

Blastomyces dermatitidis A dimorphic **fungus** which is the asexual stage of *Ajellomyces dermatitidis*. It grows as a **yeast** at 37°C and as a filamentous fungus at room temperature. **Infection** is usually by inhalation of **spores**, leading to pulmonary and systemic pyo-granulomatous lesions. See **Blastomycosis**.

Blastomycosis A **fungus** infection of skin, lungs and other viscera, caused by *Blastomyces dermatitidis*. It can produce multiple pulmonary lesions which usually heal spontaneously in healthy individuals. When required, the treatment of choice is **Amphotericin B**. The disease is **endemic** in eastern north America, parts of central and south America, and Africa.

Blastospore Round or oval, often budding, cells of **yeasts** and yeast-like **fungi**.

Bleaching In **histopathology**: 1. The chemical decolourising of pigments, especially **melanin**, in tissue sections as an aid to identification; 2. treatment of dried degreased bones for museum display.

Bleeding time The time taken for bleeding to stop following an incision or puncture in the skin. The test may be carried out on the ear lobe (**Duke's method**) or on the forearm (the **Ivy test**), but is best performed using a standard commercially-available template device to make the incision (Mielke's method). The bleeding time is a combined measure of **platelet** number and function and vessel wall integrity, and it is a useful measure of primary **haemostasis**.

Blepharitis Inflammation of the margins of the eyelids, usually caused by *Staphylococcus aureus*, and occasionally *Staph. epidermidis*.

Blepharoplast A basal granule from which the **axoneme** arises.

Block In statistics, a group of individuals identified (e.g. by sex, age or weight) so that those within a group are similar to each other. This can increase considerably the precision with which several treatment **means** are compared. See **Analysis of variance**.

Blocking antibody Any **antibody** which prevents the binding of another to an **antigen**. The term is most usually applied to **IgG** formed as a result of desensitisation of an **atopic** individual. IgG specific for an **allergen** blocks the binding of allergen to **IgE** on **mast cell** surfaces.

Blocking reaction A method of conferring greater specificity to demonstration techniques for protein groups. Sites of activity are rendered unavailable for **histochemistry** by defined chemical blocking of specific groups.

Blood agar   A solid **culture medium** consisting of **agar**, peptones and blood. In the United Kingdom the blood is usually from the horse, but sheep, cow and pig blood is used in other countries. Haemolytic organisms often show **haemolysis** only on blood from certain animals. The blood can be heated to produce **chocolate agar** for cultivation of **Haemophilus** and **Neisseria** organisms.

Blood bank   An establishment in which blood for **transfusion** is received, stored and issued.

Blood component   A product for **transfusion** prepared from **whole blood** by physical means (as in a **centrifuge**, or by freezing and thawing), and including all cellular constituents of blood.

Blood culture   Inoculation of aseptically drawn blood into a **culture medium** which is then incubated in an attempt to grow **micro-organisms**. The procedure is used in the diagnosis of **septicaemia** and **bacteraemia**. Fluid media are usually employed, but biphasic media such as Castenada's medium are sometimes used. The atmosphere in the culture bottle can be supplemented or replaced with carbon dioxide or nitrogen. Automated methods such as **BACTEC**, based on radiometry, are available.

Blood donor   One who donates a volume of his or her blood for **transfusion** to others. In the United Kingdom blood donors are healthy individuals of either sex between the ages of 18 and 65, with no history of diseases which may be transmitted by transfusion – notably certain allergic conditions, malaria, and sexually transmitted diseases (including hepatitis B and exposure to **AIDS**). Blood donors may be of four types: (i) altruistically motivated and unrewarded (as in most of Europe); (ii) those who donate on a predeposit basis, to build up credit for themselves in the event of a transfusion being needed in the future; (iii) those who donate on a replacement basis for specific transfusion needs of themselves or their friends or relatives; and (iv) paid donors who sell their blood to a **blood bank** for subsequent resale to patients requiring transfusion.

Blood film   A smear of blood on a glass slide, stained – usually with **Romanowsky stains** – to enable examination and identification of the cellular components of the peripheral blood. Films may be 'thin' for routine haematological examination, or 'thick' to aid identification of malarial parasites.

Blood fraction   A **blood product** prepared by chemical precipitation of **plasma**, usually by organic solvents. Precipitated fractions are preserved for storage by **freeze drying** or by resuspension in a buffered protein solution. See **Blood components**.

Blood group   A genetically determined characteristic expressed by

antigenic determinants found on the surface of the red cell membrane and in various body fluids and tissues.

Blood group frequency The frequency with which a **blood group** occurs in the population: it is usually quoted as a percentage. 'Blood group' in this context generally means a **phenotype** (e.g. 'the frequency of blood group A is 42%'). See **Gene frequencies**.

Blood group substance A substance (usually of human origin) which possesses the same antigenic properties as are found on some red cells. For example, B substance may be found in the saliva of some group B individuals.

Blood group system A series of **blood group antigens** determined by **genes** which are closely located to one another on the same **chromosome**.

Bloodmobile A vehicle used by a **blood bank** for the transport of equipment and personnel for the collection, in various locations, of blood for **transfusion**.

Blood product Any therapeutic product for **transfusion** which has human blood (including **plasma**) as its origin.

Blood viscosity See **Viscosity**.

Blood volume The total volume of blood in the circulatory system, comprising **plasma volume** and **red cell volume**. Plasma volume is determined by measuring the dilution of injected radioactive albumin, and in normal adults is approximately 45 ml/Kg body weight. Red cell volume is calculated following injection of **radioactive chromium**-labelled red cells and is normally around 30 ml/Kg body weight. The total blood volume can be calculated from the **red cell volume** and the **packed cell volume**, and is normally in the order of 60−80 ml/Kg body weight.

Blood warmer A device for the controlled warming of blood to body temperature prior to **transfusion**.

Blueing Mild alkali treatment to force a colour shift in **haematoxylin** staining from red to blue, with the simultaneous effect of removing free hydrogen ions and stabilising the dye/**mordant** complex. The process is usually achieved with running tap water or **Scott's tap-water substitute**.

B lymphocyte See **Lymphocyte**.

Bohr effect The effect of **pH** in altering the position of the **oxygen dissociation curve**.

Bombay phenotype The **blood group** O^h, in which there are no detectable A, B or H **antigens** on the red cells and and there is anti-A, anti-B and anti-H in the plasma. So called because the few cases reported have nearly all been found in India, around Bombay.

Bone marrow The marrow cavity of the bones, which is the site of production of all blood cells. In adults, haemopoietically-active (red) marrow is limited to the vertebrae, ribs, sternum, scapulae, skull and the extreme proximal ends of the humeri and femora. In infants, active haemopoiesis also occurs in the more distal portions of the extremities. Non-active (yellow) marrow space is filled with fat, but can be replaced with haemopoietic cells in conditions associated with long-standing increased haemopoiesis.

Booster dose An **antigen** (often in a **vaccine**) administered to raise the **antibody** level of a primed individual with pre-existing **antibody** to that antigen.

Boot In computing, an abbreviation of 'bootstrap'. Used as a verb it refers to the loading of an initialising **program** into the computer's **memory**, enabling it to read subsequent **input**. (By analogy with the computer 'pulling itself up by its own bootstraps').

Bordetella A genus of bacteria which are **aerobes**, do not exhibit **motility**, and are **catalase**-positive rod-shaped organisms which are positive by **Gram's stain** and which consist of two species. *Bordetella pertussis* and *Bordetella parapertussis* are dissimilar in some important respects and *Bordetella parapertussis* probably does not belong in the genus. *Bordetella pertussis* will not grow on media containing peptone and special media such as Bordet-Gengou or charcoal **agar** are needed. *Bordetella pertussis* is the causative agent of whooping cough, which usually affects infants and children. This is a severe respiratory tract **infection** characterised by paroxysmal coughing with a terminal whoop, and commonly lasting for weeks. There is no specific treatment for whooping cough. Vaccination of infants to achieve herd **immunity** results in a fall in incidence.

Bornholm's disease Epidemic myalgia caused by infection with some **Coxsackie** B **viruses** and characterised by malaise and chest pains.

Borrelia A genus of **bacteria** of the family of **spirochaetes**. They are negative by **Gram's stain** and strictly **anaerobic**. They have a central axial **filament** and a number of fibres in the protoplasm, contractions of which make the cell rotate. They are **parasites**, or live on mucous **membranes**, and are the cause of relapsing fever in humans and animals, being transmitted by arthropods, and sometimes by rodents.

Botulism A disease caused by **neurotoxins** produced by *Clostridium botulinum* and characterised by general and focal neurogenic weakness and paralysis, eventually leading to asphyxia. The **toxin** is elaborated in food contaminated with the organism, and intoxication follows ingestion of the preformed toxin. In wound botulism the symptoms are due to toxins elaborated in a wound infected with *Clostridium botulinum*. Infant botulism results from colonisation of the intestine by *Clostridium botulinum* and elaboration of toxin. The causative organism is widespread in soil and water and therefore is found in a variety of foodstuffs. **Outbreaks** are associated with consumption of poorly-sterilised, and particularly home-preserved, food.

Boyden chamber An item of equipment used to measure **chemotaxis**. It consists of two compartments separated by a filter. Cells under investigation are placed in the upper compartment and a chemotactic agent is placed in the lower compartment. If cells are attracted by the chemotactic agent they migrate through the pores of the filter and can be demonstrated by suitable staining of the filter.

Bradykinin A vasoactive nonapeptide formed by the cleavage of **high molecular weight kininogen** by **kallikrein**. Bradykinin forms part of the inflammatory response and may bring about increased vascular permeability, smooth muscle contraction and leucocyte **chemotaxis**.

Brain abscess An **abscess** within the parenchyma of the brain, giving rise to neurological abnormalities as a consequence of compression and displacement of central nervous system structures. The abscess may be due to direct spread of **infection** from the middle ear or from sinusitis, or occasionally it may be due to haematogenous spread in patients with **endocarditis**. The causative organisms include **Bacteroides** species, **aerobic** and **anaerobic** **Streptococci**, **Fusobacteria**, **Haemophilus**, **Actinomyces**, **Nocardia** and *Staphylococcus aureus*. Treatment is by surgical aspiration of the abscess contents and administration of **anti-microbial** drugs to cover the likely mixture of **aerobes** and **anaerobes**.

Brain heart infusion A fluid **culture medium** prepared by non-**enzymic** infusion from calf brain and beef heart, often with the addition of peptones and dextrose. It is suitable as a general medium and for cultivation of more demanding organisms. A solid version can be made by addition of **agar**.

Branhamella A genus of organisms which are obligatory **aerobes**, oxidase-positive, **catalase**-positive non-saccharolytic **cocci** which are negative by **Gram's stain**, and of which *Branhamella catarrhalis* is of human importance. **Serum** is not required for cultivation and growth occurs on nutrient **agar**. The organism has been incriminated in both upper and lower respiratory tract infections. **beta-Lactamase** is often produced.

Breakpoint The designated limit of susceptibility of a **microorganism** to an **anti-microbial** substance, beyond which it is considered resistant. The breakpoint is chosen on the basis of the clinically-achievable blood, tissue or urine levels of the drug after usual dosing, and the mean minimum inhibitory concentration of the drug for a large number of strains of that organism.

Brilliant cresyl blue A stain often used in **haematology** for the **supravital staining** of **reticulocytes**.

Brinase A proteolytic **enzyme** derived from strains of *Aspergillus oryzae*, which is capable of lysing **fibrin**. The purified enzyme may be used for **thrombolytic therapy**.

British comparative thromboplastin A carefully standardised human brain thromboplastin preparation which is used as a reference material to calibrate commercial or 'home-made' thromboplastins used in the determination of the **prothrombin time**.

British corrected ratio A means of expressing the **prothrombin time** ratio obtained with a commercial or 'home-made' thromboplastin, as an equivalent ratio to that obtained with the **British comparative thromboplastin**.

Bromelain A proteolytic enzyme sometimes used in **blood grouping** reactions. Obtained from the stem of the pineapple.

Bromination Bromine reacts with ethylene groups at the site of double bonds in unsaturated lipids to form substituted saturated compounds. These may be demonstrated with silver nitrate. Bromination also prevents **PAS** staining of unsaturated lipids and renders lecithin and free fatty acids Sudan black B positive.

Bronchial cell carcinoma See **Alveolar cell carcinoma**.

Bronchiectasis A chronic dilation of the walls of the bronchi or bronchioles. It may affect the tube uniformly, may occur in irregular pockets, or the dilation may cause terminal bulbous enlargement.

Bronchiolitis Inflammation of the bronchioles; a condition with a variety of aetiological agents. Bronchiolitis in children under 1 year of age is generally associated with **respiratory syncytial virus**.

Bronchitis Inflammation of the bronchi, usually along with other areas of the respiratory tract. The condition may be **acute** or **chronic**. Acute bronchitis varies considerably in severity depending on the cause and other factors, but rarely requires hospital admission of fit patients. Causes include influenza **virus**, adenovirus, **rhinoviruses**, and a small proportion due to **bacteria** such as *Mycoplasma pneumoniae* and *Haemophilus influenzae*. Chronic bronchitis often follows a history of acute episodes coupled with exposure to air pollution such as cigarette smoke. The proportion of mucus-secreting cells in the bronchial **epithelium** is greatly increased while there is often a decrease in ciliated cells, leading to accumulation of mucus in the bronchial lumen. Exacerbations of acute bronchitis in those with chronic bronchitis are often due to *Haemophilus influenzae*, *Streptococcus pneumoniae* and viruses.

Broth A fluid **culture medium**, usually based on an extract or infusion of animal tissue. Broth media may be enriched for special purposes or made into **selective media** by the addition of (e.g.) sodium selenite.

Brown atrophy pigment See **Lipofuchsin**.

Brucella Rod-shaped **bacteria** which are obligatory **aerobes**, non-**motile**, positive for **catalase** and **oxidase** and for **urease**, and which are negative by **Gram's stain**. They are primarily animal **pathogens** which also cause disease in humans in contact with infected animals or their products. *Brucella abortus* requires carbon dioxide for growth, and all grow relatively slowly. Biotypes of *Brucella abortus*, *Brucella suis* and *Brucella melitensis* can be distinguished on the basis of ability to grow in the presence of **dyes**.

Brucellosis The disease resulting from **infection** with **Brucella** species. Generally, *Brucella abortus* produces a less severe form of the disease, with fewer sequelae than *Brucella suis* and *Brucella melitensis*. The disease is found in farmers and their families, veterinary surgeons, abattoir workers and dairy workers. Apart from direct contact with infected animals, the ingestion of raw milk or milk products is an important means of contracting the disease. The illness may be asymptomatic, especially with *Brucella abortus*. Characteristic symptoms occur after an incubation period of weeks and include pyrexia with considerable sweating and chronic fatigue. The disease may recur within months of the first episode and it may also become **chronic**. Focal skeletal infection often occurs. Diagnosis is aided by **blood culture** and serological tests for **IgM, IgA** and **IgG** forms of **antibody**. **Tetracycline** has been the drug of choice for treatment, often combined with an **aminoglycoside**, but the relapse rate is disappointing. The addition of **Rifampicin** is said to reduce this.

Brush border A specialisation of the free surface of a cell, consisting of minute cylindrical processes which greatly increase the surface area.

Bruton-type hypogammaglobulinaemia A sex-linked **immunoglobulin** deficiency which becomes apparent when maternally derived **antibody** levels fall. Characterised by recurrent **bacterial** infections associated with low serum **immunoglobulin** levels.

BSH British Society for Haematology.

Bubble sort In computing, a **program** which sorts numerically identified data into ascending order by a selective process of exchange which systematically interchanges pairs of elements that are out of order until no more exchanges are necessary. If the records are visualised as ordered in a column, a pass is made over the records, the larger of which moves upwards in the column, the largest element moving to the top. Subsequent passes continue to move the larger records so that they 'bubble up' to their proper position in the column. The method is slow and there are better sorting methods available, but it is useful as a general purpose sorting program. See **Shell sort**.

Buccal Pertaining to the cheek or mouth.

Budding A mode of release of enveloped **virus** through cell **membranes** into intracellular **vacuoles**, or through the **cell wall**.

Buffer 1. A system comprising a mixture of a solution of a weak acid and its conjugate base, having the ability to resist changes in **hydrogen ion concentration** which would otherwise occur from the addition of another **acid** or **base**. Examples in the body include carbonic acid-bicarbonate, which helps maintain the pH of the blood. 2. A chemical system which prevents, or minimises, changes in the concentration of some chemical substance. 3. In computing, a temporary storage area for data, frequently used to hold data being transmitted between computers or **peripherals** which operate at different speeds or at different times.

Buffy coat The 'white' cellular layer between the red cells and **plasma** of blood which has been **centrifuged**.

Bulla A large blister or **vesicle**.

(alpha) Bungarotoxin A snake-derived **toxin** used in the **immuno-cytochemical** identification of acetylcholine receptors in muscle end-plates.

Bunyaviridae A large family of **RNA** viruses with **envelopes**, occurring in the tropics. All are arthropod borne.

Buoyant density The density of a particle expressed in terms of the density of a fluid **substrate** in which it neither sinks nor floats. The substrate most often used is caesium chloride. The measurement is important in differentiating **viruses** which are not **enveloped**, particularly those found in association with **gastroenteritis**.

Burkitt's lymphoma A **tumour** of **lymphoid** tissue which occurs most commonly in African children. There is a deficiency in **B cell** responses which is linked to infection with **Epstein-Barr virus** (EBV). **Antigens** of this virus have been demonstrated in the **tumour** cells of individuals with **Burkitt's lymphoma**.

Burnet's monoclonal selection theory A hypothesis which states that **antigen** entering the tissues selects (or is selected by) **B cells** carrying pre-existing **surface membrane immunoglobulin** specific for that antigen. On contact with antigen the specific B cells proliferate and differentiate into **plasma cells** which synthesise humoral **immunoglobulin**.

Burr cell A red cell showing a few spiky and irregular projections in stained **blood films**. The morphological abnormality is less severe than that seen in **acanthrocytes**. Burr cells are particularly common in cases of uraemia.

Bursa of Fabricius A sack-like lymphoid organ found attached to the cloaca of birds: first described by Fabricius in the 17th century. Neonatal **bursectomy** of birds renders them unable to synthesise **antibody**: the bursa is therefore considered to be the site at which **lymphocytes** derived from the **bone marrow** become committed **B cells**.

Bursectomy Removal of the **bursa of Fabricius** from a bird.

Burst forming unit erythroid The earliest erythroid precursors that can be identified and which give rise to haemoglobinised colonies of **erythroblasts** after 2 weeks' incubation in culture. These early cells are present in the **bone marrow** and in peripheral blood.

Bus In computing, abbreviation of 'busbar', an interconnected set of parallel electrical pathways which carry signals between a computer and its **peripherals**.

B virus A Simian herpes **virus** related to **herpes simplex**, causing cold sores in monkeys and severe central nervous system disease in man. It is a **risk group 4 pathogen**. The unexpected appearance of herpes-like cytopathic effect in primary monkey kidney cells should be investigated with considerable caution in suitable containment facilities (i.e. in a **biological safety cabinet**).

Bystander involvement The non-specific attachment of activated **complement** components to cells uncoated with complement-fixing **antibody**. These cells may be destroyed by this process due to the development of membrane lesions, or by **phagocytosis**.

Byte In computing, a **string** of eight adjacent **binary** digits. One byte contains sufficient information to represent one **ASCII** character.

C

Cabot ring   A red cell **inclusion body** which appears as a ring or 'figure 8', and stains reddish-purple with **Romanowsky** stains. These rings cannot be seen with **phase-contrast** microscopy and are considered to be an **artefact**.

Calcitonin   A calcium-mobilising polypeptide **hormone** produced by the parafollicular (or C) cells of the **thyroid**, in response to an increase in ionised calcium. It is thought to protect against hypercalcaemia and acts directly on bone to inhibit the bone's reabsorption activity.

Calcium ionophore   An agent which can cause **platelet aggregation** by directly increasing the cytoplasmic levels of free calcium ions, thereby bypassing the **arachadonic acid** pathway.

Calculus   1. Commonly called a 'stone'. An aggregation of insoluble or poorly-soluble salts precipitated out of body fluids; often, although not invariably, laid down concentrically, and sometimes formed around a central nidus. 2. Calcified plaque on the surface of the teeth.

Calibrant   The material used to standardise an analytical process, system or instrument. It is a material which has had concentration values attributed to it using, where possible, primary **standards** and reference methods. Although it may be a standard solution, it may also be an artificial material which itself plays no part in the analytical process.

Calibration   A system involving the use of a **calibrant** for measuring the response of an instrument to stimulation, and which may involve the graphical presentation of such data.

Caliciviridae   A family of **RNA** viruses without **envelopes** and with unique **capsomeres** with shallow depressions on their outer surface. They cause **gastroenteritis** in animals, and have recently been associated with human enteric disease.

Callus   1. A mass of new bone formed by direct growth, usually at the site of trauma − especially fractures. 2. A hardening of the epidermis of the skin, usually due to friction.

Calmodulin   An intracellular calcium-binding **platelet** protein which acts as a mediator of calcium's role as an intracellular messenger.

Calymmatobacterium   *Calymmatobacterium granulomatis* is the causative organism of granuloma inguinale (Donovanosis). The organism is very difficult to cultivate on artificial **culture medium**, and is usually demonstrated in direct smears using **Giemsa's stain**. The coccoid rod-shaped organisms are negative by **Gram's stain** and are usually found inside **histiocytes** and **giant cells**. Lesions appear after an **incubation** period of a few weeks, usually on the genitalia, in the groin and on the perineum, and spread is usually by sexual contact. Most cases are seen in tropical and sub-tropical areas. Treatment is by administration of **Gentamicin**, **Chloramphenicol** or **Tetracycline**.

cAMP   Cyclic adenosine monophosphate. See **Phosphodiesterase**.

CAMP test   A test for synergistic **haemolysis** by some **bacteria** on sheep or ox **blood agar**, in which the extracellular **toxin** of *Streptococcus agalactiae* (Group B streptococcus) interacts with the beta-haemolysin from *Staphylococcus aureus* to produce haemolysis. Neither organism alone is haemolytic on this **culture medium**. The toxin from the streptococcus must come into contact with the blood before that from the staphylococcus. Other organisms (such as *Pasteurella haemolytica*) may also show a positive reaction.

Campylobacter   Bacteria which exhibit **motility**, are curved **oxidase**-positive rod-shaped organisms which are negative by **Gram's stain** and which usually require an oxygen concentration of about 10%, but will not grow under **anaerobic** conditions. The **catalase**-positive thermophilic *Campylobacter jejuni* is a very common cause of **enteritis** in man and animals. Where specific anti-microbial therapy is indicated, **Erythromycin** is the drug of choice.

Canada balsam   In microscopy, a resin **mountant** of high **refractive index** (1·52) composed of terpenes, carboxylic acids and their esters, and used as a 50% solution in xylene. Obtained from the Canadian fir tree (*Abies balsamea*).

Canaliculi   Fine channels in compact bone, which radiate from central canals and through which bone cells receive metabolites.

Cancer procoagulant A   A **protein** found in several human and animal malignant cell lines and which is distinct from **tissue factor**, and is capable of directly activating **coagulation factor X**.

Candida   A genus of **yeast**-like **fungus**, of which *Candida albicans* is the main **pathogen**. In otherwise healthy people lesions occur on the mucous membranes of the mouth and vagina and are known as thrush. In the **immuno-compromised** host, including individuals suffering from **diabetes**, lesions may be more widespread and the disease may be systemic. The generalised form may also follow colonisation of an intravenous or intraperitoneal catheter. Candida species grow on ordinary types of **culture medium** at 37°C or room temperature, to give smooth or butyrous colonies which have a typical odour. The **blastospores** of which such colonies consist are positive by **Gram's stain**, oval and often budding. On corn meal **agar** large, thick-walled **chlamydospores** are formed by *Candida albicans*, which also produces short cylindrical projections known as germ tubes when **incubated** in human **serum**. In tissues and exudates, both yeasts and pseudohyphae are found.

Capillary resistance test   See **Tourniquet test**.

Capillary viscometer See **Viscometer**.

Capnocytophaga *Capnocytophaga ochracea* is a **micro-organism** which is **catalase**-negative, **fusiform** rod-shaped, and is negative by **Gram's stain**, showing gliding **motility**. It grows best as an **anaerobe** but will grow in air with added carbon dioxide, hence the generic name. It is a **commensal** of the oral cavity, but sometimes causes disease in susceptible or **immunocompromised** patients.

Capping The induction of clustering of proteins or **antigen** sites on the cell surface. This may be due to exposure of the cell to such things as **enzymes** or staining processes.

Capsomere A surface subunit of viral nucleocapsids visible in **electron micrographs**, consisting of identical **protein** molecules. Each family of **viruses** has a specific number of capsomeres of similar general morphology. There may be minor morphological differences within the family, but these are not normally identifiable in diagnostic **electron microscopy**.

Capsule An outer layer external to the **cell wall** of **bacteria**, and having a definite outer boundary consisting usually of polysaccharide, but occasionally of polypeptide. Capsulated organisms are often more virulent than their non-capsulated counterparts, largely due to protection against **phagocytosis** afforded by the capsule. Production of capsules depends upon cultural and environmental conditions.

Carbenicillin A semi-synthetic **penicillin** with activity against **Pseudomonas** and other rod-shaped organisms which are negative by **Gram's stain**. Resistance is usually due to a plasmid-mediated **beta-Lactamase**. The drug can only be administered **parenterally**. As with penicillin, side effects other than hypersensitivity are uncommon, though hypernatraemia can occur due to the high sodium content of the drug.

Carbinol A colourless compound formed by introducing hydroxyl groups into certain **chromophores**. An indicator of **pH** change which, upon dehydration, forms an anhydride which is a true dye base (for example, see **Leucodye**).

Carbohydrate An aldehyde or ketone derivative of alcohols, containing or yielding more than one hydroxyl group. Commonly called sugars, they comprise neutral polysaccharides (glycogen), **acid mucopolysaccharides** (found mainly in connective tissue), glycoproteins (**mucins**), and glycolipids.

(beta) Carboline A **fluorescent** condensation product formed by the action of formaldehyde on indoleamines. An example of **formaldehyde-induced fluorescence** is its use to demonstrate **endocrine cells** of the **diffuse neuro-endocrine system**.

Carbol xylene A mixture of phenol and xylene which has slight water tolerance and is thus suitable for **clearing** stained tissue sections susceptible to alcoholic **dehydration**.

Carbon dioxide incubator An instrument designed to maintain a constant temperature and a pre-set atmospheric level of CO_2. The successful culture of certain **bacteria**, and a number of **cell culture** methods, require carefully controlled atmospheric conditions.

Carbon film A very thin film of carbon (5−20 nm), used to support specimens in the **transmission electron microscope**.

Carborundum An **abrasive**, used either as a powder or a stone, to sharpen **microtome** knives.

Carbowax A water-soluble wax, consisting principally of polyethylene glycols. Used in **histology** where conventional **dehydration** or **clearing** is to be avoided (e.g. the demonstration of lipid in tissue sections).

(gamma) Carboxyglutamic acid Residues which are added to precursor forms of the **coagulation factors** II, VII, IX and X in a reaction catalysed by **vitamin K**, and which bestow on the parent molecule the ability to bind calcium ions. See also **Proteins induced by vitamin K absence**.

Carboxyhaemoglobin The term given to the compound formed when **haemoglobin** forms a complex with carbon monoxide. Haemoglobin has an affinity for carbon monoxide which is 200 times greater than that for oxygen. Carboxyhaemoglobin is therefore unavailable for normal oxygen transport.

Carboxylation The introduction of carboxyl groups into fixed mucosubstances. It induces strong **basophilia** of epithelial **mucins** in particular.

Carbuncle An **abscess** centred around a hair follicle, but extending to other follicles and draining to the surface by one or more sinuses. They are commonly found on the back of the neck and are caused by *Staphylococcus aureus*.

Carcino-embryonic antigen A **protein**-polysaccharide **oncofetal antigen** found in some fetal tissues during the first few months of gestation. It is also found in human cancer tissue of the colon, pancreas and liver. It can be measured in the blood and is of limited diagnostic value as a **tumour** marker.

Carcinoid Descriptive of the **enterochromaffin** cell type, commonly **argentaffin**. Due to the presence of 5-hydroxytryptamine.

Carcinoma Cancer. A **malignant** 'new growth' made up of **epithelial** cells which tend to infiltrate the surrounding tissues, giving rise to **metastases**.

Carcinoma *in situ* A **neoplasm** in which the **tumour** cells still lie within the **epithelium** of origin, without invasion of the **basement membrane**.

Cardiobacterium *Cardiobacterium hominis* is an organism which exhibits **pleomorphism**, is a facultative **anaerobe**, does not exhibit **motility**, is **catalase**-negative, **oxidase**-positive and a fermentative rod-shaped bacterium which is positive by **Gram's stain** and grows on **blood agar** to produce small colonies. Carbon dioxide is often required for primary isolation. It may be a **commensal** in the upper respiratory tract and is a cause of **endocarditis**. It is susceptible to **penicillin** and **aminoglycosides**.

Cardiolipin A lipid substance extracted from beef hearts and used (*inter alia*) as an **antigen** in tests for **antibodies** against the organism responsible for syphilis. See **TPHA test** and **VDRL test**.

Carmalum A useful red nuclear counter-stain consisting of 20 g/l carmine in a 50 g/l solution of aluminium ammonium sulphate.

Carnoy's fluid A rapidly penetrating **fixative**, consisting of ethanol: chloroform:acetic acid, in the proportion of 6:3:1. Useful for nuclear studies, *in situ* **hybridisation** and **immunocytochemistry**, this fixative may remove certain **lipids** from tissue.

Carotenoid A type of unsaturated hydrocarbon present as **lipid pigments** in adrenal cortex and *corpora lutea*. Soluble in alcohol and clearing agents, they are not found in paraffin sections and only rarely in **frozen sections**.

Caryosome A central conspicuous nuclear mass. The relative size of the caryosome may be of particular diagnostic importance in intestinal amoebae.

Cascade reaction A reaction in which activation of one element leads to sequential activation of others; for example the **coagulation** and **complement** systems. See also **Cascade theory**.

Cascade theory The term often used to describe the interaction of **coagulation factors** in which an activated factor acts on the inactive **protein**, resulting in a further enzymatic product which activates the next protein in a predetermined sequence. See **Cascade reaction**.

Casein The main protein found in milk, and used widely as a rich source of amino acids in **culture media**.

Caseinolytic assay A type of assay for **plasminogen** and **plasmin**, in which **casein** is used as a **substrate**. Now largely superseded by **chromogenic** assays.

Catecholamine A hormone with a hydroxylated benzene derivative structure, and which is synthesised primarily in the adrenal medulla. The major catecholamines are **adrenaline** (epinephrine), noradrenaline (norepinephrine) and **dopamine**.

Cathode 1. The negative electrical terminal of an electrolytic cell. 2. In **electron microscopy**, the source of electrons.

Cation See **Ion**.

Cationic dye   A dye with a positive electrostatic charge. Such dyes are attracted to tissues carrying a negative charge (**basophilia**).

Cat scratch disease   A rare, but mild, disease occuring in association with an injury inflicted by a cat. There is a pustular lesion at the site of the injury and lymphadenitis in the draining lymph glands. The disease seems likely to be caused by an infection, but no aetiological agent has yet been isolated.

Caustic pattern   A characteristic stellate pattern seen in the **transmission electron microscope** when the **intermediate lens** is close to the crossover point.

CEA   See **Carcinoembryonic antigen**.

Ceftriaxone   A **cephalosporin** type of **anti-microbial** substance which has activity against most rod-shaped **bacteria** which are negative by **Gram's stain**, with the exception of **pseudomonas**. It has an exceptionally long half-life in the body.

Cefuroxime   A **cephalosporin** type of **anti-microbial** substance which has activity against most rod-shaped **bacteria** which are negative by **Gram's stain**, with the exception of **pseudomonas** and **bacteroides**. Activity against **staphylococci** is higher than with most other cephalosporins, although **methicillin**-resistant *Staphylococcus aureus* is not susceptible. **Enterococci** are resistant.

Cell-associated virus   A **virus** which remains within the cell in large numbers at the completion of its replication cycle.

Cell culture   The *in vitro* cultivation of cells disaggregated from their original tissue using **enzymes**. Many of the most useful cell types grow in a single layer (**monolayer**) attached to a suitable glass or clear plastic surface. Some cells (e.g. **lymphoblasts**) do not become **attached** to any surface and grow naturally in suspension. Others may be induced to grow in this way by constant agitation. All cell cultures require highly enriched culture media, and are highly susceptible to contamination. Monolayer cell cultures provide the optimal medium for the demonstration of **cytopathic effects** caused by **viruses** and some bacterial **toxins**.

Cell-mediated immunity   **Immunity** which is dependent upon the activity of **T-cell** lymphocytes (e.g. **Allograft** rejection, **delayed hypersensitivity**, viral **immunity**).

Cell membrane   The **membrane** surrounding the **cytoplasm** of the **bacterial** cell, and lying between it and the **cell wall**. It is a lipoprotein bilayer which, apart from being an osmotic barrier, is the site of many **enzymic** reactions and transport systems.

Celloidin   Cellulose tetranitrate, or gun cotton. Used in **histology** as an alternative **embedding** medium to **paraffin wax**. Its use avoids the application of heat during **processing**. Low viscosity nitrocellulose is preferred by some workers.

Cellular pathology The microscopic study of disease in cells and tissues, including chemical and physical structure, morphology, metabolism and **immunology**. See also **Histology, Histopathology, Histochemistry, Immunocytochemistry** and *In situ* **hybridisation**.

Cellulitis An **infection** of the skin and subcutaneous tissue which tends to spread superficially and does not usually involve the deep fascia. However, spread is rapid and can give rise to **septicaemia** and thrombophlebitis, especially in the elderly. The usual causative agent is either *Streptococcus pyogenes* or *Staphylococcus aureus*.

Cell wall The rigid layer surrounding most **bacteria**, conferring a definite shape on the cell. The cell wall is external to the **cell membrane**. In cells which are positive with **Gram's stain** the wall is about 80 nm thick and consists mainly of **peptidoglycan**. The cell wall in organisms which are negative by **Gram's stain** is about 20 nm thick and has only a thin layer of peptidoglycan situated between the cell membrane and the outer membrane which, like the inner cell membrane, consists mainly of lipoprotein, phospholipid and specialised proteins such as porins.

Cell wall-active antibiotic An **anti-microbial** substance which interferes with the **cell walls** of **bacteria**, and particularly with their synthesis. Examples are the **beta Lactams**, which bind to **penicillin**-binding proteins, thus preventing incorporation and cross-linking of muramic acid pentapeptides, and **Vancomycin**, which binds to **bactoprenol** and prevents it from rejoining the cycle.

Cement line The junction resulting either from a quiescent period during sequential bone growth, or where adjacent areas of bone growth meet. The line is uncalcified and relatively rich in connective tissue **mucopolysaccharide**.

Cementum Calcified hard tissue covering the roots of teeth. It is morphologically indistinguishable from bone.

Central processing unit The part of a computer which acts as a calculator and which controls the computer's other functions. In a **microcomputer** the central processing unit is contained in the **microprocessor**.

Centrifugal analyser An automated analytical device which uses centrifugal force to transport and mix samples and reagents, and concludes the reaction phase of the test by centrifugation of the mixed reactants prior to end point measurement by optical reading.

Centrifuge A device used to separate particulate from non-particulate material, or materials of differing densities, by the application of centrifugal force. The extent of the force exerted (the **relative centrifugal force**) depends upon the radius of the instrument (i.e. the distance from the spindle of the instrument to the position of the interface between the materials being separated) as well as upon the speed of rotation.

Centrosome See **Caryosome**.

Cephaloridine A semi-synthetic **cephalosporin** type of **anti-microbial** substance which has activity against most rod-shaped **bacteria** which are negative by **Gram's stain**, with the exception of **pseudomonas**, indole-positive **proteus**, **serratia**, **enterobacter** and **bacteroides**. Cephaloridine is also more active against **staphylococci** than some other cephalosporins, but is inactive against **methicillin**-resistant strains and against **enterococci**. High serum levels can give rise to **nephrotoxicity**.

Cephalosporin A group of **beta lactam** type of **anti-microbial** substances which have a similar anti-bacterial action to the **penicillins**, but differ markedly in their spectra of activity. Cephalosporins are usefully active against a wide range of rod-shaped **bacteria** which are negative by **Gram's stain**, due mainly to their greater resistance to beta lactamases, and in some instances to a more efficient penetration of the **cell membrane**. They are traditionally classified in 'generations'. **Cephaloridine** and **Cephradine** are examples of the first, **Cefoxitin** and **Ceforoxime** of the second, and **Cefotaxime**, **Ceftriaxone** and **Ceftazimide** of the third. Few are active against **pseudomonas**, and **Ceftazidime** is an exception in this respect. Most cephalosporins, like the penicillins, are non-toxic and safe in clinical use but some, such as **Cephaloridine** and **Cephalothin**, are nephrotoxic.

Cephalothin A semi-synthetic **cephalosporin** with a spectrum of activity similar to that of **Cephaloridine**.

Cephamycin A naturally-occurring **anti-microbial** substance produced by the **Streptomyces** species and structurally closely related to the **cephalosporins**. An example of a semi-synthetic cephamycin, derived from cephamycin C, is **Cefoxitin**.

Cephradine A 'first generation' **cephalosporin** which can be administered both orally and parenterally. It is active against **penicillinase**-producing **staphylococci**, but not **methicillin**-resistant strains. **Enterococci** are resistant. Among the rod-shaped bacilli which are negative by **Gram's stain** most **proteus**, **enterobacter** and **serratia** are resistant, as is **pseudomonas**. The drug has poor activity against **haemophilus**.

Cercaria A larval stage in the life cycle of **flukes**. The larval stage in some species of flukes may be infective to the definitive host, but usually not until it has developed to the metacercarial form. Numerous species of flukes found throughout the world are infective to man.

Cerebrospinal fluid (CSF) A normally clear fluid which is produced in the choroid plexuses of the cerebral ventricles, and which circulates through the ventricular system and the subarachnoid space of the central nervous system, to be absorbed by the arachnoid villi. It normally has a protein content of about 0·4 g/l and up to five **leucocytes** per cubic mm. In bacterial **meningitis** the content of **protein** and the **polymorphonuclear** leucocyte count are raised and the glucose level is low.

Ceroid A yellow **lipid** pigment at an early stage of oxidation that may be found in **frozen sections** of tissue. May be demonstrated as fat, and **autofluoresces** yellow.

Certified cell line A cell line which is fully defined and has been listed by the American Cell Culture Committee.

Cervicitis Inflammation of the *cervix uteri*, caused by a variety of **infectious** and non-infectious agents.

Cestoda Tapeworms. Segmented worms which have complex life cycles and intricate host/parasite relationships. Taenia, Hymenolepis, Diphyllobothrium and Echinococcus cause human disease, the last being a cause of **hydatid cysts** which are seen in farmers due to the passage of parasite from dogs to humans and to sheep and cattle. Of the species infective to man, the most common in European countries are *Taenia saginata* and *Taenia solium*, both acquired from eating under-cooked meat − beef and pork respectively.

CFU-C See **Colony forming unit cell**.

CHAD See **Cold haemagglutinin disease**.

(kappa) Chain A type of **light chain** found in **immunoglobulin** molecules. Immunoglobulin monomers have either two kappa chains or two **lambda chains**.

(lambda) Chain A type of **light chain** found in **immunoglobulin** molecules. Immunoglobulin monomers have either two lambda chains or two **kappa chains**.

(mu) Chain The **heavy chain** of **immunoglobulin M**.

Chancre The first lesion to appear in **syphilis**, about 3 weeks after exposure. The typical ulcer has a different appearance to that of **chancroid**, but might readily be confused with it. **Treponemes** can be seen in scrapings from the chancre, using **dark ground microscopy**.

Chancroid Also known as soft **chancre**, this sexually transmitted disease is caused by *Haemophilus ducreyi*, and occurs in the form of an ulcer on the genitalia. The causative organism requires **X factor** and its growth is encouraged by carbon dioxide. **Erythromycin** and **Trimethoprim** are the most useful drugs for treatment.

Charcot-Leyden crystals Crystalline material seen in **eosinophil**

granules by **electron microscopy**, and which may be deposited in secretions or exudates following the disintegration of large numbers of **eosinophils**.

Chediak-Higashi syndrome An **autosomal** recessive condition affecting the structure and function of **lysosomes** in **neutrophils**. Individuals with the condition suffer from infections with **pyogenic** bacteria.

Chelating agent An organic compound with the power to bind certain metals (e.g. the di-sodium salt of **EDTA**, which binds calcium). Uses include **decalcification** of bone, copper binding to **azo dyes** formed by **simultaneous coupling** in enzyme **histochemistry**, and removal of calcium from blood to prevent clotting.

Chemiluminescence The emission of light by molecules in excited states, as a result of a chemical reaction (e.g. as in fireflies).

Chemoautotroph A **bacterium** which can utilise carbon dioxide as a source of carbon and can obtain energy by oxidation of inorganic chemicals. Such organisms are rarely encountered in medical **bacteriology**.

Chemography In **autoradiography**, reactive tissue groups which produce a latent image in the silver halide (positive chemography) or cause the latent image to fade (negative chemography).

Chemoorganotroph A **bacterium** which depends on organic compounds for energy and sources of carbon. Those of medical importance belong to this group.

Chemoprophylaxis The use of **anti-microbial** substances in order to prevent, rather than treat, **infection**. Often only one or two doses are administered if the risk of infection is associated with surgery.

Chemotaxis The directional migration of cells − primarily **neutrophils**, **macrophages** and **monocytes** − under the influence of an attractant stimulus. See also **Cytotaxin** and **Cytotaxigen**.

Chemotherapy 1. The treatment of **malignant** disease with **cytotoxic** drugs. 2. The use of **anti-microbial** substances to treat existing **infection**. The anti-microbials and the dose used are often different from those used in **chemoprophylaxis**.

Chimera A creature which has two or more genetic lineages. Named after a mythical creature which had a goat's body, a lion's head and a serpent's tail. For example, as a result of an apparent uterine vascular anastomosis a very few examples have been reported of dizygotic (dissimilar) twins who each had a mixture of two different sets of **blood groups**, so that instead of one being group O and the other group A, each may be a mixture of O and A. Such chimeras are recognised by the mixed-field **agglutination** of the red cells given by some **antibodies**, and by the lack of reciprocal ABO **antibodies** in the serum.

Chip A piece of semi-conductor material, such as silicon, which has microscopic integrated circuits etched upon it.

Chi-squared test In statistical analysis, a **hypothesis** test using the chi-squared **distribution**. It is used when observations are put into classes and the observed frequencies in the classes are to be compared with those expected, given a particular hypothesis.

Chitin A neutral polysaccharide containing N-acetyl-glucosamine, used to inhibit **lectin** binding, and thus demonstrate **specificity**.

Chlamydia A type of obligate intracellular **pathogen** of man and animals, resembling **bacteria** but having an unusual replication cycle. Their obligate intracellular pathogenicity is due to their defective energy pathways. While unable to reproduce outside **prokaryotic** cells, they contain both **RNA** and **DNA**, have **peptidoglycan** in their **cell walls** and have ribosomes in their **cytoplasm**. The drug of choice for Chlamydia infections is **tetracycline**. *Chlamydia psittaci* is the species causing **psittacosis** and **ornithosis**. The organism is **zoonotic** in man, infection almost invariably being associated with contact with a pet bird. The species has many serotypes, those causing the most severe disease coming from psittacine birds. Laboratory diagnosis is by isolation of the organism in **cell cultures** or fertile hen eggs, or by serological methods. *Chlamydia trachomatis* is another species which infects man and causes a wide variety of diseases. Originally associated with the blinding eye disease **trachoma**, and with **neonatal conjunctivitis**, it is now known to be a common venereal disease. Chlamydia is a proven cause of **urethritis** in men and **cervicitis** in women. Chronic infection is thought to be at least contributory to the level of male and female infertility. Pelvic inflammatory disease and perihepatitis are severe complications of infection in women. Three of the 15 serotypes cause *Lymphogranuloma venereum*. Diagnosis of the infection is by isolation in **cell culture**, or by demonstration of **elementary bodies** by **immunofluorescence**. **Enzyme immunoassays** may replace isolation methods, and may prove essential as the number of tests required increases.

Chlamydospore A thick-walled asexual spore produced by some **fungi**, including *Candida albicans*. The spores are relatively resistant to unfavourable growth conditions. Candida chlamydospores are best demonstrated on corn meal **agar**.

Chloramphenicol Originally a naturally-occurring **anti-microbial** substance produced by **Streptomyces** species, the drug is now manufactured synthetically. A wide range of rod-shaped **bacteria** which are negative by **Gram's stain**, including **anaerobes** and many Gram-positive bacteria, are susceptible. **Rickettsiae, chlamydia, mycoplasma** and **coxiella** are also susceptible. Some strains become resistant due to **plasmid**-mediated production of acetyl transferase which inactivates the drug. Chloramphenicol is well-absorbed when taken orally, but can also be used parenterally. When given by either route it is one of the few drugs to penetrate into the **cerebrospinal fluid**, even in the absence of meningeal inflammation. It is the treatment of choice for **typhoid** fever, although resistant strains have been reported. Toxicity gives rise to **aplastic anaemia**. The drug exerts its antibacterial effect by binding to the 50s sub-unit of the ribosome, thus inhibiting protein synthesis.

Chlorhexidine A chlorophenol with activity against vegetative **micro-organisms** staining both positive and negative with **Gram's stain**, other than **pseudomonas** and some strains of **proteus, enterobacter** and **flavobacterium**. It is inactive against **spores** and **mycobacteria** and poorly active against most **fungi**.

Chloroform sensitivity In a **virus**, indicates the presence of essential lipid, usually contained in an envelope. The use of chloroform provides a relatively safe alternative to ether when investigating this feature. See also **Ether sensitivity**.

Chlortetracycline This **anti-microbial** substance, produced by **Streptomyces** species, was the first **tetracycline** discovered. It is suitable for oral administration only.

Chocolate agar A **culture medium** made by heating a mixture of horse blood and nutrient **agar**, during which the red blood cells disrupt to release their contents, including **haemoglobin** and the related substance haemin or **X factor**. The medium is useful for the isolation of fastidious organisms including **haemophilus**, meningococcus and **gonococcus**.

Cholecystitis Inflammation of the gall bladder, often associated with gall stones. Infection is usually secondary to obstruction and stasis, and is caused by enteric organisms.

Cholera An **acute** enteric intoxication with **toxin** produced by *Vibrio cholerae*, which causes rapid loss of body water and electrolytes into the lumen of the gut. Hypotension, hypoglycaemia and electrolyte depletion follow rapidly and, if untreated, death can occur within hours of the onset of symptoms. Treatment is by administration of dextrose and electrolyte solutions, of which many litres are often required. The administration of **tetracycline**, **chloramphenicol** or other **anti-microbial** substances shortens the duration of fluid loss.

Cholesterol 1. Crystals. Envelope-shaped or square alcohol soluble crystals with one corner missing, seen in unstained smears and having a macroscopically characteristic glistening appearance. 2. Clefts. Characteristically shaped spaces in **paraffin wax** sections from which this **lipid** has been lost during **processing** for **histology**.

Cholinesterase (EC 3.1.1.8) Sometimes called pseudo-cholinesterase, this substance acts on a number of esters of choline to give choline and acetic acid. It plays an important part in the physiology of the nervous system and destroys acetylcholine after the transmission of an impulse. It is found in liver, pancreas, heart and brain, and is active against benzoylcholine.

Chondroitin sulphate An **acid mucopolysaccharide** of connective tissue origin, subdivided into types A, B and C.

Chorioepithelioma A **tumour** formed by **malignant** proliferation of the chorionic villi of the placenta.

Christmas disease The congenital deficiency of **coagulation factor IX**. This sex-linked condition is clinically similar to **haemophilia A** and is also known as **haemophilia B**.

Christmas factor See **Coagulation factors**.

Chromaffin Dark brown granular material found in cells of the adrenal medulla after chrome **fixation**, and derived from adrenalin and noradrenalin.

Chromate deposit Salts which are formed in tissue if chromate **fixation** is followed immediately by alcohol **dehydration**. It can be prevented by washing in water, and removed by alcoholic hydrochloric acid.

Chromatic aberration Describes a defect resulting from 'white' light, split into its component spectral colours on passage through a lens, failing to re-form at a common focus. In particular, blue rays (of shorter wavelength) come to a focus before the (longer wavelength) red rays, producing an image fringed with colour haloes.

Chromatid One of the two spiral filaments making up a **chromosome** and which separate in cell division, each going to a different pole of the dividing cell. One strand of a **metaphase** chromosome.

Chromatin The protoplasmic substance in the nuclei of cells. It is readily stainable with basic dyes and consists of **deoxyribonucleic acid** attached to a protein structure base. It is the carrier of the **genes**.

Chromatography The separation of molecules from a mixture according to their polarity, and by partition between two phases. There is a variety of chromatographic techniques including adsorption, gas-liquid and high performance liquid chromatography.

Chromatoid body Also known as chromatoid bar and chromatoid mass. An aggregate of **RNA** seen in young **cysts** by **light microscopy,** or dispersed and only seen by **electron microscopy** in **trophozoites** of the *Entamoeba* species.

Chrome-gelatin A useful section **adhesive** prepared as 1 g/l chrome alum in 10 g/l aqueous gelatin, into which acid-washed slides are dipped and then dried prior to use.

Chromobacterium Rod-shaped organisms which exhibit **motility**, are **oxidase** and **catalase** positive and are negative by **Gram's stain**. *Chromobacterium violaceum* is a facultative **anaerobe**, is mesophilic and produces a violet pigment. *Chromobacterium lividum* is strictly an **aerobe**, is psychrophilic and produces a less pronounced violet pigment. The organisms are occasionally involved in human infection.

Chromocentre A condensation of dark **chromatinic** material appearing as a granule in the nuclear chromatin structure, and composed of **DNA**.

Chromogen A coloured compound produced by introducing certain chemical groups (**chromophores**) into the benzene ring by substitution. With the addition of an **auxochrome**, the coloured compound becomes a dye.

Chromogenic substrate Increasingly used in blood **coagulation** testing, chromogenic substrates are short (3–4 amino acid) synthetic **peptides**, joined via an amide bond to an indicator group. When an enzyme cleaves the amide bond, the chromophore is released and may be detected by **spectrophotometry**. See also **Amidolytic assay**.

Chromolipid See **Carotenoids**.

Chromophobe A cell type of the pituitary, so-called because it fails to stain with **acid** and **basic dyes** used to differentiate other cells of this gland.

Chromophore A chemical group which, when introduced into a benzene ring by substitution, produces a coloured compound – a **chromogen**.

Chromoprotein Protein combined with coloured pigment (e.g. **haemoglobin**) in tissue section.

Chromosome A structure within the cell nucleus, composed of **DNA**, upon which the **genes** are arranged.

Chronic Persisting over a long period of time.

Chronic granulomatous disease A sex-linked condition affecting the **neutrophils** of young males. The neutrophil **lysosomes** are deficient in lysosomal NADH oxidase, which makes the neutrophils unable to kill **phagocytosed** bacteria.

Chronic leukaemia A **malignant** proliferation of **leucocytes** which may be of myeloid or lymphoid origin. The disease is characterised by increased numbers of immature **leucocytes** in the peripheral blood and **bone marrow**, and a relatively **chronic** course which may terminate in **acute leukaemia**. See **Blast cell crisis**.

Chronic mucocutaneous candidiasis A condition in which there is a defect in **cell-mediated immunity** to infection by *Candida albicans*. The condition is characterised by persistent *C. albicans* infection of the mucuous membranes, nails and skin.

Chyle 1. A milky fluid taken up by the lymphatic ducts from the intestine, consisting of lymph and triglycerides in emulsion. It enters the blood by way of the thoracic duct. 2. Lymph in urine, giving a milky appearance. Syn. Chyluria. A feature of the chronic obstructive stage of **filariasis**, when the lymphatics become blocked by worms. **Microfilariae** can sometimes be demonstrated in the urine.

Chylomicron A **lipoprotein** which contains mostly exogenous triglycerides. Chylomicrons are the least dense of the lipoproteins and float to the top of **serum** when allowed to separate out. They often remain at the point of application on **electrophoresis**.

CIEP See **Counter immunoelectrophoresis**.

Cilia Specialised hair-like locomotor **organelle** structures attached to the free surface of a cell. Fundamentally similar to a **flagellum**, but typically much more numerous and not restricted to the anterior region. They maintain passage of fluid over the surface **membrane**.

Ciliocytophthoria Destruction of **cilia**-covered respiratory **epithelial** cells. Pinching off the distal ciliated portion of the cells results in the formation of anucleated ciliated tufts, and of nucleated **cytoplasmic** sects.

Ciprofloxacin A 4-**quinolone** type of **anti-microbial substance** with high activity against a wide range of rod-shaped bacteria which are **aerobes** staining negative by **Gram's stain**, including **pseudomonas**. It also has high activity against many aerobic Gram-positive bacteria including **methicillin**-resistant **staphylococci** and multi-resistant **coryneforms**, but activity against **streptococci** is variable.

Circadian rhythm Rhythmic repetition, at regular times of night or day, of activities or processes of living organisms. For example, the appearance of **microfilariae** in peripheral blood. (See **Filariasis**).

Circulating anticoagulant Substances in the peripheral blood which interfere with blood **coagulation**. They are especially common in **haemophilia**, disseminated lupus erythematosus, and following pregnancy.

Cirrhosis Chronic interstitial inflammation of an organ, characterised by destruction of the **parenchyma** and hardening due to the overgrowth of the connective tissue.

***Cis* position** In genetics, the location of two **alleles** on the same **chromosome** of a **homologous** pair.

Cistron The unit of genetic function. Loss of any part of a cistron results in the complete loss of its function.

Citrate phosphate dextrose An **anticoagulant**/preservative solution used for the collection and storage of blood for **transfusion**. There are a number of formulations and the solution often has **adenine** added to further retard **glycolysis**.

Citrobacter   Rod-shaped bacteria which exhibit **motility**, are facultative **anaerobes** which are **oxidase** negative, **catalase** positive, ferment lactose and are members of the family **Enterobacteriaceae**. They differ from *Escherichia coli* in being able to use citrate as their sole carbon source and in being unable to decarboxylate lysine. There are serological cross-reactions between *C. freundii*, *Escherichia coli* and **Salmonella**. *C. freundii* is found in the healthy intestine and is also found in food and water.

Class I antigen   A **Human Leucocyte Antigen** (HLA) of type A, B or C. These antigens are carried on a transmembrane glycoprotein of 44 000 D, which is associated with **beta₂ microglobulin**.

Class II antigen   A **Human Leucocyte Antigen** (HLA) coded for by the D loci on **chromosome** 6 in man. These antigens are carried on a transmembrane glycoprotein heterodimer consisting of an alpha chain (34 000 D) and a beta chain (28 000 D).

Class I exhaust protective cabinet   An enclosed ventilated cabinet providing safe working conditions, and in which air is drawn in through the front from the room and exhausted either (i) via a single **HEPA** filter and through ducts to the outside of the building, or (ii) via two HEPA filters in sequence and back into the same room. These cabinets are suitable for manipulation of **risk group 3 pathogens** and are not normally fitted with glove ports. Class I cabinets must be sited in rooms having negative air pressure relative to adjacent rooms and corridor space. Their primary function is to protect workers from aerosols produced by their work. See also **Class II cabinet** and **Class III exhaust protective cabinet**.

Class II cabinet   An enclosed ventilated cabinet providing safe working conditions. **HEPA** filtered air is passed over the working surface and, through vents in it, back through the HEPA filter. Some exchange of air takes place at the front opening of the cabinet. The primary function of these cabinets is to protect work from **aerosols** in the room. See also **Class I exhaust protective cabinet** and **Class III exhaust protective cabinet**.

Class III exhaust protective cabinet   An enclosed ventilated cabinet providing safe working conditions, similar in mode of action to **Class I exhaust protective cabinets**. The working area is completely sealed and is reached through gauntlets fixed to glove ports on the front. Exhaust air must be passed through **HEPA** filters and ducted to the outside of the building. Input air is also passed through a HEPA filter. These cabinets are essential for all work with viable **risk group 4 pathogens**, and must be sited in purpose-built accomodation.

Classical pathway One of the main pathways by which the **complement** system may be activated. In the presence of calcium ions C1qrs is converted to C1 esterase, which converts C4 and C2 into a C4b2a complex. C4b2a converts C3 into C3a and C3b.

Clauss technique A rapid method for the estimation of plasma **fibrinogen**, based on the **thrombin clotting time** of diluted **plasma**.

Clavulanic acid A **beta Lactam** type of **anti-microbial** substance which has little useful anti-microbial activity but high **avidity** for **beta Lactamases**. Once clavulanic acid has bound to beta Lactamases they are irreversibly inactivated. Clavulanic acid is used clinically in conjunction with either **amoxycillin** or **ticarcillin** in order to overcome beta lactamase-mediated resistance to these agents.

Clearance The quantity of material cleared or removed from the body, and a measure of physiological activity. For example, the clearance of creatinine from the blood is a measure of kidney glomerular filtration rate.

Clear cell A literal description of cells surrounded by an apparent space, found scattered in several organs including the alimentary tract, leading to the concept of a **diffuse neuroendocrine system**.

Clearing In **histology**, literally, to render tissue transparent. The preliminary to infiltrating tissue with **paraffin wax** during **processing**, or to mounting tissue sections. Treatment of tissues with a medium compatible with both **dehydrating** agents and wax or **mountant**.

Clindamycin A semi-synthetic derivative of lincomycin which is an **anti-microbial** substance produced by **Streptomyces** species. Clindamycin is active against most **aerobic** organisms which are positive by **Gram's stain**, with the exception of **enterococci**. It is also active against most **clostridia** and **bacteroides** but inactive against aerobic Gram-negative rods. The drug acts by binding to the 50s sub-unit of the bacterial ribosome, thus inhibiting protein synthesis. The main side effect of the drug is the development of **pseudomembranous colitis**, a potentially fatal disease. This is now known to be due to toxigenic strains of *C. difficile*, and Clindamycin is only one of many antibiotics which predispose to the condition.

Clinistix℠ A plastic test strip for testing urine. There is an absorbent area at one end, impregnated with glucose oxidase and o-tolidine, and this is dipped into the sample. In the presence of glucose, peroxidase is formed and the o-tolidine is oxidised to a blue dye.

Clinitest℠ A proprietary tablet test containing copper sulphate, sodium hydroxide, sodium carbonate and citric acid, used for estimating reducing substances in urine. A dropper is used to add a known volume of urine and water to the tablet; heat is generated as the tablet dissolves and copper-reducing substances – particularly glucose concentrations in the urine – can be measured by assessing colour changes.

Clonal selection theory   A theory which hypothesises that an individual has an array of **lymphocytes** each capable of responding to a different **antigen**. During fetal and early neonatal life, lymphocytes capable of responding to an individual's own tissue antigens are suppressed or deleted. In later life, on exposure to foreign antigen, the lymphocytes capable of responding to that antigen are 'selected' by the antigen and stimulated to undergo proliferation, transformation, production of **antibody**, or to take part in **cell-mediated immunity**.

Clone   Genetically identical progeny of a single cell, **gene** or organism.

Clostridium   Rod-shaped **bacteria** which usually exhibit **motility**, are usually **spore**-forming, **catalase**-negative, obligatory **anaerobes** which are positive by **Gram's stain** and are members of the family Bacillaceae. Some species, such as *Clostridium tertium*, *Clostridium carnis* and *Clostridium histolyticum* are oxygen-tolerant. A variety of **enzymes** are produced by most strains and some of these act as **toxins** in humans, causing conditions such as necrotising tissue infections (e.g. *Clostridium perfingens*), enterocolitis (e.g. *Clostridium difficile*) and neuro-intoxication (e.g. *Clostridium botulinum*, *Clostridium tetani*). Clostridia are found in soil and water, animal and human excreta and animal products.

Clot retraction   After blood has been allowed to clot in a glass tube for approximately 1 hour the clot begins to shrink and clear **serum** is expressed. This process depends upon the presence of a sufficient number of **platelets**.

Clotrimazole   A synthetic **anti-microbial** substance of the **imidazole** group, used topically to treat superficial **mycoses**. Most medically important **fungi** are susceptible.

Clot solubility test   A simple screening test for **factor XIII** deficiency in which **plasma** is clotted in the presence of calcium ions and the clot resuspended in a solution of either 5 mol/l urea, 2% acetic acid or 1% monochloracetic acid. Normal clots are insoluble in these reagents, but clots deficient in **fibrin stabilising factor** will dissolve within a few minutes.

Clotting time   See **Partial thromboplastin time** and **Prothrombin time**.

CMLM   Certificate in Medical Laboratory Management. Awarded from 1972 to 1983 by the Institute of Medical Laboratory Sciences (**IMLS**). Now replaced by the **DMLM**.

CMV   See **Cytomegalovirus**.

CNP 30Ⓣᴹ Proprietary industrial cleaning agent used in **histopathology** for **clearing** tissue.

Coagulase An extracellular **enzyme** produced by *Staphylococcus aureus*, but not by other species of staphylococci of human origin. The **substrate** is coagulase-reacting factor in **plasma**, which forms a **thrombin**-like substance which then polymerises **fibrinogen** to form a **fibrin** clot. The reaction is independent of Ca^{++}. When citrated plasma is used other organisms can cause clot formation by utilising the citrate **anticoagulant**. Bound coagulase or clumping factor acts directly on fibrinogen without the need for coagulase-reacting factor, causing clumping aggregation of the cells. Neither enzyme has a proven role in pathogenesis.

Coagulation The process by which a fluid (e.g. blood) changes to a clotted state with the cellular elements enmeshed in a fibrinous clot surrounded by exuded **serum**.

Coagulation factors Plasma **proteins** which form part of the **coagulation** mechanism. Each factor is assigned a Roman numeral by international convention, but may also be referred to by its synonym:

Factor	I	**Fibrinogen**
Factor	II	Prothrombin
Factor	III	**Tissue factor**
Factor	IV	Calcium ions
Factor	V	Labile factor
Factor	VII	Stable factor
Factor	VIII	Anti-haemophilic factor
Factor	IX	Christmas factor
Factor	X	Stuart-Prower factor
Factor	XI	Plasma prothrombin antecedent
Factor	XII	Hageman factor
Factor	XIII	Fibrin stabilising factor

See also **Cascade theory**, **Intrinsic system** and **Extrinsic blood coagulation system**.

Coated cells See **Sensitised cells**.

COBOL An acronym for 'COmmon Business-Orientated Language'. In computing, a **high level language** usually used for business applications.

Cobra venom Venom from the Indian cobra, *Naja naja*. It contains a factor which resembles the **complement** activation product C3b. The cobra venom factor activates the **alternative pathway** of the complement sequence.

Coccidia A sub-class of **parasites** which contains many examples which occur in laboratory and domestic animals. Apart from the very rare occurrence of two species known to infect man, the other animal species – including some from fish – may occur as spurious infections. This parasite appears as the **oocyst** in faeces and is approximately the same size as amoebic cysts.

Coccidioides *Coccidioides immitis* is a filamentous **fungus** whose **spores** are inhaled with dust. It is commonest in the south-western United States of America. Most cases of coccidioidomycosis are asymptomatic but some progress to self-limiting pneumonitis, and some of these to fatal disseminated disease. Cultures are dangerous to laboratory workers due to release of **arthrospores**.

Coccus A **bacterium**, the cell of which is roughly spherical. **Staphylococci** have spherical cells and *Streptococcus pneumoniae* has lanceolate cells.

Codabar(TM) A popular commercial system of **bar codes**. This is the system used in the UK and America for identification of blood and **blood components** for **transfusion**.

Codon A group of three consecutive bases on a nucleic acid molecule which specify a particular amino acid during translation from **messenger RNA**.

Coefficient of variation A standardised statistical measure of variability in a **sample**, being the **standard deviation** of the sample divided by the sample **mean**.

Co-enzyme An organic co-factor which ensures maximum activity of a particular **enzyme**.

Coherence Relates to the size of the electron source in the **transmission electron microscope**. High coherence results from a very small source.

Cold agglutinin A type of **antibody** that agglutinates **erythrocytes** at low temperatures (e.g. 4°C), and loses activity at higher temperatures. These antibodies occur frequently in certain infections (e.g. **primary atypical pneumonia** due to *Mycoplasma pneumoniae*), where they may provide a means of rapid preliminary diagnosis of the infection. When having **blood group** specificity they may be the cause of **haemolytic anaemia**. They may also occur without apparent stimulus in the **plasma** of healthy individuals.

Cold antibody An **antibody** active below body temperature. Often more active around 4°C but sometimes as high as 30°C. See **Cold agglutinin**.

Cold antibody lysis test **Erythrocytes** are suspended in dilutions of a high-titre **cold agglutinin** in the presence of fresh human serum **complement**. Under appropriate conditions, cells from patients with **paroxysmal nocturnal haemoglobinuria** undergo **haemolysis**, whereas normal red cells do not.

Cold finger A trap upon which sublimed water molecules from frozen tissue condense as ice during **freeze drying**. Commonly, a small tube filled with liquid nitrogen within the drying tube and situated close to the tissue.

Cold haemagglutinin disease A form of **auto immune haemolytic anaemia** caused by a high **titre** of **cold antibodies** acting as **agglutinins**. The specificity is usually that of anti-I.

Coliform A term in common use, but having no taxonomic validity, and which refers to members of the **Enterobacteriaceae**.

Colistin A member of the **polymixin** group of **anti-microbial** substances, produced by *Bacillus polymyxa*. Colistin is polymyxin E. Most rod-shaped **bacilli** which are facultative **aerobes** and negative by **Gram's stain** are susceptible, including **pseudomonas**, but **proteus**, **serratia** and *Bacteroides fragilis* are resistant. *Neisseria* and almost all Gram positive bacteria are also resistant. The site of action is the cell membrane, where the drug binds and causes leakage of vital cytoplasmic constituents. The drug is nephrotoxic and ototoxic. It can also cause neuromuscular blockade.

Colitis A general term covering several inflammatory conditions of the colon with different pathologies and causes. When the colitis is caused by **bacteria** the lesions may consist of erosion of the mucosa, or they may also include ulceration and **necrosis** of the submucosa, and possible perforation of the wall of the colon, leading to **peritonitis**. Colitis is seen in infections with *Clostridium difficile*, *Salmonella typhi*, *Yersinia enterocolitica* and *Entamoeba histolytica* among others. Ulcerative colitis and Crohn's disease do not have a known infective aetiology.

Collagen An acellular product of **fibroblasts**, which forms the bulk of many connective tissues. Occurring as single fibres or in bundles, it is composed of smaller fibrils and microfibrils 40 nm in diameter, with characteristic ultrastructural cross-banding at a frequency of 64 nm. At least five separate site-specific types have been identified.

Colloidal gold Dispersed gold particles of selected size in a colloidal sol. Used as a marker of **antibody** reactivity in **immunocytochemistry**. By judicious choice of particle sizes it may be used to detect binding of more than one antibody in a single section at the ultrastructural level.

Colloidal iron Dispersed iron in a colloidal sol. The iron is present as ferric hydroxide which acts as a **cationic dye**, used to demonstrate free acidic groups in **mucopolysaccharides**.

Colonisation The production of communities, or colonies, of **microorganisms** in a new environment. As this requires multiplication it implies that more than a simple attachment of organisms is involved. In colonisation the introduction of an organism to a new environment is followed by attachment or adhesion to the available surfaces, which is then succeeded by multiplication to produce micro-colonies. The whole process often involves several complex mechanisms. It is the basis on which the normal flora of the human body, as well as other animate and inanimate environments, are established and maintained.

Colony unit forming cell A **pluripotential** haemopoietic precursor cell that is capable of giving rise to **neutrophils, megakaryocytes** and **eosinophils**.

Colorimeter An optical instrument which measures the absorbance of light transmitted through a sample. A filter is used to limit the light passing through the sample to a range of frequencies suitable for the band of the spectrum represented by the sample.

Colostrum The first breast milk passed by female mammals. It is rich in **immunoglobulins** and provides a source of **passive immunity** to the offspring of ruminants, but not man.

Colour Index A list of unique numbers assigned to **dyes** by the Society of Dyers and Colourists and the American Association of Textile Chemists and Colorists, and which includes preferred names and synonyms.

Columbia agar A solid **culture medium** containing a special blend of **peptones** designed to give a wide range of peptides, trace elements and other nutrients. The medium is especially useful for cultivation of fastidious organisms and as a base for **blood agar**.

Columnar cell An **epithelial** cell which is taller than it is broad. A general secretory cell, some of which may contain **cilia** arising from the flattened exposed surface.

Column chromatography A technique for the separation of molecules of different sizes from a mixed solution, such as **serum**. The mixture is allowed to flow down a column of a molecular sieve such as **Sephadex**℠, which allows the rapid passage of large molecules while retarding the progress of smaller ones. This results in the components separating into bands down the column, so that they can subsequently be **eluted** by washing through with successive volumes of a suitable solvent or solvents. Alternatively, there is a continuous flow of the mobile phase through the column, the sample being injected at one end and the separated components quantitated by a suitable detector at the other end.

Combined immunodeficiency syndrome An autosomal recessive or X-linked condition in which **cell-mediated** immunity and **antibody** production are defective. One type is known as 'Swiss-type' **hypogammaglobulinaemia**.

Combining site That portion of the **antibody** molecule which combines specifically with the corresponding **epitope** on the **antigen**. It is found on the **Fab fragment**.

Comma   In microscopy, a form of aberration producing a 'comet-like' tail to an object when viewed in the image plane.

Commensal   A **micro-organism** which is commonly found in association with a particular species – in this case, man – and which does not cause harm. Members of the normal flora of the human body are commonly referred to as commensals to distinguish them from **pathogens**, but in this context both terms require careful qualification and probably should be avoided.

Common cold   A very common upper respiratory tract disease caused by **rhinoviruses**, and also by **coronaviruses** and **adeno-viruses**, and characterised by a watery nasal discharge. The symptoms are due to the viral destruction of nasal **ciliated** epithelial cells, and the resulting inflammatory response.

Compatibility test   An *in vitro* test in which the serum of a person who is to receive a **transfusion** is incubated with red cells of the **blood donor**, using a variety of techniques, to determine whether there is any **antibody** present which may cause an adverse *in vivo* reaction to the transfusion.

Compensating eyepiece   A microscope eyepiece lens which is designed to compensate for residual **chromatic aberration** remaining in **semi-apochromat** and **apochromat** objective lenses.

Compensation   The physiological response to maintain equilibrium after assault. For example, the response to an increase in **hydrogen ion concentration** as a result of respiratory distress is for the kidney to reabsorb bicarbonate, which increases in the blood in an attempt to maintain the **pH** within normal limits.

Competitive binding assay   See **Enzyme-linked immunosorbent assay**.

Compiler   A computer **program** which translates programs written in a **high level language** into **machine code**.

Complement   A complex system of proteins and glycoproteins present in freshly drawn serum, which is essential for the completion of certain **antigen-antibody** reactions (e.g. haemolysis). Complement is thermolabile and may only be preserved by storage below $-30°C$ or by freeze drying.

Complementary strand   A single stranded nucleic acid molecule complementary in base sequence to the single stranded form from which it was transcribed, and with which it is capable of **hybridisation**. All viruses with single stranded **RNA** use complementary strands in their replication cycle.

Complement fixation test   A procedure which provides a means of **assay** of an **antibody**, using the activity of **complement**. The test system consists of known **antigen** and dilutions of unknown antibody, which are allowed to react together in the presence of a standard dose of **complement**. After **incubation**, a second antigen/

antibody system (usually comprising sheep **erythrocytes** coated with anti-sheep erythrocyte antibody) is added to the mixture. **Lysis** of the erythrocytes indicates the presence of complement, and therefore lack of specific antibody. Lack of lysis indicates absence of complement, due to its utilisation in the test system. The test may also be used with known antibody to identify an unknown antigen.

Complete antibody An obsolete term for an **antibody** which causes agglutination of red cells in any suspending medium. See **Immunoglobulin, IgM**.

Compound lipid A **lipid** containing products other than fatty acids and alcohol (i.e phosphoric acid or sugar with sphingosine).

Con A See **Concanavalin A**.

Concanavalin A A **lectin** present in extracts of the Jack bean *Concanavalia ensiformis*, which agglutinates **erythrocytes** and acts as a **mitogen** on **T-cell** lymphocytes.

Concentrated red cells A product for **transfusion** prepared by removing **plasma** from a donation of **whole blood** to leave a **haematocrit** level of 70%.

Concentration The measurable quantity of a solute in a given volume of solvent.

Condensation reaction The formation of water as a product when molecules react and join together.

Condenser lens Part of a microscope system used to focus the illuminant in the object plane. In **electron microscopes**, an electromagnetic lens which projects an image of the electron source in the plane of the specimen.

Condyloma acuminatum A **papilloma** caused by a filterable **virus** found in the vulva, the cervix and the vagina, which may occasionally shed large **squamous** cells with slight to moderate nuclear enlargement and slight **hyperchromasia**.

Condylomatous cell An intermediate epithelial **squamous cell** varying in size from two to three times normal, with a poorly defined cell border and vacuolated uneven polychromatic **cytoplasm**.

Confidence interval A statistical method of measuring the accuracy of an **estimated** quantity. A 95% (or 99%) confidence interval for a quantity (e.g. the **mean** or the slope of a **regression** line) is an interval which, on average, will contain the true value of that quantity 95% (or 99%) of the time.

Confounding In a statistical sense, two **parameters** (e.g. the effects of **factors**, or **interactions** between **factors**) are confounded if it is impossible to **estimate** them separately. This may be an intentional part of the design of an experiment, or due to a poorly designed experiment or to missing data.

Conglutinogen Obsolete term used to describe a property of in-activated **complement** component C3b.

Conidiophore In **mycology**, a filament which is part of the vegetative form of a **fungus**, and which carries one or more asexually-derived **spores**.

Conjugate A union between **proteins**, especially **antibodies,** and a marker which may be visualised or measured yet does not interfere with the **antigen**/antibody reaction. Examples of markers include **fluorescent** dyes, **enzymes,** and **colloidal gold.**

Conjugation The process by which genetic material is transferred from one **bacterium** to another, and which requires direct contact between the donor and recipient cells. The ability of the donor cell to carry out this process is governed by a large conjugate **plasmid,** which also encodes for its own transfer. In rod-shaped organisms which are negative by **Gram's stain** the process appears to depend on **pili** ('sex pili'), but conjugate transfer occurs in Gram positive **cocci** in the absence of pili. Conjugation is one of the ways in which resistance to **antibiotics** − as well as other medically important characteristics, such as **colonising** ability − are spread among bacteria.

Conjunctivitis Inflammation of the **membrane** covering the globe of the eye and the inner surfaces of the eyelids. It may involve **oedema,** hyperaemia and suppuration. Most cases are caused by **bacteria** but 10−20% are due to **viruses,** notably **Adenoviridae.** The most common bacterial causes are *Streptococcus pneumoniae, Haemophilus influenzae* and *Chlamydia trachomatis,* though *Neisseria gonorrhoea* − often along with *Chlamydia trachomatis* − gives rise to conjunctivitis (*ophthalmia neonatorum*) in babies born to mothers with venereal disease.

Constant region An area of the **heavy chains** and **light chains** of **immunoglobulin** molecules which has a similar amino acid composition from molecule to molecule. See **Domain.**

Consumption coagulopathy See **Disseminated intravascular coagulation.**

Contact activation The process by which the **coagulation** mechanism is initiated by contact with a foreign surface (e.g. **collagen,** glass, kaolin). It is thought to involve **coagulation factors** XI and XII, together with **high molecular weight kininogen** and **prekallikrein.**

Contact hypersensitivity A reaction of either **immediate hypersensitivity** or **delayed hypersensitivity** provoked by **antigenic** chemicals to which the skin is exposed.

Contact inhibition The cessation of movement or growth seen in tissue culture when cells come into contact with another cell. This may be an important process in tissue differentiation. Cancer cells may not cease division or movement on contact with another cell, and this may lead to the formation of a **tumour** or invasion of other tissues by the cancer cells.

Contact plate An **agar** plate prepared so that when the lid is removed the agar surface is slightly proud of the sides of the **Petri dish**. The plate can be pressed onto a surface which it is wished to sample, such as a kitchen work surface or operating theatre wall, then removed and incubated. Where organisms have been collected from the surface samples, colonies will appear which can be counted and tested further.

Contamination 1. The introduction, whether deliberately or accidentally, of a foreign material into a supposedly pure substance, or onto a surface. For example, the accidental introduction of **bacteria** into a supposedly sterile **culture medium**. 2. In **electron microscopy**, carbonaceous deposits formed by the action of the electron beam on organic molecules in the system.

Contingency table A statistical method of displaying the relationship between two **variables**, both of which can be categorised. For example, for samples **assayed** by two methods with the results categorised as abnormal, indeterminate and normal, a two-way table can be formed showing the number of samples for which each possible pair of results (e.g. if both are abnormal) were obtained. **Independence** between the **variables** is tested using a **Chi-squared test**.

Continuous ambulatory peritoneal dialysis A method of dialysis using the peritoneum as the exchange membrane, in which the dialysis fluid is introduced into the peritoneal cavity and later removed from it while the patient leads a relatively normal life outside hospital. The patient is responsible for changing the dialysis fluid and for maintaining the equipment between hospital visits. **Peritonitis** is a significant problem in this form of treatment for renal failure. It is often associated with **colonisation** of the peritoneal catheter by **coagulase** negative **staphylococci**, although other organisms (such as **pseudomonas**) are also responsible.

Continuous cell line A cell line with the capacity for an infinite number of **passages** *in vitro*.

Continuous flow analyser A form of instrumentation for the analysis of fluids, which are driven by means of peristaltic pumps through lengths of coiled tubing, separated into small segments by the injection of air. Reagents are added, and the tubing may be subjected to **incubation**, at appropriate points. The reaction may be measured optically by a **colorimeter** (or, in some older systems, by deposit of the reaction mixture onto a continuously moving roll of filter paper). The first example of this type of instrument was the **Auto-Analyser**Ⓣᴹ.

Contrast 1. The difference in tone between light and dark parts of an image. 2. In **transmission electron microscopy**, variations in intensity in an image formed by **electron scattering** in the specimen.

Control A standard of comparison. 1. In a laboratory procedure, a test set up in parallel with the test on an unknown material, using the same reagents and test conditions but with reactants of known composition or quantity, in order to validate the results obtained with the unknown materials. 2. In statistics, a control group is one which is given a standard treatment and against which a treated group or groups are to be compared. It is important that the control group is handled in exactly the same way as the treated group, apart from receiving the treatment(s) being studied. See also **Placebo**, **Quality Assurance** and **Quality Control**.

Controlled chromation A method of demonstrating **phospholipids** by **pH** and time-controlled **fixation** in dichromate, and subsequent staining with buffered **haematoxylin**.

Convalescent serum A **serum** sample obtained from an individual approximately 21 days after the onset of an infection. If the specific **antibody** level in this serum is significantly higher than that of a sample obtained soon after the onset of the disease, then this provides supportive diagnostic evidence for infection by a specific agent. Convalescent serum has also been used to provide other individuals with **passive immunity** to particular **microorganisms**.

Coombs, Robert (born 1921) English immunologist who adapted the 1908 antiglobulin concept of Moreschi to **blood group** serology – the so-called Coombs' test. See **Antiglobulin Test**.

Coombs' test See **Antiglobulin test** and **Coombs, Robert**.

Coproporphyrinogen III The precursor of protoporphyrinogen III, and which is catalysed by coproporphyrinogen oxidase. Urinary excretion is increased in hereditary and acute intermittant porphyrias. The excretion of faecal coproporphyrin is greatly increased in hereditary coproporphyria.

Cord blood Blood obtained from the umbilical vein. Cord blood is from the infant's circulation, not that of the mother.

Cornification Maturation of a cell by hormonal activity.

Cornification Index The percentage of superficial cells in a vaginal smear which have **nuclei** exhibiting **pyknosis**, expressed as a percentage of the total squamous cells. The Cornification Index is indicative of the level of **oestrogen** activity. Also known as the Karyopyknotic Index.

Cornified cell An epithelial **squamous cell** with a **nucleus** which exhibits **pyknosis**.

Coronaviridae A family of enveloped **RNA** viruses, 60–200 nm in diameter and exhibiting **pleomorphism**. They have unique club-shaped projections over the surface of the **virus**. The coronoviridae seem to fall into two groups: acid-labile viruses, which are associated with **common cold**-like illnesses; and acid-stable viruses associated with both human and animal **gastro-enteritis**. There are many serotypes, mostly fastidious and difficult to grow in **cell culture** systems.

Corpora amylacea Circular or oval bodies, often with a laminar structure, most commonly found in the central nervous system but also in lung and prostate. They have a common property of staining with iodine.

Corpus albicans A mass of fibrous tissue found in the ovary, replacing the **corpus luteum**.

Corpus amylacea Small hyaline masses found in prostatic secretions and in sputum.

Corpus luteum A yellow body found in the ovary, formed by an ovarian **follicle** that has matured and discharged. The colour is due to the presence of many lipid-filled cells. The *corpus luteum* secretes **progesterone**.

Correct value In **clinical chemistry**, the estimated value found by the use of a particular method. It may not be the true value and may not compare with values found by another method.

Correlation coefficient A statistical method of measuring the strength of the straight line relationship between two **variables**. It always lies between minus one and plus one, the former occuring if observations lie exactly on a line with negative slope and the latter if they lie exactly on a line with positive slope. Independent **variables** have a zero correlation coefficient. See **Regression**.

Corticosteroid A generic term encompassing the steroid **hormones** secreted by the adrenal cortex.

Corticotrophin Adrenocorticotrophic hormone (ACTH). A generic term describing **hormones** produced by the anterior pituitary and which have adrenocorticotrophic activity.

Cortisol The major glucocorticoid controlling the **metabolism** of carbohydrates. It is secreted by the *zona reticularis* in the adrenal cortex, under the control of the hypothalamus and the anterior pituitary gland. It promotes gluconeogenesis, has anti-inflammatory effects when used in pharmaceutical doses, and depresses glucose utilisation. About 90% is bound to **protein** in **plasma** to enable transportation. Increased levels of cortisol are found in pregnancy, obesity, women taking oral contraceptives, and in

Cushing's syndrome and adrenal carcinoma. There are decreased levels in Addison's disease. Also known as hydrocortisone.

Corynebacterium Rod-shaped **bacteria** which do not exhibit **motility** nor produce **spores**, are **aerobes**, positive for **catalase**, non acid-fast, positive by **Gram's stain**, and are wide-spread in nature. Some corynebacteria, such as *C. xerosis* and *C. pseudodiphtheriticum* form an important part of the normal body flora. *C. diphtheriae*, when toxigenic, causes diphtheria in susceptible people. 'JK' corynebacteria, which appear to belong to a previously unrecognised species, cause **septicaemia** and disseminated infections in the **immunocompromised** host. Corynebacteria, and particularly 'JK' types, can be resistant to a wide range of **anti-microbial** substances.

Coryneform A collective term for rod-shaped **bacilli** which are **aerobes**, do not form **spores** and are positive by **Gram's stain**, and which are members of, or are similar to, the **corynebacterium** species.

Cotrimoxazole An **anti-microbial** preparation consisting of a mixture of **Trimethoprim** and sulphamethoxazole, a **sulphonamide**. It is widely used in infections of the chest and urinary tract.

Coulombic forces The affinity between opposite ionic groups that gives rise to **electrostatic bonding**, and which is the commonest mechanism of the **mordant** dye process.

Coulter counter™ An electronic device for counting particles or blood cells. The cell or particle suspension flows through a small orifice across which is passed an electric current. Each cell or particle causes a resistance to the current, and results in a brief voltage pulse with an amplitude proportional to the size of the particle.

Counter immunoelectrophoresis A double diffusion technique in which **antigen** and **antibody** are placed in opposing wells cut into an **agarose** gel. An electrical direct current is applied across the wells, with the positive pole to the well containing the antibody. The antigen will migrate towards the antibody-containing well and the antibody moves towards the antigen by electroendosmosis. If an antigen/antibody reaction occurs a line of precipitate develops where the antigen and antibody meet.

Counting chamber A glass chamber used for counting blood cells, **bacteria** or other particles, having an etched ruling of known dimensions covered with a thick coverslip at a known fixed height. A suspension of blood or particles is introduced into the gap between ruling and coverslip and the number of cells in a given area is counted. From the dimensions of the ruled area and the height of the coverslip, the number of cells in a given volume can be calculated. Two types of chamber in common use are the **Neubauer** and Fuchs-Rosenthal. In **haematology** these have mostly been replaced by electronic counters. See **Coulter counter**.

Covalent bonding The sharing of electrons between atoms of two elements to satisfy valency. An important mechanism of the **mordant** dye process.

Cow pox An **orthopoxvirus** of cattle, of the type thought to have been used by **Jenner** as a **vaccine** against **smallpox**. It is possible that the **Vaccinia** virus was derived from a strain of cowpox. Though originally thought to have been a disease of cattle, it now seems likely that wild rodents are the natural host, infection in them being asymptomatic. Infection in man is **zoonotic**, with transmission from man to man being unusual. Diagnosis is by **electron microscopy** of the contents of the **vesicles**, and by inoculation of the chorioallantoic membrane of the fertile hen egg, characteristic haemorrhagic pocks 1–3 nm in diameter being produced within 72 h.

Coxiella burnettii A **bacterium** which exhibits **pleomorphism** and is an obligate intracellular **parasite**. To some extent it resembles the **Rickettsiae**, though there are important differences, one of which is its resistance to dessication and the lack of an insect **vector** in human disease. It is the cause of **Q fever**, as well as a relatively rare **endocarditis** of poor prognosis. The organism occurs naturally in ungulates and is **zoonotic** in man. Domestic, farm and wild animals are susceptible and **abortion** is a feature of the **zoonosis**. **Infection** is acquired by contact with infected cattle and their excreta, or by consumption of infected milk or milk products. Control has been achieved by pasteurisation of milk. Laboratory diagnosis is usually by serological methods such as **complement fixation tests**. The organism is a **risk group 3 pathogen**: isolation techniques, usually using guinea pigs, should be undertaken with care.

Coxsackie viruses A group of **enteroviruses**. The coxsackie A viruses are associated with a variety of diseases, notably **hand, foot and mouth disease** and **meningitis**. Only a few **serotypes** grow readily in **cell culture; suckling mice** are the most sensitive laboratory material. The Coxsackie B viruses are associated with **Bornholm's disease**, meningitis, **pericarditis** and **myocarditis**. There seems to be a causal association between some **serotypes** and the type of **diabetes** mellitus with juvenile onset. All the six serotypes grow well in various cell cultures.

CPA See **Cancer procoagulant A**.

CPD See **Citrate phosphate dextrose**.

CPE See **Cytopathic effect.**

CP/M™ An abbreviation of 'Control Program for Microprocessors'. The most commonly used **operating system** for **eight-bit** computers, although a version for **sixteen-bit** computers (known as CP/M 86) is also widely used.

CPSM Council for Professions Supplementary to Medicine. In Britain, the statutory body charged with regulating training and maintaining a register of practitioners for each of a number of professions supplementary to medicine. One of the Council's Boards is responsible for a medical laboratory scientific officers' register.

CPU See **Central Processing Unit.**

Crash A computer is said to crash when a program which is running can not be continued nor restarted.

C-reactive protein A non-**immunoglobulin** protein present in small amounts in health but produced in the **acute** phase of the inflammatory response, increasing dramatically in concentration in the **plasma** following infection or tissue injury. Within hours of the onset of the inflammatory response its level rises rapidly, and falls rapidly when the reaction is over. It is released from the liver in response to endogenous **pyrogen** derived from **endotoxin**-stimulated **macrophages**. The protein binds to the cell wall of certain micro-organisms and may activate **complement** by the **classical pathway**. It can easily be detected qualitatively or quantitatively in **serum** and has proved useful in the diagnosis of bacterial infections such as **meningitis**, **peritonitis** and **pneumonia**. It is nonspecific and surgery, trauma and non-infective **necrosis** can all cause a rise in **titre**.

Creatine The immediate precursor of creatinine. It is synthesised in the liver and taken up almost entirely by muscle.

Creatine kinase (EC 2.7.3.2) A substance which catalyses the reversible transfer of phosphate from creatine phosphate. It is found in skeletal muscle, the brain and heart muscle. There are three iso-**enzymes** − BB, MB and MM − of which MB is the one most frequently used to detect heart muscle damage. BB is seldom found in the blood because it cannot pass the blood/brain barrier.

Creatinine clearance A measure of glomerular filtration rate: the amount of blood cleared of creatinins in one minute by the kidneys. It is an endogenous clearance test and is estimated by measuring the serum creatinine level and the amount of creatinine excreted in the urine in a carefully timed period.

C region See **Constant region.**

Crenation Irregular variation in the outline of **erythrocytes** in stained **blood films**. This may occur in some disease states but can also be produced as an **artefact** by (for example) slow drying of the blood smear.

Creutzfeldt-Jakob disease A sub-acute spongiform encephalopathy occurring sporadically throughout the world. It is caused by an agent of remarkable stability which may survive boiling and treatment with **formaldehyde**. The disease is progressive and fatal. The natural route of infection is unknown; **nosocomial** infection from corneal grafts has occurred. The main pathological feature is the presence of large numbers of **vacuoles** in neurones. One feature remarkable for its absence is the apparent total lack of any **immune response** to the infection.

Crimea-Congo haemorrhagic fever virus A **risk group 4 pathogen** causing a generalised disease of high mortality. The infection is **zoonotic** in man, with little man-to-man spread, the **vector** being ticks.

Critical electrolyte concentration The point at which staining is inhibited by the presence of added salts in the dye bath competing for dye-binding sites on the tissue **substrate**. Commonly used to differentiate **mucopolysaccharide**, using alcian blue with magnesium chloride as the competing salt.

Critical illumination In microscopy, a system of illumination in which the condensing lens is used to focus an image of the light source in the object plane. Applicable to large homogeneous light sources (e.g. an opal lamp), but with modern small intense light sources (e.g. a quartz-iodine lamp) **Kohler illumination** is preferred.

Critical point drying A preparative technique for biological specimens for microscopical examination. The point at which, at a given temperature, vapour and liquid density are equal so that there is no interface − and thus no surface tension − between the two phases. Critical point drying exploits this phenomenon to convert the liquid phase of tissue directly to the vapour phase, thus avoiding tissue disruption.

Cross infection The transmission of an **infection**, or (more loosely expressed) its causative organism, from an infected patient to a non-infected one in the same ward or institution by direct or indirect means. The most common vehicle for cross infection is the hands of staff, but utensils, medicines, clothes, dust, etc., can all be responsible.

Cross match An old term for a **compatibility test** prior to **transfusion**. The term is outmoded as it reflects the now obsolete concept of testing both recipient's serum with donors' cells and donors' sera with recipient's cells.

Cross reaction The reaction of an **antibody** with an **antigen** that is structurally related to the antigen which elicited the formation of the antibody.

Cross resistance The exhibition by a **micro-organism** of resistance to two or more **anti-microbial** substances, so that when resistance to one is demonstrated it can also be predicted in the other(s). Cross-resistance occurs usually between anti-microbials which have the same target sites or which are affected by the same resistance mechanisms.

Cross striation 1. In muscle, microscopic bands which traverse skeletal and cardiac muscle and which have varying optical characteristics. 2. In **collagen**, characteristic cross-banding of microfibrils at a frequency of 64 nm when viewed by **electron microscopy**.

Cryofibrinogen Complexes containing **fibrin degradation products** X and Y, **fibrinogen** and soluble **fibrin monomers**, and which precipitate in the cold. **Fibronectin** is necessary for the cold precipitation of these complexes.

Cryoglobulin Serum **proteins** or protein complexes that undergo reversible precipitation in the cold and are commonly seen in **myeloma, macroglobulinaemia, autoimmune** disorders and infections. See **Cryofibrinogen**.

Cryoprecipitate A preparation for **transfusion** made from fresh **whole blood** by separating the **plasma** and freezing it rapidly at $-80°C$ or below and then thawing it slowly not above $+5°C$. The precipitate so formed will contain some 60–70% of both the **factor VIII** and the **fibrinogen** of the original donation. If stored at $-30°C$ or below, suspended in 5–10 ml of its supernatant plasma, the factor VIII activity of the cryoprecipitate will remain at therapeutically useful levels for 3–6 months, and the fibrinogen levels for much longer.

Cryopreservation A method of preparing and maintaining specimens at low temperatures for examination in the **scanning electron microscope**.

Cryostat A refrigerated cabinet containing a **microtome** fitted with remote controls so that tissue sections may be cut at, or below, 0°C.

Cryo-ultramicrotome An **ultramicrotome** adapted to provide a knife cooled with liquid nitrogen, and a cooling system to freeze the tissue block so that **ultra-thin sections** (e.g. of tissue) may be cut at temperatures below the tissue freezing point.

Cryptococcus The single species *Cryptococcus neoformans* is a **yeast**-like **fungus** whose yeast phase is heavily encapsulated and reproduces by budding. It is widely distributed in nature, being found particularly in soil and pigeon droppings. However, human **infec-**

tion is usually caused by inhalation of the **spores** of *Filobasidiella neoformans*, which is the sexual stage found in nature. Cryptococcus is usually an asymptomatic, self-limiting pulmonary infection which produces an active pulmonary process during which the patient's sputum and bronchial washings can produce positive cultures. In some individuals, particularly if they are **immunocompromised**, the infection progresses to involve the central nervous system and sometimes other sites. Death may ensue from respiratory insufficiency. The treatment of choice is a combination of **5-flucytosine** and **amphotericin B**.

Cryptogram A code used to record stable basic properties of **viruses** in symbolic form. The code takes the form of four pairs of symbols: (i) relating to the nucleic acid type and its number of strands; (ii) describing the molecular weight of the nucleic acid in millions of **Daltons**, and its percentage of the complete cell-free virus; (iii) identifying the general outline of the particle and the shape of the **nucleocapsid**; and (iv) the host infected, and any animal **vector**. Thus **polio virus** is described as R/2 2·5/7 S/S M/O, and **Influenza** A virus is R/2 5·5/7 S/H M/O. While the original concept is quite informative, the proliferation of known viruses means that the method provides less discriminatory information than was once the case.

Cryptosporidium A unicellular **protozoan** of the phylum Apicomplexa, sub-order Eimeriorina, with a thick-walled **cyst**-like body. It causes **enteritis** in animals and humans, with a massive watery diarrhoea which may be self-limiting, except in **immuno-compromised** subjects in whom it becomes uncontrollable and can be fatal. The typical **oocysts** can be demonstrated in the stool by various staining methods. There is no known effective **chemotherapy**.

CSF See **Cerebrospinal fluid**.

Cuboidal cell A cell from the transitional **epithelium**, in which the transverse and vertical diameters are equal.

Culture medium A mixture of chemicals which will support the growth of **micro-organisms**. There are two main types, liquid and solid, the latter generally produced in the form of a gel by the addition of **agar**. The nutrients added depend on the requirements of the organisms to be grown, but might include peptones as a source of nitrogen, carbohydrates as a carbon source, and minerals and other growth factors such as **vitamins** or **serum**. All culture media contain water, which must be available to the organisms. Inhibitory substances can be added to make the medium selective, and indicator systems can also be incorporated to detect the ability to utilise certain compounds. A defined medium is one consisting only of chemicals of known composition.

Cumulative sum A calculation in **statistics** which may be used to plot changes in the **accuracy** of a method. The mean value is subtracted from the value obtained; ideally this should be zero, and it is added to the accumulation of previously obtained values and plotted. The plot should be a straight line and a change in direction indicates a change in accuracy.

Curschmann's spirals Mucinous **fibrils** sometimes seen in sputum.

Curvature of field In microscopy, a form of aberration resulting in the periphery of the image field being out of focus. Modern practice is to introduce a flattening component to correct this defect, as with the **planachromat** series of objective lenses.

Cusum See **Cumulative sum**.

Cuvette A small container which holds liquid, the light absorption of which is to be measured. The cuvette may be round or square in section and may be made of a variety of materials including glass and plastic.

Cyanmethaemoglobin When blood is diluted in a solution containing potassium cyanide and potassium ferricyanide, the **haemoglobin** is converted to a stable derivative called cyanmethaemoglobin (HiCN). The **absorbance** of this solution at 540 nm is directly proportional to the haemoglobin concentration.

Cyanocobalamin See **Vitamin B12**.

Cyanophilia Staining blue or purple with basic dyes (i.e. **basophilic**).

Cyclic AMP Formed by conversion of **ATP** by **adenyl cyclase**. In **platelets**, adenosine$-3,5'$-cyclic monophosphate (cyclic AMP $-$ cAMP) is an important regulator of aggregation and secretion. Increased cAMP levels inhibit aggregation while decreased levels stimulate aggregation.

Cyclohexamide An anti-mitotic substance employed in some laboratories to potentiate the isolation of *Chlamydia trachomatis* in **cell culture**, by arresting cell division without causing cell death. An enlarged **cytoplasm** results, facilitating the development of chlamydial **inclusions**.

Cyclooxygenase An important **enzyme** in the synthesis of **prostaglandins**, catalysing the conversion of **arachadonic acid** to unstable prostaglandin intermediates. It is irreversibly inhibited by aspirin (acetylsalicylic acid).

Cycloserine A naturally-occurring **anti-microbial** substance produced by **Streptomyces** species and showing activity against *Mycobacterium tuberculosis* and other mycobacteria, including *Myco. intracellulare*. Cycloserine is a structural **analogue** of D-alanine and competes for two enzymes which convert D-alanine to D-alanine-D-alanine and L-alanine to D-alanine; thus it interferes with **cell wall** synthesis. Resistance, when it develops, is due to genetic **mutation** which produces a variant of the **enzymes** affected. Neurotoxicity occurs in the form of headache, tremors, convulsions and psychoses.

Cyclosporin A   A fungal metabolite which is used to supress **B cell** and helper **T cell** activity in recipients of tissue grafts, to help prevent rejection of the graft.

Cyst   1. A closed, bag-like thin-walled structure, usually containing a liquid or semi-solid material and often lined by connective tissue, epithelium or bone. 2. The resting phase or infective stage in the life cycle of some **protozoa**, during which they are contained within a protective sac (e.g. the cysts of *Entamoeba* species).

Cysticeroid   The larval stage of tapeworms, ingested by man – most commonly from under-cooked meat. Maturation of the larva occurs in the alimentary canal and the head of the young worm passes to the small intestine, where it fixes to the gut wall.

Cystine aminopeptidase   An **enzyme** produced by the placenta. It hydrolyses **oxytocin** and thus prevents uterine contractions and prevents the onset of labour.

Cystitis   A urinary tract **infection** involving the bladder and giving rise to frequency and urgency of micturition, often with pain over the bladder and a burning sensation when passing urine. The condition is much more common in women than in men due to the shortness of the female urethra, which is colonised by a variety of organisms, which become introduced into the bladder either spontaneously or during instrumentation or sexual activity. The most common organisms are *Escherichia coli* and *Staphylococcus saprophyticus*, though in hospitalised patients the range is much greater.

Cytapheresis   An **apheresis** procedure to obtain only cellular elements from the **blood donor**.

Cytocentrifuge   A device for depositing cells from suspension directly on to a microscope slide by centrifugation.

Cytochrome oxidase   A bacterial **enzyme** which oxidises reduced cytochrome using molecular oxygen. Tests for the enzyme are important in identification of **bacteria** and reagents based on tetramethyl-p-phenylenediamine dihydrochloride, which changes from colourless to blue.

Cytogenetics   The study of the structure and abnormalities of chromosomes, and the effects of these.

Cytology   The study of cells, including their structure, origin and function.

Cytolysis   The dissolution or destruction of the **cytoplasm** of cells, usually by the action of **bacteria**.

Cytomegalovirus An ubiquitous member of the **Herpetoviridae**. In **neonates** it may be a cause of cytomegalic inclusion disease, usually as a result of **intrauterine infection**. It is also a common cause of less severe central nervous system disease in neonates, resulting in varying degrees of mental retardation. Infected neonates excrete large amounts of virus in the urine. In adults it is a cause of an **infectious mononucleosis**-like disease which sometimes follows blood **transfusion**. **Infection** of the **immunocompromised** host may be severe and possibly fatal, with pneumonia and generalised infection. It seems likely that infected individuals carry the virus for life, in their **lymphocytes**. The **virus** can be grown *in vitro* only in lines of human embryo fibroblast cells, for which the lines must be chosen with care since they are not all sensitive. Use of **immunofluorescence** tests may accelerate diagnostic procedures. Presence of **antibody** against cytomegalovirus is indicative of infectivity and a number of tests have been devised to test for the presence of antibody, this being especially important in **blood donors** whose blood may be given to neonates or to immunocompromised patients. Virus specific **IgM** antibody is present in acute infections with cytomegalovirus, and various techniques have been devised for demonstration of this. The virus can also be grown in human **fibroblasts**, although the typical **cytopathic effect** may take several weeks to appear.

Cytopathic effect A morphological change in the appearance of a **monolayer** in **cell culture**. The discovery that **viruses** caused specific cytopathic effect in cell culture was an important step in the development of modern virology. The cytopathic effect shown by some viruses provides a means of presumptive diagnosis, while other effects are shown by a number of usually related species. It may also be caused by numerous non-infectious agents, including bacterial **toxins**.

Cytoplasm The protoplasm of a cell, which surrounds the nucleus.

Cytosis The **absorption** of particulate matter by cells. See **Pinocytosis** and **Phagocytosis**.

Cytoskeleton A filamentous system within cells that is intermediate in size between microtubules and microfilaments (diameter 7−11 nm). See **Intermediate filament**.

Cytostome A permanent 'mouth' opening found in most ciliates. See **Cilia**.

Cytotaxigen A substance which is not itself directly **chemotactic**, but which gives rise to **cytotaxins** after interacting with plasma or **complement** components.

Cytotaxin A substance which has a direct **chemotactic** effect on cells (e.g. certain **complement** components).

Cytotoxic Harmful − usually lethal − to cells. Though many **infectious** agents and **toxins** are cytotoxic, the term is usually applied to drugs and to certain classes of **lymphocyte**.

Cytotoxic T cell A **T cell** subset which can lyse cells expressing specific **antigens**.

Cytotoxin A **toxin** which is active − usually lethally − against mammalian cells. Examples are the alpha-toxin of **staphylococci**, which is lethal to **neutrophils**, and the enterocytotoxins of ***Clostridium** difficile* and *Clostridium perfingens*.

D

DAB See **Diamino-benzidine**.

DAG Direct **Antiglobulin Test**. An antiglobulin test applied directly to red cells which may have been sensitised *in vivo* (as in **auto immune haemolytic anaemia** – AIHA – or **haemolytic disease of the newborn** – HDN), and not requiring prior incubation of the cells *in vitro* with an antibody. A positive DAG is diagnostic of both AIHA and HDN.

Dalton 1. John Dalton. (1766–1808). English chemist who proposed the atomic theory of matter. 2. A unit of measurement representing a mass of one-sixteenth that of an oxygen atom (i.e. approximately that of a hydrogen atom), usually abbreviated to D.

Dansylcadaverine A fluorescent amine which may be incorporated into casein by the transamidase activity of **fibrin stabilising factor**. This forms the basis of an assay method in which the intensity of the fluorescent casein substrate is proportional to the factor XIII level.

Dapsone A synthetic sulphone used in the treatment of **leprosy**. Its mode of action is similar to that of **sulphonamides**.

Dark ground microscopy A system employing a hollow cone of light to illuminate the object, either by the introduction of patch stops into the light path of the condensing lens or by the employment of a specially constructed dark ground condenser. The former are used with low power objective lenses and the latter with high power objectives. Of particular value for the observation of biological specimens in the living state, which appear as illuminated objects against a dark background.

Database In computing, a series of files containing a collection of organised data required to perform a task or to supply information.

Davis cytopipette A pipette containing fixative, designed to be used by the patient herself for collection of vaginal secretion and cells for laboratory study.

DCM Abbreviation of the procedure used to **dehydrate**, **clear** and **mount** tissue sections.

DCT Direct **Coombs' test**. See **DAG**.

DDAVP See **Deamino-D-arginine vasopressin**.

D-dimer A **fibrin degradation product** formed by **plasmin**-mediated cleavage of cross-linked **fibrin**, and consisting of a pair of D fragments covalently linked by the action of **fibrin stabilising factor**.

Deamination Treatment of sections of tissue, usually with nitrous acid, to block the reactivity of amino acid groups.

Deamino-D-arginine vasopressin A synthetic derivative of **vasopressin** which, when administered to normal individuals or to patients with **von Willebrand's disease** or mild **haemophilia**, brings about an increase in the level of circulating **coagulation factor VIII**.

Decalcification Removal of calcium salts from tissue to facilitate **microtomy**. May be achieved by use of mineral acids, organic acids, **chelating agents** or appropriate buffers.

Decarboxylase A group of **enzymes** which have the ability to catalyse the release of carbon dioxide from organic compounds by decarboxylation. An example is malate dehydrogenase (EC 1.1.1.38). The reaction is used in **bacteriology** to differentiate between some closely-related **bacteria** staining negative by **Gram's stain**.

Decidual cells **Stromal** cells of the **endometrium**, modified by **progesterone** during pregnancy. They occur singly or in sheets, usually as large mononucleated cells with abundant **cytoplasm**, sometimes diffusely **vacuolated** and with **vesicular** nuclei containing **nucleoli**.

Decline phase The phase in the growth of **bacteria** immediately following the **stationary phase**. The number of viable organisms begins to fall due to exhaustion of stored nutrients and the activity of toxic metabolites.

Decoy cells **Benign** cells mimicking **tumour** cells, having hyperchromatic round or oval nuclei, course **chromatin** and little **cytoplasm**. They may be found in urine from seminal **vesicles**.

Deep vein thrombosis The term given to the formation of a blood clot consisting mainly of **erythrocytes** and **fibrin**, occuring in the deep venous circulation. Most commonly seen in the deep veins of the calf.

Default In computing, an assumption made by a computer when it is not given specific instructions by a **program** or by the operator. For example, when a **microcomputer** has more than one **disc drive**, one of these is normally designated as the default drive, to which the computer automatically refers unless instructed otherwise.

Defective interfering virus When present in large numbers this **virus** occupies so many receptors on cells that the access of infectious particles may be severely hampered, greatly reducing the amount of virus produced by the cells.

Defective virus A **virus** which is unable to replicate due to some natural or acquired deficiency in its structure or nucleoprotein. Naturally defective viruses such as **adeno satellite viruses** require a helper virus in order to complete their replication cycle. A proportion of progeny virus from any infected cell will be defective; inoculation of high multiplicities into cells may result in a majority of the progeny being defective.

Defibrination A term given to the therapeutic reduction of plasma **fibrinogen** levels by the administration of drugs such as **Ancrod** in order to prevent thrombosis. See also **Disseminated intravascular coagulation**.

Defibrination syndrome See **Disseminated intravascular coagulation**.

Definition In microscopy, the ability of a lens to render the outlines of an image distinct. It is a property which varies directly with the **numerical aperture** of the objective lens employed, and is associated with the **resolving power**.

Deformability A property of cells — applied mainly to **erythrocytes** and **leucocytes** — which governs their ability to distort while negotiating blood vessels or inter-cellular spaces smaller than the diameter of the cell concerned.

Degreasing 1. Of bones: removal of fat by immersion in chloroform prior to bleaching and dry-mounting as a museum specimen. 2. Of sections: treatment with trichlorethylene prior to staining by **trichrome** methods, with a view to achieving more brilliant results.

Degrees of freedom These are statistical values which need to be calculated before using the **Chi-squared test**, **t-test** or **F-test** for **distribution**, and when making an **analysis of variance**. Essentially, degrees of freedom are the numbers of **independent** quantities needed to calculate certain functions of the observations.

Dehydration Removal of water from tissue blocks during **processing**, or from tissue sections prior to staining.

De-ionised water Water purified by removal of cations and anions by passage through ion-exchange resins.

Delayed hypersensitivity The cell-mediated response of an individual to an **antigen** to which (s)he has previously been exposed, some 24−48 h after repeated exposure to certain antigenic materials, e.g. chemicals, minerals, topical ointments. The reaction is mediated by **T cells** and has been classified as a **Type IV reaction** hypersensitivity state. See also **Immediate hypersensitivity**.

Delesse principle A geologist's definition applied to **quantification** in microscopy. Appropriately translated it infers that by measuring area fractions on tissue sections, volume fractions may be estimated.

Delta chain The heavy chain of **IgG**.

Demethylation The reversal of **methylation** of tissue sections by sequential treatment with potassium permanganate and oxalic acid. **Saponification** is more often employed to hydrolyse methyl groups.

Dendrite Fine branching fibres extending from nerve cells, and which transmit impulses from the peripheral organ to the nervous system. They form sensory or receptor nerve endings.

Dendritic 1. Branching. Having extensions which divide and subdivide into two or more, like a tree. 2. Descriptive of something possessing **dendrites** (e.g. dendritic cells – see **Langerhans' cell**).

Dengue virus A group of four related members of the **flaviviridae**, occurring in the tropics and sub-tropics, and occasionally in parts of eastern Europe. The **vector** is the mosquito. Primary infection often results in a moderately severe febrile illness; further infection with another serotype may induce a severe **haemorrhagic fever** – dengue shock syndrome.

Dense bodies Granules found in blood **platelets** which appear dense on **electron microscopy** and which contain **ADP, ATP, 5-hydroxytryptamine** and calcium ions.

Density The mass per unit volume of a substance.

Density gradient centrifugation A method of separation of molecules on the basis of their size and molecular weight. Separation is achieved by high-speed centrifugation of a mixed suspension through a gradient of an inert **substrate** more concentrated at the proximal than the distal end of the centrifuge tube. Popular substrates include caesium chloride, sucrose and sodium tartrate. The method has proved useful for the separation of **IgM** from other **immunoglobulins**, and for measuring the **bouyant density** of viruses of similar morphology.

Dentine Hard tissue of the tooth, which surrounds the pulp and extends through both the root – where it is covered by **cementum** – and the crown, where it is covered by **enamel**. Normally tubular and carrying **odontoblast** processes.

Deoxycholate A **bile salt** of deoxycholic acid. 1. Used in bacteriological **culture media** as a selective **inhibitor** to prevent the growth of organisms which are positive by **Gram's stain**, and **spore**-forming organisms, while permitting growth of Gram negative enteric **bacilli**. 2. Used to measure **virus** sensitivity for purposes of classification, the results closely paralleling **ether sensitivity** and **chloroform sensitivity**. (Also spelled 'desoxycholate').

Deoxyribonucleic acid Genetic material of high molecular weight, which is the main component of the nucleoproteins in **chromatin** and which stains with basic dyes.

Dermatophyte A type of filamentous **fungus** of the genera Trichophyton, Epidermophyton and Microsporum, which are responsible for ringworm, a superficial **mycosis** of animals and humans. Dermatophytes grow relatively slowly on laboratory **culture media** at room temperature, usually producing filamentous colonies of characteristic appearance, and usually producing structures such as **macrospores** and **microspores**, which help in their identification.

Desmosome Point of cohesion between adjacent cells, seen as a stratum of thickened **cytoplasm** between and adjacent to the two cell membranes at this site, demonstrated by **electron microscopy**.

Desoxycholate See **Deoxycholate**.

Detector The part of an instrument that converts light or other energy into electrical energy, as (for example) in a **spectrophotometer** or gamma counter.

Deuterium lamp A source of ultraviolet light used in a **spectrophotometer**.

Dexamethasone suppression test A measure of the suppression of **ACTH** secretion after the administration of a powerful exogenous glucocortoid (dexamethasone).

Dextran A high molecular weight de-polymerised polysaccharide used in solution as a **plasma expander** in **transfusion**.

Dhobie's itch Syn. *Tinea cruris*. A fungal infection of the skin; although the term is usually used to describe itching infections comprising some form of **epiphytic** disease of the crutch or axilla. Several species of fungus may be responsible.

DHCC See **1.25-Dihydroxycholecalciferol**.

DHSS Department of Health and Social Security. In the United Kingdom, the government department with overall responsibility for health care services.

Diabetes A general expression to describe conditions in which there is an abnormal increase in the amount of urine produced and excreted by an individual. See **Diabetes mellitus**.

Diabetes mellitus A chronic condition in which a malfunction of the pancreas causes inadequate secretion of insulin, leading to impaired metabolism of carbohydrates, fats and proteins. Treatment is by insulin injection, but this needs to be balanced by a **diet** which controls the intake of carbohydrates, etc.

Dialysed iron See **Colloidal iron**.

Diamino-benzidine A commonly used reagent to detect **antigen/antibody** reactions by reacting with **conjugated** horse-radish peroxidase to form a brown deposit.

Diamond knife Diamond, polished to a sharp cutting edge, used to cut **ultra-thin sections** in an **ultramicrotome**.

Diarrhoea The frequent and excessive discharge of unformed stool from the bowel, due to failure to absorb water from − or its active secretion into − the intestinal contents. In severe cases dehydration results, and in chronic states malabsorption may also occur.

Diastase An enzyme used for the **selective** removal of glycogen from tissue sections. Available as an extract of malt, it is also present in saliva. See **Amylase**.

Dibucaine number A parameter indicating the degree of inhibition of **cholinesterase** activity for a given **substrate** in the presence of a standard **concentration** of the compound Dibucaine. Inhibition may be reduced in some patients due to a genetic variant, and such patients are sensitive to the use of particular muscle relaxants such as suxamethonium (scoline).

DIC See **Disseminated intravascular coagulation**.

Dichroic mirror A device employed in **fluorescence microscopy**, using **incident light**. Introduced into the optical train, the dichroic mirror reflects short wavelength exciting radiation into the objective lens, which acts as its own condenser, focusing the radiation onto the object. The longer wavelength emission emanating from the object then passes back through the objective and through the dichroic mirror, which is transparent to the longer wavelength emission.

Dichroism The property of a substance to show a change in colour when viewed in **polarised light**, due to destructive interference by induced phase differences in the light. Characteristic of Congo red-stained **amyloid**.

Diet The type and quality of food and drink ingestion, which should be appropriately balanced to form a normal diet.

Differential leucocyte count The classification, by examination of stained blood films or automated analysers, of peripheral blood **leucocytes** into the individual cell types (e.g. **neutrophil, eosinophil, basophil, monocyte** or **lymphocyte**). The results may be expressed as a percentage of the total leucocyte count or in absolute numbers.

Differentiation Literally, the distinguishing of one thing from another. 1. In staining, the process of selectively removing a dye from some structures while leaving it in others; often achieved by alteration of the **pH**. 2. In cytology, development from the immature to a mature stage, or from a general to a specific nature. In the **squamous epithelium** this refers to the change from the small, undifferentiated basal cells to fully mature large superficial cells.

Diffraction 1. The spreading of rays passing through an opening. 2. In **transmission electron microscopy**, an image formed from an electron beam scattered by a crystalline specimen.

Diffuse neuro-endocrine system A diffuse system of polypeptide secreting **endocrine cells**. The enzyme **neuron-specific enolase** is common to all components. See **APUD**.

Diffusion pump A high vacuum pump which operates by the diffusion of molecules under the influence of a stream of oil or mercury vapour.

Di George's syndrome A condition in which there is an inborn absence of the **thymus** and consequent defects in **cell-mediated immunity**. The condition is also called hypoplasia.

Digital 1. In anatomy, relating to a finger or toe. 2. In mathematics, relating to numbers. A single number is one digit. 3. In connection with electrical systems, a digital signal is one which has a finite number of discrete values, as distinct from an **analogue** signal. **Computers** are automated digital electronic calculating machines.

Dihydrofolate reductase An **enzyme**, important in folate metabolism, which catalyses the conversion of **folic acid** to tetrahydrofolic acid.

Dihydroisoquinoline A **fluorescent** product of the **formaldehyde-induced fluorescence** method for **biogenic amines**, representing primary and secondary catecholamines.

1.25-Dihydroxycholecalciferol A **hormone** which, in the presence of parathyroid hormone and a low ionised calcium concentration, promotes osteoclastic activity and the release of calcium ions from bone.

Dilute whole blood clot lysis time A modified version of the **whole blood clot lysis time**, in which the blood is diluted to minimise the effect of fibrinolytic inhibitors. The diluted blood is then clotted and the time taken for lysis of the clot is noted.

Dimethyl sulphoxide A liquid used in **cell culture** growth medium, at a concentration of 10%, to reduce greatly the formation of ice crystals in cell suspensions during slow freezing prior to storage in **liquid nitrogen**, so greatly improving the survival of the cells. Its solvent and penetrating properties have led to its use as a suspending medium for topically applied drugs.

Dimorphic anaemia A term given to the peripheral blood film appearance when two different types of **erythrocyte** are seen. Most commonly this results from a mixture of **hypochromic** and **normochromic** cells (e.g. during treatment of iron deficiency).

2,3-diphosphoglycerate An organic phosphate ester, commonly known as **DPG**, formed during **glycolysis** in **erythrocytes**. DPG binds specifically to **haemoglobin** and lowers oxygen affinity with disturbing haem-haem interaction, (the **Bohr effect**).

Diphtheria A condition caused by toxigenic strains of *Corynebacterium diphtheriae*. The organism is usually spread by direct contact with an infected person. Within a few days **pyrexia** and malaise develop, followed by sore throat and cervical **oedema** and **lymphadenopathy**, and a leathery membrane appears over the pharynx. The **toxin** acts on cells to prevent **protein** synthesis. Neuropathy affecting cranial and peripheral nerves, and **myocarditis** and **pneumonitis** are direct results of the toxaemia. Treatment involves administration of diphtheria **anti-toxin**, and **penicillin** or **erythromycin**.

Diploid   Having two sets of **chromosomes**, as normally found in the **somatic** cells of higher organisms.

Dip.Med.Tech   Diploma in Medical Technology. A higher qualification awarded from 1972 to 1977 by the Institute of Medical Laboratory Sciences. See **IMLS**.

Disc   See **Floppy disc**.

Disc diffusion   A technique in which discs of absorbent paper which have been impregnated with **anti-microbial** substances are placed on the surface of an **agar** plate which has been inoculated with the test organism. The anti-microbial substances diffuse out radially into the agar, causing corresponding zones of growth inhibition of susceptible organisms.

Disc drive   In computing, a device used to read data from, or write data to, a **floppy disc**.

Discrete analyser   An automatic analyser that is capable of handling each sample separately in individual vessels, in contrast to a **continuous-flow analyser**. Samples and reagents are transported so that there is a physical separation of each sample from the others. This may be achieved by using a rack or chain which holds **cuvettes** or reaction tubes.

Discretionary analyser   An automatic analyser which is able to measure several analytes but where the operator can select a single test or group of tests from the repertoire available; in contrast to a **continuous-flow analyser**, in which all samples have all analytes determined, without any selection.

Disinfectant   An **anti-microbial** substance which inhibits the multiplication of organisms, usually in a concentration of several grams per litre. Disinfectants are usually too irritant to be used in contact with skin or tissue, and may actually be corrosive. Often they are reliably lethal to **bacteria** only within a narrow range of dilution, and they may be inactivated by **protein** or other organic substances.

Disseminated intravascular coagulation   A potentially severe disorder in which the blood **coagulation** and **fibrinolytic** mechanisms become activated within the circulation. This results in depletion of **platelets** and **coagulation factors**, elevation of **fibrin degradation products** and, ultimately, haemorrhage. Also known as **consumption coagulopathy**.

Dissociation   A method of preparing thin pieces of tissue for microscopy by gently teasing apart with needles.

Distilled water   Water purified by distillation. For many chemical and biological laboratory purposes the distillation needs to be in a glass still in order to avoid metallic impurities.

Distortion   1. A twisting deformation. 2. In **electron microscopy**, assymetrical images produced by lens defects.

Distribution   In statistical usage, the **distribution** of a **variable** describes how likely it is that certain values will occur. Certain distributions are encountered frequently and can be described mathematically, the most common being the **Normal distribution**.

Distribution-free test   See **Non-parametric test**.

Disulphide bond   A covalent bond ($-S-S-$) often present in **proteins**. This type of bond forms intra-chain, inter-chain and inter-unit linkages in **immunoglobulin** molecules and can be disrupted by sulphydryl reagents such as **2-mercaptoethanol** or **dithiothreitol**.

Dithiothreitol   A sulphadryl compound used in **serology** to reduce human **IgM** molecules so as to abolish the ability of the **antibody** to behave as an **agglutinin**, thus distinguishing IgM from **IgG** antibodies.

Diuresis   Increased excretion of urine from the kidney, which may be as a result of administration of a **diuretic**, excess drinking of fluids, or other causes such as renal disfunction, etc.

Diuretic   A substance which stimulates or promotes the output of urine from the kidney.

DMLM   Diploma in Medical Laboratory Management, awarded by the Institute of Medical Laboratory Sciences (**IMLS**). See also **CMLM**.

DNA   See **Deoxyribonucleic acid**.

DNA Hybridisation   The process by which complementary single strands of DNA from different cells are formed into stable double-stranded molecules (**hybrids**).

DNA Probe   An analytical technique using **DNA hybridisation**, in which the test sample is denatured and immobilised on a solid support (such as nitrocellulose). A single strand of DNA is radio-labelled (using, for example, **tritiated thymidine**) and this (the DNA probe) is hybridised with complementary strands. Positive signals are detected by **autoradiography** or scintillation counting, the strength of the signal being a measure of the concentration of the target sequence. Use of such probes may provide a highly sensitive method of detecting the nucleic acid of **pathogenic** agents.

DNES   See **Diffuse neuro-endocrine system**.

Dohle bodies   Small elliptical bodies, staining bright blue with **Romanowsky stains**, found in the **cytoplasm** of **neutrophils** and **eosinophils**. These inclusions are typically seen in the **May-Hegglin anomaly**, but may also occur in some cases of infection.

Dolichos biflorus   The tropical horse grain, extracts from the seeds of which are used as an anti-A_1 **lectin** in **blood group** serology.

91

Domain An area of the **heavy chain** or **light chain** of an **immuno-globulin** molecule, delineated by an intra-chain **disulphide bond**. Each domain has a particular function. See **V region**.

Dominant gene A gene which in the **heterozygous** state masks the manifestation of its **allelomorph** on the other chromosome of the pair.

Donath Landsteiner antibody A cold-active, **complement**-fixing IgG **antibody** which may occur in up to 10% of cases of **syphilis**, but also in a number of patients without evidence of syphilis. This antibody binds to **erythrocytes** in the cold and causes complement-mediated **haemolysis** when the cells are warmed to 37°C. See also **Paroxysmal cold haemoglobinuria**.

Donath Landsteiner test A test for **paroxysmal cold haemoglobinuria** in which two samples of blood are taken from the patient. One sample is placed immediately at 37°C and the other in crushed ice. After 30 minutes the cooled sample is warmed to 37°C. In paroxysmal cold haemoglobinuria **haemolysis** will be evident in the previously cooled sample, but not in the blood maintained at 37°C throughout.

DOPA Dihydroxyphenylalanine. Originally thought to be the precursor of **melanin**.

Dopamine One of the **catecholamines**. An intermediate substance in the formation of adrenaline from tyrosine. Its excretion is often greatly increased in some cases of neuroblastoma and **malignant** phaechromocytoma.

DOPA-oxidase The **enzyme** responsible for the conversion of tyrosine to melanin. More properly called tyrosinase.

Doppler flowmetry A method of measuring blood flow in which an **ultrasonic** beam is directed at a blood vessel. The beam is reflected back to the detector at an altered frequency (the so-called Doppler shift), which is proportional to the velocity of blood flow.

Dosage effect A state when the reactivity of an antigen determined by a gene in the **homozygous** state is greater than in the **heterozygous** state. (e.g. With a given anti-c, red cells of **genotype** c/c will react more strongly than will cells of genotype C/c).

Double diffusion test A **gel diffusion test** in which **antibody** and soluble **antigen** are allowed to diffuse and react in an **agar** gel. Where the antigen and antibody meet in **optimal proportions**, lines of precipitation are formed.

Double embedding A method of combining the advantages of both **paraffin wax** and **celloidin** by infiltrating tissue with celloidin before **embedding** in wax prior to **microtomy**. See also **Peterfi**.

DPG See **2,3-diphosphoglycerate**.

DPX A synthetic polystyrene **mountant**.

Drabkin's solution A solution of potassium cyanide and potassium ferricyanide used to dilute blood samples for measurement of **haemoglobin** concentration by the **cyanmethaemoglobin** method.

DR antigen A type of **antigen** coded by **genes** of the **major histocompatibility complex** on chromosome 6 in man. They are present on **B cells** and are detected by serological means using **complement**-mediated **lymphocytotoxicity**. See **Class II antigen**.

Dried plasma (Obsolete). **Plasma for transfusion**, separated from **whole blood**, pooled (generally in 10-donor pools) and freeze-dried. When reconstituted with **distilled water**, used as a blood volume expander in treatment of massive haemorrhage and oligaemic shock. Now superceded by **plasma protein solution**.

Dry ice Solid carbon dioxide, which sublimes to the gas at $-79°C$. A white crystalline solid.

dsDNA Double stranded deoxyribonucleic acid.

Dubin-Johnson pigment A **lipofuchsin** found in a type of chronic idiopathic **icterus** in otherwise normal livers.

Duke's method See **Bleeding time**.

Duplex In computing, a system which can transmit data in two directions along a communications link between two computers. In full duplex, data can be transmitted simultaneously and independently from each terminal. In half duplex, transfer of data is in one direction at a time only, from either computer.

Duplicate Results from two analyses of the same sample for the same component, carried out simultaneously or on different occasions, with the object of comparing the results to see by how much they differ. The results may be used to assess the **precision** of the analytical process. See **Quality control**.

DVT See **Deep vein thrombosis**.

Dye A coloured compound that will stain tissue and be resistant to simple washing.

Dyserythropoiesis A condition associated with anaemia and low numbers of peripheral blood **reticulocytes**, despite evidence of **erythrocyte** production in the bone marrow (dyserythropoietic anaemia). Also known as ineffective **erythropoiesis**.

Dysfibrinogenaemia The presence in the peripheral blood of a qualitatively abnormal type of plasma **fibrinogen**. The congenital condition is due to an **amino acid** substitution in one of the constituent polypeptide chains, and by convention each variant is named after its place of discovery (e.g. Fibrinogen Paris I). More commonly, the condition is acquired, usually in association with liver disease, and is due to an increase in the **fibrinogen**-bound **sialic acid** content.

Dyskaryosis Having an abnormal nucleus, manifested by increase in size, **hyperchromatism** and irregularity of form, with little or no modification of **cytoplasmic differentiation**.

Dyskeratosis Abnormal keratinisation of individual epithelial cells, associated with irregular maturation of the **epithelium**.

Dysplasia A disorder of the differentiation of **squamous epithelium** covering the surface and the glands. It is pre-**malignant**.

Dysproteinaemia The presence in the peripheral blood of an abnormal type of plasma **protein**. The term is usually applied to the abnormal **immunoglobulins** found in cases of **myeloma** and **macroglobulinaemia**.

Dysprothrombinaemia The presence in the peripheral blood of a qualitatively abnormal form of plasma **prothrombin**. As with the congenital **dysfibrinogenaemias**, these conditions may be due to an **amino acid** substitution and are named after their place of discovery. See also **Coagulation factors**.

E

EACA See **Epsilon amino caproic acid**.

Ebola virus A **filovirus** of unknown natural history, responsible for widespread outbreaks of **haemorrhagic fever** in east Africa. It is a **risk group 4 pathogen**.

EB virus See **Epstein-Barr virus**.

ECCLS European Committee for Clinical Laboratory Standards.

ECF-A Abbreviation for **eosinophil** chemotactic factor of **anaphylaxis**. It is liberated from **mast cells** during **immediate-type hypersensitivity** which is **IgE**-mediated, and 'attracts' eosinophils.

Echovirus Obsolescent name for a group of **viruses**, derived from the acronym of Enteric Cytopathic Human Orphan virus. They are **enteroviruses** of man which, when first isolated, were not immediately associated with any clinical condition. Some types are proven causes of **meningitis** and **exanthema**, as well as severe neonatal disease. They grow readily in **cell culture**, but rarely cause any lesions in **suckling mice**. Recently isolated related viruses have been named **enterovirus**, with an identifying number, the title Echovirus being retained only by those familiarly known in this way.

ECLT See **Euglobulin clot lysis time**.

Ectoparasite A **parasite** living on the outside of its host (e.g. a flea).

Ectopic An abnormality of position or situation, e.g. an ectopic pregnancy is one in which the **fetus** develops other than in the uterus, for example in the Fallopian tube or the abdominal cavity.

Ectoplasm The outer layer of the **cytoplasm** of a cell.

Ectromelia virus A **poxvirus** of mice, closely related to **variola**, **vaccinia** and **cowpox**. The virus causes a severe, often fatal, **haemorrhagic fever** in mice and may occasionally prove a severe problem in animal houses.

Edema See **Oedema**.

EDTA See **Ethylene diamine tetra-acetic acid**.

Edwardsiella Rod-shaped **bacilli** which exhibit **motility**, are **catalase** positive, facultatively **anaerobic**, **oxidase** negative, **indole** positive and which are negative by **Gram's stain**, differing little from *Escherichia coli* in their biochemical reactions. Edwardsiella produces hydrogen sulphide in some circumstances and does not produce beta-galactosidase: some workers prefer to consider it a species of **Escherichia**.

Ehrlich, Paul (1854−1915) German doctor who founded the modern sciences of chemotherapy and haematology, was a pioneer immunologist, and undertook widespread research into the chemical basis of stains and their actions on tissues and bacteria.

Ehrlich's test A test which uses *p*-dimethylaminobenzaldehyde as a reagent. A red colour is produced in the presence of urobilinogen and some precursors of **porphyrin** in urine.

EIA See **Enzyme immunoassay**.

Eight bit computer A computer which handles data in units of one **byte** (i.e. a **word** of eight **bits**) at a time.

Eikenella Rod-shaped bacteria which do not exhibit **motility**, are **oxidase** positive, weakly **catalase** positive, asaccharolytic and which are negative with **Gram's stain**. They do not hydrolyse urea and do not grow on MacConkey **agar**. They are **aerobes** and facultative **anaerobes** which grow on **blood agar** or **chocolate agar**, requiring haemin for growth. Pitting of the agar under the colonies is often seen. *E. corrodens* is distinct from the urease-positive obligate anaerobe *Bacteroides corrodens*, now known as *B. urealyticus*.

Elastin Branching fibres or sheets of amorphous **protein** containing microfibrillar glycoprotein with a molecular structure permitting it to stretch, and subsequently return to a relaxed configuration.

Electron deflector In **electron microscopy**, a system of electromagnetic coils used to impart lateral translocation of an electron beam.

Electron detector An electronic device to collect electrons from the surface of specimens in the **scanning electron microscope**.

Electron gun In **electron microscopes**, the combination of a **filament** assembly and **Wehnelt cylinder**, insulated from the instrument, which produces the electron beam.

Electron micrograph A photograph produced in an **electron microscope** by projecting the image onto photographic film. These photographs are always in black and white.

Electron microscope See **Scanning electron microscope** and **Transmission electron microscope**.

Electron scattering In **electron microscopy**, the deflection of beam electrons by interaction with atoms in a specimen.

Electropherotype A form of classification used to delineate a **virus** distinguishable from its close relatives by the relative mobility on **electrophoresis** of segments of its nucleic acid.

Electrophoresis A technique for separating mixtures of charged particles by differences in their rates of migration through a stationary gel or liquid when subjected to an electric field.

Electrophoretic decalcification A method of removing calcium ions from tissue by immersion in an electrolytic solution. In the presence of an electric current, calcium ions migrate to the cathode.

Electrostatic bonding The affinity between radicles of opposite ionic charge, which is the major mechanism of most staining reactions between tissues and **dyes**. See also **Anionic dye** and **Cationic dye**.

Elementary body The infectious particle of organisms of the *Chlamydia* species.

ELISA See **Enzyme linked immunosorbent assay**.

Ellagic acid A substance sometimes employed as the **contact activation** agent in estimation of the **activated partial thromboplastin time**. As it is not opaque, it may be useful for automated procedures.

Elliptocytosis An inherited abnormality of **erythrocyte** morphology in which a large proportion of the cells appear elliptical. It is usually asymptomatic, but is sometimes associated with a **haemolytic anaemia**.

Elution The process of removing into solution an **antibody** which has been **adsorbed** onto **antigens** (e.g. on a cell surface). Generally effected by the use of heat, freezing, or organic solvents.

Embedding Positioning tissue in the plane appropriate for **microtomy**, and its subsequent solidification in a mould containing liquid casting material (e.g. molten **paraffin wax, celloidin**).

Embden-Meyerhof pathway A metabolic pathway of anaerobic **glycolysis** used by **erythrocytes** to convert glucose, via a series of phosphorylated intermediates to **lactate**. As far as red cells are concerned, the major products of this activity are nicotinamide adenine dinucleotide (NAPH), **ATP** and **DPG**.

Embolism Cessation of the flow of blood within a blood vessel as a result of blockage by a clot, clumps of bacteria, etc., or by bubbles of air.

Embryo A fertilised ovum, from the 3rd to the 12th week of gestation.

EMIT See **Enzyme Multiplied Immunoassay Technique**.

Empty magnification The limit of **magnification** above which image quality, in terms of **resolving power** and **definition**, is lost. This limit is approximately 1000 times the **numerical aperture** of the objective lens.

Emulsion The suspension of an insoluble solute in a solvent which does not separate out into its phases.

Enamel Hard tissue covering crowns of teeth. Composed of 98% inorganic material − primarily long hydroxyapatite crystals − bound by small amounts of **acid mucopolysaccharide**.

Encephalitis Strictly, inflammation of the brain. The term is applied to a number of inflammatory diseases affecting all or part of the brain.

Endemic Describes a disease which occurs frequently within a defined community but is found much less often outside it. Limiting factors are racial or cultural characteristics, social practices, geographical barriers and **vectors**.

Enders, John F. (1897−   ) American virologist who was the first to demonstrate the replication of **poliovirus** in non-neurological cells. His work laid the foundations for much of modern **virology**.

Endocarditis Inflammation of the lining of the heart and its valves, and usually classified as infective endocarditis or prosthetic valve endocarditis. Infective endocarditis is a relatively rare disease with a poor prognosis. Underlying factors include rheumatic heart disease, congenital cardiac anomalies, compromised **immunity** and intravenous drug abuse. Symptoms include sweating, weakness, malaise and weight loss. The organisms responsible for most cases are **streptococci** − particularly of the viridans group − with *Staphylococcus aureus*, *Pseudomonas aeruginosa* and **fungi** being found mainly in intravenous drug abusers. In prosthetic valve endocarditis the organism responsible for most cases is the **coagulase** negative staphylococcus, with *Staphylococcus aureus* and viridans streptococci also being important. Some infections are associated with the original cardiac surgery whereas others are almost certainly due to haematogenous spread of organisms from a site such as the oral cavity or urethra following instrumentation or manipulation. In both types of endocarditis treatment consists of prolonged intensive **anti-microbial** therapy, often with surgical removal and replacement of cardiac valves.

Endocrine A ductless gland which secretes directly into the blood stream. Examples are the **pituitary**, adrenal and **thyroid** glands.

Endocrine cell A polypeptide and/or amine-secreting cell of the **diffuse neuroendocrine system**. These cells contain neurosecretory bodies of characteristic **ultrastructure**.

Endocrine gland A ductless gland which secretes its product directly into the blood or the lymphatic system. See **Exocrine gland**.

Endogenous Describes a naturally-occuring substance formed in the body.

Endogenous pigment Granular material of intrinsic origin which may be present in both normal and pathological tissues. Classified as being of haematogenous, tyrosine or **lipid** derivation.

Endogenous virus A **virus** existing with its nucleic acid incorporated into the **DNA** of host cells. The virus may be passed from cell to cell, and vertically from host to progeny, without any expression of complete virus particles. **Retroviruses** are particularly notable for this feature.

Endometrial glandular cells Small columnar to cuboidal cells with scanty **cytoplasm** which is finely **vacuolated** and **cyanophilic**, and with eccentrically placed nuclei displaying a finely uniform **chromatin** pattern.

Endometrial stromal cells Small cells with tiny dark nuclei and scanty **cytoplasm**, occurring in tightly packed clumps. Typically found as the centre of a core of cell groups, surrounded by

endometrial gland cells during the late phase of the menstrual cycle.

Endometritis Inflammation of the lining of the uterus, associated with caesarian section, instrumentation, **abortion** or the insertion of intrauterine contraceptive devices. The organisms encountered are **streptococci**, **chlamydia** and **anaerobic** rod-shaped **bacilli** which are negative by **Gram's stain**; **Actinomyces** species are associated particularly with intrauterine contraceptive devices. Anti-microbial **chemotherapy** should include **metronidazole**.

Endometrium The glandular lining of the body of the uterus.

Endomitosis Reproduction of nuclear elements, not followed by **chromosome** movement and **cytoplasmic** division.

Endoplasm Internal **cytoplasm**, between the **nucleus** of a cell and the **ectoplasm**.

Endoplasmic reticulum A network of cavities in the cell **cytoplasm**, which acts as a circulatory system involved in the import, export and intracellular circulation of various substances.

Endosome See **Caryosome**.

Endospore A non-sexual **spore** produced by some **bacteria** and **fungi**, and representing a resistant 'resting' phase. The spore is produced within the body of the organism, which then atrophies. **Bacteria** which commonly produce endospores are those belonging to the genera **Bacillus** and **Clostridium**. The term is also used to refer to spores found in **dermatophyte** infections which lie within the hair shaft rather than on its surface.

Endothelium The layer of cells of the **epithelium** that line the cavities of the heart, and the blood and lymph vessels and **serous** cavities of the body.

Endotoxin A **toxin** which is retained within the organism and released only on its death and lysis. In practice, the term is applied to the **lipopolysaccharide** of the cell wall of bacteria which are negative by **Gram's stain**. When released into the circulation these endotoxins give rise to a complex cascade reaction resulting in inflammation, hypotension, intravascular coagulation and fibrinolysis, known as toxic shock. See **Toxic shock syndrome**.

End point method A reaction that is terminated at a fixed point and where no more product is formed under the conditions prevailing.

Energy dispersive spectroscopy A system in **X-ray microanalysis** which permits the simultaneous display of X-rays collected in a single analysis period.

England finder An engraved microscope slide used to relocate sites within a preparation by carefully noting and subsequent repositioning of the alignment of the mechanical stage.

Enoxacin A 4-**quinolone** type of **anti-microbial** substance which has activity in terms of MIC against susceptible organisms, which is about one order of magnitude less than **Ciproflaxacin**.

Entamoeba A genus of **protozoa** of the sub-phylum Sarcodina, of which only *E. histolytica* is capable of causing human disease. The organism is ingested as a **cyst** containing four nuclei, which germinates to release eight **trophozoites** in the gut. Ulceration of the colon follows, sometimes with further spread to the liver. Amoebic dysentry affects an estimated 10^7 people annually and causes tens of thousands of deaths. **Metronidazole** is commonly used to treat the condition.

Enteric fever An enteric **infection** characterised by fever, headache, abdominal cramps, vomiting, **diarrhoea** or constipation and a rash ('rose spots'). While the condition can be caused by a variety of organisms, *Salmonella typhi* is the most common. This organism can be isolated from the blood, urine and stools at different stages of the illness. **Chloramphenicol** is the **anti-microbial** substance of choice.

Enteritis Inflammation of the small and/or large intestine, resulting in **diarrhoea**, sometimes with vomiting and abdominal cramps. The stools may be watery or may contain blood and mucus. A variety of organisms cause the condition including **Salmonella**, **Yersinia**, **Campylobacter**, **Shigella** and **Escherichia**. For treatment, **anti-microbial** substances are not generally indicated and correction of hydration, hypoglycaemia and electrolyte balance are more important.

Enterobacter Rod-shaped **bacteria** which exhibit **motility**, are facultatively **anaerobic** and **catalase** positive, **oxidase** negative and members of the **Enterobacteriaceae**. They produce **indole** and ferment lactose. The species usually encountered are *E. aerogenes*, *E. agglomerans* and *E. cloacae*, and infections are found almost exclusively in hospitalised patients.

Enterobacteriaceae A family of **bacteria** consisting of approximately 15 genera, including **Escherichia**, **Citrobacter**, **Enterobacter**, **Klebsiella**, **Shigella**, **Yersinia** and **Salmonella**. All either exhibit **motility** with peritrichate flagellae, or are non-motile, and all are **oxidase** negative. Almost all are **catalase** positive. Some cause **diarrhoea** and some cause **enteric fever**, while others are **commensals** and only cause disease when introduced into distant parts of the body.

Enterobius A **helminth**. *E. vermicularis* (or pinworm) infection is very common, especially among children. The worm is about 1 cm long and lives in the caecum. Female worms leave the gut at night and deposit large numbers of eggs on the anal and perineal skin, causing pruritus. The drug of choice is mebendazole.

Enterochromaffin Granular material found in Kultschitsky cells of the intestine which **fluoresces** characteristically following **fixation** with **formaldehyde**. Previously called **argentaffin** cells, they contain 5-hydroxy-tryptamine, and are the cell type of **carcinoid** tumours.

Enterococcus A group term which includes *Streptococcus faecalis* and *Strep. faecium*, both of which are capable of growth in **culture media** containing 65 g/l sodium chloride. Both have Lancefield group D **antigen**, but other streptococci with this antigen which are not included in the enterococci are found in stools.

Enterocolitis Inflammation of both the small and large intestines. This is often, but not always, due to infection with **bacteria** or **protozoa**.

Enterotoxin A **toxin** produced by a **micro-organism** which acts on enterocytes to influence their secretion and/or absorption of water and electrolytes. The action is not usually lethal to the enterocytes. An example is **cholera** toxin, which causes outpouring of water into the gut lumen due to activation of adenylate cyclase, which causes accumulation of cyclic adenosine monophosphate (**CAMP**). In turn, this causes excretion of electrolytes and water from the cell.

Enterovirus A genus of the **picornaviridae**, comprising three **polioviruses**, 21 **coxsackie A viruses**, six coxsackie B viruses, 29 **echoviruses** and enteroviruses types 68−74. Newly isolated enteroviruses will be given sequential numbers from 74 onwards.

Entomology The aspect of zoology concerned with the study of insects, particularly those known to be the definitive hosts of **parasites** which cause disease in man, and those acting as **vectors**.

Envelope A cell envelope consists of the **cytoplasmic** membrane, **capsule**, slime layer and appendages such as **fimbriae** and **flagellae**.

Enzyme immunoassay An **immunoassay** method in which one of the reagents is labelled with an enzyme, such as horseradish peroxidase or alkaline phosphatase, in contrast with **radioimmunoassays**, which use a radioactive label. See **Enzyme linked immunosorbent assay**.

Enzyme Linked Immunosorbent Assay An immunological technique for measuring or detecting **antigen** or **antibody**. In a test for antigen (for example), a known **antibody** is bound to a plastic surface − usually a well in a **microtitre plate**, in which the subsequent reactions are carried out. An **enzyme** conjugated to the complementary antibody is added and the antigen/antibody reaction is visualised by incubation of the antigen/antibody/enzyme complex with a suitable **substrate**; this leads to development of a coloured pigment which can be measured spectrophotometrically.

The most commonly used enzymes are horseradish peroxidase and alkaline phosphatase. The method can be extremely sensitive, and does not have the potential disadvantage of **radioimmunoassays** (RIA) of using radioisotopes, although it is more susceptible to interference (particularly by minute traces of heavy metals), and is a less 'robust' methodology than RIA. Various modifications of the technique are practised, including tests with bound antigen to detect free antibody, and competitive binding assays. In the latter, in a test for antibody a known antigen is bound to the solid phase and the unknown test serum added. After washing, a known antibody conjugated to an enzyme is then added to the wells and this will be bound to any well in which a reaction has not previously taken place, thus leading to colour development in negative tests, lack of colour indicating a positive test.

Enzyme multiplied immunoassay technique (EMIT℗). An automated competitive method of quantitation of **antigen**. It is used (for example) for the assay of drugs, and depends on the change in activity of an **enzyme** bound to the drug to be assayed, when combined with **antibody** to the drug. The difference in product concentration after reaction with a **substrate** relates to the drug concentration. The method solves the difficulty of separating bound **enzyme**-labelled antigen by inhibiting the enzyme activity in one or other form − usually the bound form − and the antigen is labelled in such a way that the enzyme retains its activity.

Eosin A series of rose-coloured acid dyes used as biological stains.

Eosinopenia A reduction in the number of circulating peripheral blood **eosinophils** below normal levels; classically observed in Cushing's syndrome.

Eosinophil A member of the **polymorphonuclear leucocyte** family characterised by the presence of distinctive eosinophilic granules when stained by **Romanowsky stain**ing methods. This cell normally comprises from 1% to 5% of the peripheral blood **leucocytes**.

Eosinophilia 1. Characteristic of a cell which is readily stained with **eosin**, showing various shades of red or pink. 2. An increase in the number of circulating peripheral blood **eosinophils**, seen primarily in **allergic** reactions, infections by **parasites** and skin disorders.

Eosinophilic Index A differential count of **squamous cells**, according to the staining characteristics of the **cytoplasm**.

Epidemic A sudden increase in the incidence of cases of a particular disease, rapidly reaching a peak and then declining to low or undetectable levels. There is usually a spread of cases beyond the population in which the disease is normally **endemic**.

Epidemiology The study of factors which influence the occurrence, frequency and distribution of **infection** within a given population. See also **Epidemic**.

Epidermophyton One of the three genera which, with **Trichophyton** and **Microsporum**, constitute the **dermatophytes**. *Epidermophyte floccosum* rarely causes hair or nail infections; it produces club-shaped **macrospores**.

Epiglottitis Inflammation of the epiglottis, which can be fulminating resulting in asphyxia. It is usually caused by *Haemophilus influenzae* type B, although other bacteria are occasionally involved. Most patients have positive **blood cultures**. After measures directed toward maintenance of the airway, the treatment of choice is **chloramphenicol**.

Epimastigote The development stage of the **trypanosomes** which cause African trypanosomiasis (**sleeping sickness**) and South American trypanosomiasis (Chaga's disease). Found in the **vector** or may be produced in laboratory culture.

Epinephrine A **hormone** which is synthesised in and secreted by the adrenal medulla. It is released into the circulation in response to stress, and itself stimulates glycogen breakdown. In **haematology** epinephrine has two main uses: (1) administration of the drug results in the re-entry of marginating **neutrophils** to the circulating pool, and may therefore be used to assess the size of the **marginating** pool; (2) it is useful for **platelet aggregation** studies.

Epiphysis A part of a bone which is derived from a centre of ossification other than the main one for that bone.

Epiphyte A fungus growing on the skin. Not a true parasitic condition.

Epiphytic Describes an organism which is **parasitic** upon another organism.

Epithelioid Morphological description of cells of epithelial appearance seen in many granulomas – especially in tuberculosis and sarcoid – but which are in fact **macrophages**. See **Epithelium**.

Epithelium The covering of internal and external surfaces of the body, including the lining of vessels and other small cavities. Epithelium is classified into types on the basis of the number of layers and the shape of the superficial cells: **squamous**, columnar, cuboidal, stratified, pseudo-stratified or simple.

Epitope The combining site of an **antigen** which reacts with the corresponding combining sites of the specific **antibody**.

EPROM Acronym for **Erasable Programable Read Only Memory**.

Epsilon amino caproic acid An anti-fibrinolytic agent which may be used therapeutically to treat hyperfibrinolysis. It is also useful in the laboratory in **anticoagulants** and **buffers** to prevent **fibrinolysis** occuring *in vitro* following blood collection or subsequent processing.

Epstein-Barr virus A member of the **herpetoviridae**, and probably the most important cause of **infectious mononucleosis**. It is probably involved in the **pathogenesis** of **Burkitt's lymphoma** in Africa, and nasopharyngeal **carcinoma** in the far east. The virus will grow only *in vitro* in **cell cultures** of **lymphoblasts**. Diagnosis of **acute** infection is achieved by the detection of virus-specific **IgM**, and by the demonstration of **heterophile** types of **antibody** using the **Paul-Bunnell-Davidsohn test**.

Equilibrium   A state of reaction when the rate of formation of products is equal to the reverse process, which is the formation of the reactants. The rate of the forward reaction is equal to that of the reverse.

Erasable Programmable Read Only Memory   In computing, a **chip** which can be fed with a **program** which is stored in **Read Only Memory**, but which can be erased by exposure to ultraviolet light and the chip subsequently reprogrammed.

E-rosette   A complex formed between a **lymphocyte** and sheep **erythrocytes**. The capacity to form an E-rosette is accepted as a **T cell** lymphocyte marker in man.

Erwinia   Rod-shaped **bacteria** which do not exhibit **motility**, are microaerophilic, do not produce **spores**, are positive by **Gram's stain**, **oxidase** negative and which produce a yellow pigment on **culture media**. Like the **Proteae** they are capable of de-aminating phenylalanine. Many strains cause diseases of plants. Like the other members of the **Enterobacteriaceae**, *Erwinia herbicola* causes infection of the lungs, urinary tract, meninges and elsewhere.

Erysipelothrix   Rod-shaped **bacteria** which do not exhibit **motility**, are non-**sporing**, microaerophilic and are positive by **Gram's stain**. *Erysipelothrix rhusiopathiae* produces small colonies showing alpha **haemolysis** on **blood agar**. The organism is a **commensal** of the intestine in many animals, birds and fish and causes serious disease in pigs and sheep. Butchers, fishermen, animal products process workers and farmers are at risk of developing infection following abrasions. The cutaneous lesion is purplish in colour and painful, but does not suppurate. It is usually self-limiting but can take weeks or months to resolve. Occasionally, **endocarditis** develops. The treatment of choice is **penicillin** or **erythromycin**.

Erythrasma   A skin infection characterised by pigmented (pink or brown) scaly lesions, usually in intertriginous areas and caused by *Corynebacterium minutissimum*. The treatment of choice is oral **erythromycin**, but relapse often occurs.

Erythroblast   A general term given to nucleated red blood cells of any developmental stage. See also **Normoblast**.

Erythroblastosis   The appearance in the peripheral blood of nucleated red cell precursors. This is particularly characteristic of

haemolytic disease of the newborn, also known as *erythroblastosis fetalis*.

Erythroblastosis fetalis Literally, an increase in the number of circulating immature cells of the erythrocyte series in the fetal circulation. As this is a sign of **anaemia** the term was formerly used to describe the milder form of **haemolytic disease of the newborn**, in which there is anaemia but not jaundice.

Erythrocyte A fully mature red blood cell which circulates as a biconcave disc and appears in **blood films** stained by **Romanowsky stains** as a pink circular disc staining more deeply at the edge of the cell. It has a diameter of approximately 7×10^{-6}m, a volume of 85 fl and survives in the circulation for about 120 days. In **virology**, erythrocytes of various species are used to detect the presence of viral **antigens** with an affinity for receptors on their surfaces by **haemagglutination** or **haemadsorption**. Specific **antibodies** may be demonstrated by the inhibition of these effects. Labelled erythrocytes are the indicators in **passive agglutination tests** and **reverse passive agglutination tests**. They are also visible reactants in **complement fixation tests** and **radial haemolysis tests**.

Erythrocyte sedimentation rate The rate at which the cellular components of a column of blood sediment in a fixed period of time – usually 1 hour. The most commonly used method is that of Westergren, when the normal values are 3–5 mm/h (males) or 4–7 mm/h (females).

Erythrocytosis An increase in the number of circulating **erythrocytes** which may be primary, or secondary to other conditions. See also **Polycythaemia**.

Erythroleukaemia A **malignant** proliferation of the **erythrocyte** series of blood cells; also known as Di Gugliemo's disease.

Erythromycin A **macrolide** type of **anti-microbial** substance produced by the **Streptomyces** species of **micro-organism**. It is active against many strains of **staphylococci**, *Streptococcus pyogenes*, *Strep. pneumoniae*, *Strep. viridans* and **Enterococci**, as well as **Corynebacteria**, **Listeria** and most other rod-shaped **bacteria** staining positive by **Gram's stain**, with the exception of **Nocardia**. Among the Gram negative bacteria, **Neisseria**, **Haemophilus**, **Campylobacter** and **Bacteroides** are susceptible, but the **Enterobacteriaceae** are not. **Mycoplasma** and **Chlamydia** are also susceptible. The drug binds to the 50s subunit of the ribosome and disrupts **protein** synthesis. There are no serious toxic effects of treatment with erythromycin other than reversible hepatotoxicity associated with the use of erythromycin estolate.

Erythron A term given to the combined population of **erythrocytes** and their precursors in the peripheral blood or **bone marrow**, which emphasises the functional unity of red blood cells wherever they are in the body.

Erythrophagocytosis The process of **phagocytosis** of **erythrocytes** by **monocytes** or, less commonly, by **neutrophils**.

Erythropoiesis The process of **erythrocyte** production and maturation occurring in the **bone marrow**.

Erythropoietin A **glycoprotein**, synthesised mainly by the kidney, produced in response to anoxia and/or falling **haemoglobin** concentrations. Erythropoietin stimulates certain marrow stem cells to produce increased numbers of **normoblasts** and increases maturation rate, haemoglobin synthesis and release of **erythrocytes** into the peripheral blood.

Escherichia Rod-shaped **bacteria** which exhibit **motility**, are facultative **anaerobes** which are **catalase** positive, **oxidase** negative and negative by **Gram's stain**. Their natural habitat is the large intestine. *Esch. coli* produces **indole** from trytophan, fails to grow in the presence of potassium cyanide, cannot utilise citrate as a carbon source and produces beta galactosidase. Atypical strains fail to ferment lactose and some are not motile. Many **serotypes** are known based on somatic flagellar and other **envelope** antigens. Certain strains are entero-toxigenic, producing a **toxin** which causes loss of water and electrolytes from the enterocytes; others are entero-invasive and invade the mucosa and sub-mucosa of the gut wall, causing thrombosis and necrosis and giving rise to the presence of blood and mucus in the stools. Others cause intestinal disease by different means. Most strains, however, are **commensals**, but they can cause serious infection if introduced into the body at sites other than the alimentary tract.

ESR See **Erythrocyte sedimentation rate**.

Esterase An **enzyme** which catalyses hydrolysis of an ester to an alcohol and acid. An example is **lipase** (EC 3.1.1.3), which is glycerol ester hydrolase.

Esterified Describes compounds that have been converted to an acid or ester. For example, cholesterol forms an ester with fatty acids and about 70% of the total cholesterol is esterified.

Ester wax A mixture of stearate esters formulated to facilitate **microtomy** of hard and dense tissue blocks.

Estimation In statistical usage, any method by which observations from a **sample** are used to find a likely value of an unknown **parameter**. For example, the **population** mean is usually **estimated** by the sample **mean**.

Estrogen See **Oestrogen**.

Ethambutol A synthetic **anti-microbial** substance active against **mycobacteria**, including most 'atypical' strains. Other organisms are resistant. Though its precise mode of action is not known, Ethambutol probably interferes with **RNA** synthesis. The most important toxic effect is retrobulbar neuritis which leads to potentially serious, but usually reversible, visual deterioration. As with other anti-tuberculous drugs, ethambutol should not be used alone to prevent development of resistance.

Ethanol gelation test   A simple test for the demonstration of soluble **fibrin monomer** complexes in **plasma** which depends on the gelation of the plasma, due to **fibrin** formation, after addition of ethanol.

Ether sensitivity   A property of **viruses** containing essential **lipid**, usually in the form of a cell-derived **envelope**. Sensitive viruses, after **incubation** for 1 hour in ether, suffer **virolysis** and cannot be recovered from the suspension.

Ethionamide   A synthetic **anti-microbial** substance active against *Mycobacterium tuberculosis*, but having no useful activity against other species. Gastro-intestinal disturbance, peripheral neuropathy, psychiatric disturbance and hepatotoxicity are among the adverse effects of its use. It is also teratogenic and must be avoided in pregnancy.

Ethylene diamine tetra-acetic acid   In common usage, reference is usually to the di-sodium or di-potassium salt of the acid, each of which is used as an **anticoagulant** and is anti-complementary (see **Complement**). The substance is a chelating agent and is also used in the disruption of **bacterial** cells for **DNA** studies.

Ethylene oxide   A gaseous, toxic, explosive **disinfectant** used to sterilise equipment such as endoscopes which cannot be heated. It dissolves in rubber and plastic and articles made from such materials must be stored in a vented aerator after sterilisation to allow escape of residual gas. The substance is active against both vegetative **bacteria** and **spores**.

Eubacterium   Rod-shaped **bacteria** which are **anaerobes** which do not form **spores**, do not exhibit **motility**, do not branch and which are positive by **Gram's stain**. They are common **commensals** of the large intestine.

Euglobulin clot lysis time   When plasma is diluted and acidified, a white precipitate forms (the euglobulin fraction), which contains **fibrinogen, plasminogen**, and **plasminogen activator**. The precipitate is redissolved and clotted with **thrombin**. The time taken for the resultant clot to lyse is noted. (This is normally greater than 150 minutes.)

Eutectic point   The temperature at which, on cooling, a mixture of two liquids solidifies. The eutectic point varies with the presence of salts in one of the constituents.

Eversion   Literally, a turning outwards. In **cytology**, a condition in which the lining **epithelium** of the cervical canal rolls out over the ectocervix.

Exanthum   A skin rash or eruption.

Exchange transfusion   A procedure in which the entire circulating blood volume is replaced with donor blood by a process of continuous dilution. Used as a form of treatment for severe **haemolytic disease of the newborn**, blood being alternately infused and removed in small volumes (of approximately 20 ml) at a rate of around 80 ml per Kg of body weight.

Excitation   The process of rendering an atom or molecule unstable by stimulating it to absorb energy. This will occur, for example, in flame emission and atomic absorption spectroscopy.

Excited state   The relatively unstable state of an atom or molecule which has absorbed energy and may be in the process of giving up this energy and returning to the ground state.

Excretion   The process of elimination. This may be from an organ or from the body, as with the excretion of urine.

Exfoliation   The shedding of cells from a surface.

Exocrine gland   A gland which secretes outwardly (e.g. a salivary gland). See **Endocrine gland**.

Exodus   Literally, a going out. In **cytology**, a **histiocyte** 'shower' that occurs normally toward the end of the endocervical canal leading into the vagina.

Exogenous   A substance which does not occur naturally in the body, but which can be measured after it has been introduced into a living body.

Exogenous pigment   Material which has been introduced into tissue, rather than resulting from a biological process. Examples include **artefact** (**fixation** pigment), minerals (e.g. carbon, silica) and tattoo pigment.

Exogenous virus   A **virus** derived from a source other than the cell in which it is found.

Exospore   A little-used term to denote **spores** formed on the spore-bearing structures separate from the vegetative cell, as in **Actinomyces** and some **fungi**.

Exotoxin   A substance which is typically **protein** in nature, which is released from living bacterial cells and which has a toxic effect on cells or systems in the host. Examples are the **toxins** of *Corynebacterium diphtheria*, *Clostridium tetani* and *Vibrio cholerae*. Many exotoxins have a similar structure, being composed of two units, one of which mediates binding to the receptor sites and cell penetration, while the second exerts the toxic effect intracellularly.

Explanatory variable   See **Regression**.

External quality assessment A system of retrospective objective checking of the **quality** of laboratory results by an external agency.

Extinction See **Absorbance**.

Extinction coefficient The degree of extinction, or absorbance, under defined conditions with a path length of 1 cm.

Extrinsic blood coagulation system The term given to the pathway of **coagulation factor X** activation, which is dependent on **tissue factor** and factor VII.

Exudate Fluid which has passed into a **serous** cavity as a result of tissue damage (e.g. by infection or trauma). See **Transudate**.

Eyepiece graticule A glass disc with ruled lines, or a grid, placed in the eyepiece of a microscope and used in conjunction with a **stage micrometer** in **micrometry**.

F

FAB classification   See **French-American-British classification**.

Fab fragment   Fab is the abbreviation for 'fragment, **antigen** binding', which is the area of an **immunoglobulin** molecule responsible for specific interaction with antigen. If an intact immunoglobulin molecule is treated with **papain**, two Fab fragments are liberated, consisting of an entire **light chain** and the N-terminal half of a **heavy chain** joined by a **disulphide bond**.

F(ab)₂ fragment   A fragment liberated from an intact **immunoglobulin** molecule by pepsin treatment. It consists of two **Fab fragments** joined by at least one **disulphide bond** between the **heavy chains**.

Facet   The bevels either side of a **microtome** knife, which converge to form the cutting edge.

Factorial experiments   An experiment where two or more statistical **factors** are studied to see which are important in affecting a certain **variable**, and also to see whether there are any important **interactions** between the factors. It is usually analysed using **Analysis of variance**.

Factors   Statistically, quantities which can take certain predetermined values (e.g. drug dose or sex) and which may affect the value of a **variable** being studied.

Faecal-oral route of transmission   A route of transmission of **infection** implying the consumption of faeces. The term is correctly applied to the spread of disease by ingestion of infected food or fluids.

Faeces   The material expelled from the bowel.

Family antigen   A **blood group antigen** found only in the members of a closely related group of individuals. Also referred to as a 'low incidence' antigen.

Farmer's lung   A respiratory condition, mainly seen in farm workers, caused by the inhalation of *Micropolyspora faeni*, spores of which may be present in mouldy hay. The condition is mainly due to a **type III reaction** of **hypersensitivity**.

Farr test   A **radioimmunoassay** method for assessing the amount of **antibody** bound to an **antigen**. Excess radio-labelled antigen is added to antibody. Antibody bound to antigen is then precipitated with ammonium sulphate, leaving unbound antigen in solution. The method can only be used in conjunction with antigens which are soluble in 500 g/l ammonium sulphate.

Fasciitis   Infection of the fascia, or subcutaneous sheets of connective tissue. The infection often progresses very rapidly, laterally along the planes of the superficial and/or deep fascia, the over-

110

lying skin breaking down to become gangrenous. Predisposing conditions are **diabetes** and alcoholism and the causative organisms are a mixture of **Bacteroides** species, **Enterobacteriaceae** and anaerobic **Streptococci**; sometimes *Streptococcus pyogenes* and *Staphylococcus aureus* are involved. Treatment involves prompt surgical debridement and administration of broad-spectrum **antimicrobial** substances and **Metronidazole**.

Fat The generic term used to describe lipids and lipoproteins. It includes fatty acids, neutral fat and phospholipids.

Fatty acids The generic term for saturated and unsaturated fatty acids. The former have the general formula C_nH_{2n+1} COOH and includes acetic and palmitic acids; the latter have the formula C_nH_{2n-x} COOH and include oleic and linoleic acids.

Favism A type of **haemolytic anaemia** which follows ingestion of the fava bean by individuals with congenital deficiency of **glucose 6-phosphate dehydrogenase**.

Fc fragment The C terminal part of the **heavy chain** of an **immunoglobulin** molecule. It can be released from the intact molecule by papain hydrolysis. The abbreviation stands for 'fragment crystallisable'.

Fd fragment The N terminal region of the **heavy chain** of an **immunoglobulin**. It consists of the **variable domain** and the C_H1 **domain**.

FDP See **Fibrin degradation products**.

Febrile Characterised by a **fever**.

Feedback 1. Return of part of the output of an electrical or electronic amplifier to the input, causing either increased distortion of the signal (positive feedback) or reduction of distortion (negative feedback). 2. The mechanism of modulation of **hormone** release from a gland. The release is stimulated by a change in level of a circulating substance (e.g. glucose), or by the increase in blood levels of a trophic hormone.

Femtolitre The **SI** unit of measurement used for **mean cell volume**: equal to 10^{-15} litres. Abbreviated fl.

Fermentation A metabolic process used by **bacteria** and **fungi** to produce energy in the form of **adenosine triphosphate** by **substrate** level phosphorylation. Substrates are usually carbohydrates or organic acids and end products vary considerably, but many include fatty acids, carbon dioxide, hydrogen and alcohols. The process usually takes place **anaerobically**, metabolism switching to **aerobic** respiration in the presence of oxygen.

Ferritin A form of storage iron consisting of a protein shell (**apoferritin**) surrounding a ferric core which comprises about 23% of its dry weight.

Ferritin labelling The chemical attachment of the radio-opaque substance **ferritin** to **antibody**. Antibody so labelled can be detected by **electron microscopy**.

Ferrokinetics In **haematology**, the study of iron absorption, transport or excretion following administration of radio-labelled iron. See also **Iron turnover**.

Fetal fibrinogen A form of plasma **fibrinogen** with a higher concentration of phosphorus and **sialic acid**. Occurs normally in newborn infants, and has a longer **thrombin clotting time** than adult fibrinogen.

Fetal haemoglobin See **Haemoglobin**.

(alpha) Fetoprotein A glycoprotein, an $alpha_1$-**globulin** which is synthesised in the fetal liver and present in the **serum** of the **fetus**, the newborn and women in pregnancy. Synthesis is almost completely repressed in normal adults. It diffuses through capillary membranes into the fetal urine and then into amniotic fluid and maternal plasma. Raised levels in the amniotic fluid or serum of pregnant women are indicative of severe neural tube defects in the fetus, and its measurement in maternal serum can be used to screen for these abnormalities. High concentrations in the non-pregnant adult are diagnostic of some forms of **carcinoma**. Alpha fetoprotein is demonstrated in serum by **radioimmunoassay** techniques, and in tissue sections by **immunoperoxidase** methods.

Fetuin A **glycoprotein** found in calf serum; closely related to orosomucoid.

Fetus A fertilised ovum, from the 12th week of gestation to birth.

Feulgen's reaction A **cytochemical** test for **deoxy-ribonucleic acid** which depends on the liberation of free pentose aldehyde groups from DNA after **hydrolysis** with HCl, and their subsequent interaction with leucobasic fuchsin.

Fever Disturbance of temperature regulation with elevation − and sometimes lowering − of body temperature. The cause of the fever is often the cause of infection, but fever can also be due to non-infective causes such as cerebral haemorrhage or trauma, drug toxicity and endocrine disorders. The pattern of the rise and fall, or constant elevation, of temperature is useful in diagnosis of its cause. **Pyrogens** are important in causing fever. These substances may be derived from drugs or organisms, an instance being **endotoxin**. They may also be produced by **leucocytes**.

FFP See **Frozen fresh plasma**.

F_1 hybrid A **heterozygous** first generation offspring from genetically dissimilar parents.

Fibril A thread-like structure, smaller than the fibre of which it is a part.

112

Fibrin An insoluble protein formed during **coagulation** of blood to form a clot.

Fibrin degradation products Fragments which result from the breakdown of **fibrin** or **fibrinogen** by the **fibrinolytic** enzyme **plasmin**.

Fibrin monomer The term given to the molecule remaining after removal of **fibrinopeptides** from **fibrinogen** by **thrombin** or **Reptilase**ᵀᴹ, but before **fibrin polymerisation** has occurred.

Fibrinogen A plasma **protein**, and member of the **coagulation factor** family, which is converted to an insoluble fibrin clot by the action of **thrombin** in the final stage of the blood coagulation **cascade**.

Fibrinogen titre A semi-quantitative test for the measurement of plasma **fibrinogen** in which **thrombin** is added to serial dilutions of test plasma. Normally, fibrin clots will be seen up to dilutions of 1 in 128. A lower **titre** suggests **hypofibrinogenaemia** or **hyperfibrinolysis**.

Fibrinoid Hyalin material which has similar staining reactions to fibrin, yet is immunologically different.

Fibrinolysis The process in which **plasminogen activators** convert **plasminogen** to the active enzyme **plasmin**. The biological function of this pathway is to convert fibrin into **fibrin degradation products**.

Fibrinopeptides Small **peptides** which are released from the N-terminal ends of the A alpha- and B beta-chains of the **fibrinogen** molecule by **thrombin**. The resultant molecule is known as **fibrin monomer**.

Fibrin plate test **Fibrinogen** solution is poured into a **petri dish** and clotted with **thrombin**. Test **plasma** or **euglobulin** fraction is placed in wells punched into the surface of the fibrin layer. After incubation the areas of lysis are measured and are proportional to the concentration of **plasminogen activator**. Fibrin plates may also be used to detect free **plasmin** if the plates are heated to destroy **plasminogen activator** before use.

Fibrin polymerisation The process by which **fibrin monomers** spontaneously aggregate, or polymerise, to form a visible clot.

Fibrin stabilising factor See **Coagulation factors**.

Fibroblast The commonest type of tissue cell, responsible for the production of **collagen** − the major acellular component of connective tissue.

Fibromyoma A **benign tumour** composed of fibrous tissue and muscle fibres.

Fibronectin A large **glycoprotein** found in blood and other body fluids, previously known as cold-insoluble globulin, which mediates the adhesion of cells to the extracellular connective tissue matrix. Fibronectin may also be cross-linked to **collagen** by **fibrin stabilising factor** and may act as an **opsonin**.

Ficin   A proteolytic **enzyme** sometimes used in serological reactions. Obtained from figs.

Field   In microscopy, the area of observation seen through the eyepiece.

Field's stain   A method for staining **blood films** for **malarial** parasites using polychromed methylene blue and counter-stained with **eosin**.

Field stop   A diaphragm located within the eyepiece of a microscope, at the primary plane of the objective lens. It limits the field of view and is useful in supporting an **eyepiece graticule**.

FIF   See **Formaldehyde-induced fluorescence**.

FIGLU   See **Formiminoglutamic acid**.

Filament   In **electron microscopy**, generally a hairpin-shaped tungsten wire, heated to produce electrons.

Filariasis   A condition produced by some nematode (filarial) worms. The adults live in the lymphatics, skin, connective tissue or serous membranes, producing live **embryos** (microfilariae), and can be demonstrated in blood, skin snips, serous fluid and urine.

File   In computing, an organised collection of information treated as a single item and usually stored on a **floppy disc** or on magnetic tape.

Filoviridae   A family of **viruses** comprising (to date) **Marburg virus** and **Ebola virus**. They are **risk group 4 pathogens** causing severe **haemorrhagic fever**. They may be isolated in **vero cell** culture, their presence being demonstrated by **immunofluorescence**.

Filtration   The removal of particles from fluids by passing them through a matrix or membrane which does not allow the passage of the particles, while permitting the fluid to pass freely. Depending on the pore size of the matrix or membrane, large particles such as precipitated chemicals, **bacteria** and **fungi** can be removed from solutions. A pore size of 0·45 micrometre will remove most bacteria and fungi but will pass **viruses** and **mollicutes**.

Fimbriae   Filaments of **protein** protruding from the bacterial **cell wall**. They are hollow and are shorter than **flagellae**. Their functions include attachment to inanimate and animate surfaces and to other **bacteria**, and the exchange of genetic material. Fimbriae each have a particular function in this respect. Cultural conditions are important in their expression. Strains which possess fimbriae often have enhanced **virulence**. Examples are *Neisseria gonorrhoeae* and certain strains of *Escherichia coli*.

FIMLS   Fellow of the Institute of Medical Laboratory Sciences. See **IMLS**.

Fine needle biopsy   A method of obtaining small amounts of cellular fragments from a living person, for laboratory investigation, by aspiration with a syringe and negative pressure into the core of a fine-bore needle.

Firmware   In computing, a **program** stored in a **Read Only Memory** chip, and which cannot normally be erased.

First order kinetics   The rate of activity of an **enzyme** becoming dependent on **substrate** concentration only, because other conditions (such as temperature, time, etc.) remain constant.

First set rejection   A rejection mechanism seen following grafting of incompatible tissue to an individual previously unexposed to such tissue.

FITC   See **Fluorescein isothiocyanate**.

Fitzgerald factor   See **High molecular weight kininogen**.

Fixation   Treatment of tissue to prevent autolysis and putrefaction, yet retain reactivity and localisation of components as closely to the living state as possible.

Fixed point method   See **End point method**.

Flagellum   An organ of motility in some **micro-organisms**. A long whip-like structure composed of a central **axoneme** consisting of helical fibrils of the **protein** flagellin, covered by a sheath which is an extension of the cell **membrane**. There is a structure at the base of the flagellum, extending through the cell **membrane** into the **cytoplasm**, which appears to supply the motive force. Where several flagellae are present they move in a co-ordinated manner. There may be one or more flagellae on the cells of flagellated **bacteria**, and these may be placed at the poles of the cell − in which case they are said to be polar − or arranged in groups over the whole of the cell surface, in which case they are said to be peritrichous. Flagellae are one of the four basic means of movement of **protozoa** (flagellum, **cilia**, **pseudopodium** or undulating ridges).

Flame photometry   A system which causes atomic excitation by flame and atomisation, followed by measurement of the level of emitted radiation as light.

Flaujeac factor   See **High molecular weight kininogen**.

Flaviviridae   A large family of arthropod-borne **RNA** viruses, including the **viruses** of **yellow fever** and **Dengue**. Many of them cause **zoonotic** diseases in man in tropical and sub-tropical areas.

Flavobacterium   Rod-shaped **bacteria** which usually do not exhibit **motility**, are **catalase** positive and **oxidase** positive, staining negative by **Gram's stain** and growing on ordinary **culture media** with production of a yellow pigment. *F. meningosepticum* produces **indole** from tryptophan and oxidises glucose, lactose and maltose. It occasionally causes **meningitis** in infants.

Fletcher factor   See **Prekallikrein**.

Flocculation test   An **antigen/antibody** reaction involving a soluble antigen which undergoes flocculation (the formation of downy masses of precipitate) when combined with antibody.

Flocloxacillin   A semi-synthetic **beta lactam** type of **anti-microbial** substance which is resistant to staphylococcal **penicillinase** and to gastric acidity. The drug is classified as an isoxazolyl **penicillin** and it differs from **cloxacillin** in having a fluorine atom. It has very useful activity against **staphylococci** but a small proportion of strains show intrinsic resistance which is not mediated by **beta lactamase**. Toxicity in use is comparable to that of other penicillins.

Floppy disc   A flexible circular disc permanently housed in a stiff envelope, and with a magnetic coating, used to store data which has been entered into a computer. Standard disc sizes are 8, 5¼, 3½, 3¼ and 3 inches in diameter.

Flucytosine   A synthetic **anti-microbial** substance, active against **Candida** and **Cryptococcus** species, and other **yeasts**, but significantly less so against filamentous **fungi**. It acts mainly by replacing uracil in fungal **RNA**, thus interfering with protein synthesis, and partly by interfering by another route with **DNA** synthesis. Resistance, when it develops, is due to modification to the permease, which allows the drug into the cell, or to the various **enzymes** involved in the conversion and incorporation of 5-fluorocytosine as 5-fluorouracil into fungal RNA. The drug is used in combination, usually with **Amphotericin B**.

Fluke   Synonyms: Diagenetic trematode; Flat worm. Among the most common and abundant of parasitic worms. The life cycle involves at least two hosts. Some species are parasitic in man and in domestic animals, where their presence is of economic importance. The schistosoma alone − particularly *S. mansoni* and *S. haematobium* − account for over 200×10^6 human infections around the world. **Swimmers itch**, caused by bird schistosomes penetrating the skin of swimmers bathing in ponds and rivers in Europe, is not uncommon. However, these species cannot complete their life cycle in man, and consequently are of nuisance value only.

Fluorescein isothiocyanate   A fluorochrome **dye** notable for the ease with which it may be bound to **immunoglobulin**. It is commonly used in **fluorescence** techniques to label **antibodies**, e.g. in **immunocytochenistry** and for **fluorescence activated cell sorting**. When illuminated with ultraviolet light, stained objects appear apple green in colour.

Fluorescence   A molecule in which one electron is elevated to an anti-bonding orbital on excitation. It exists with its original spin and, on its return to the ground state, radiation is emitted in the form of light.

Fluorescence microscopy A system of microscopy used to exploit the phenomenon of fluorescence, and in which certain substances absorb light of short wavelength which is emitted at a longer wavelength within the visible spectrum. An ultraviolet (or near ultraviolet) light source is employed, either as **transmitted light** together with appropriate excitation and barrier filters, or as **incident light** using a **dichroic mirror** and appropriate barrier filters.

Fluorescence polarisation immunoassay A technique developed to assay a variety of substances including **anti-microbial** substances. It depends on excitation of the drug-antibody complex by polarised light to produce fluorescence which is of the same polarisation plane. With increasing drug concentration there is a decrease in fluorescence polarisation.

Fluorimetry The measurement of light emitted as a result of fluorescence. Since this is emitted in all directions the detector is moved at right angles to the path of exciting incident radiation to avoid stray incident light.

Fluorochrome A **dye** which absorbs light of short wavelength (400 nm and below), loses energy and emits light of a longer, visible wavelength (about 500 nm).

Foam cells Large round cells with small round or oval nuclei and abundant finely **vacuolated cytoplasm**. Seen in breast secretions.

Foamy viruses Members of a sub-family of the **retroviridae**, known as spumavirinae. They are frequent contaminants of primate **cell cultures** in the laboratory, causing large **vacuol**ated multinuclear **giant cells**. Their presence greatly reduces the usefulness of the cell cultures for virus isolation.

Focal length The distance from the focal point to the central point of a lens.

Foetus See **Fetus**.

Folic acid The trivial name for pteroylmonoglutamic acid, the parent compound of the group of substances collectively known as folates. Folic acid is an essential cofactor in **DNA** synthesis, and its deficiency leads to **megaloblastic anaemia**.

Follicle A pouch-like cavity, or sac.

Follicle stimulating hormone One of several specific **hormones** secreted by the anterior pituitary which stimulate or inhibit specific target glands. The targets for this hormone are the ovary and testis.

Follicular cervicitis An inflammatory disorder with formation of mature lymph **follicles** located beneath the **epithelium** and characterised in **cytology** by clusters of mature and immature **lymphocytes**.

Folliculitis Suppurative inflammation of the hair follicles, which may become chronic. The causative organism is almost always *Staphylococcus aureus*, though the folliculitis associated with the use of whirlpool baths (**Jaccuzi rash**) is caused by **Pseudomonas**.

Fomites Items of clothing, bed linen, towels and dressings — as well as larger objects such as mattresses — on which infectious agents may collect, and from which organisms may be spread to others. They may be a source of **nosocomial** infection.

Forbidden clone A **clone** of **lymphocytes** which has become suppressed during fetal or early neonatal life. The clone may regain reactivity during later life and cause **auto immunity**. See **Burnett's monoclonal selection theory**.

Formaldehyde An astringent smelling highly toxic gas, highly soluble in water and commercially available as a 40% aqueous solution commonly called **formalin**. Its commonest laboratory use is as a general agent for **fixation** of tissue prior to **histology** processing, when it is diluted to 4% in water or **normal saline** and is then known as (e.g.) Formal saline or Formalin saline. It reacts by cross-linking protein and end-groups, and by forming methylene bridges. Aqueous solutions may also be used, with care, as a disinfectant for surfaces, metallic objects, etc., as the solution is not corrosive; it can be used safely on clothing and furniture as well as walls and floors, although it is irritant to skin and mucous membranes. Both vegetative **micro-organisms** and **spores** are killed rapidly. Formaldehyde acts by denaturing cell proteins. (NB When used as a **fixative** in **histology**, formalin penetrates tissues slowly and fixed tissues should not be assumed to be free from viable organisms.) Formaldehyde vapour is used to fumigate **Class I exhaust protective cabinets** and **class III exhaust protective cabinets,** and also rooms which may be infected with pathogens or potential contaminants of (e.g.) **cell cultures**. See also **Formalin**.

Formaldehyde induced fluorescence A powerful and accurate method of demonstrating catecholamines and indoleamines by treating tissue with either the water or gaseous phase of **formaldehyde**. The reaction is visualised by **fluorescence** microscopy.

Formalin A 40% solution of **formaldehyde** gas in water. In widespread use for tissue **fixation** and as a **disinfectant**. See **Formaldehyde**.

Formalin pigment An **endogenous** pigment formed in tissue by the action of acidic **formalin** solutions on **haemoglobin**. Dark brown, small **birefringent** crystals. Removed by treatment with alcoholic picric acid.

Formal-sublimate Mercuric chloride-**formalin** mixture used for tissue **fixation**, giving good results with **acid dyes**. Causes tissue shrinkage and hardening. Also gives rise to **mercury pigment**.

Formazan An insoluble coloured product resulting from the reduction of **tetrazolium salts**.

Formiminoglutamic acid (FIGLU). A breakdown product of histidine formed in a reaction catalysed by **folic acid**. In the absence of folic acid, FIGLU accumulates and is excreted in the urine, providing the basis of a test for folic acid deficiency. See also **Histidine loading test**.

Formvar Polyvinyl formal, used as an electron-luscent support film, 10−20 nm thick, for sections on **grids** for **electron microscopy**.

Forsmann antibody A **heterophile** antibody found in normal human sera and directed against the **Forsmann antigen**, which is widely distributed in nature. It is to be distinguished from the heterophile **antibody** of **infectious mononucleosis** and that found in **serum sickness**.

Forsmann antigen A **heterophile** antigen found in many animals, and some bacteria, but not in man or in the rabbit. On injection into the rabbit the antigen stimulates a **haemolysin** for sheep **erythrocytes**.

FORTRAN Acronym for 'FORmula TRANslation'. A **high level language** in computing, used especially in scientific applications.

Fosfomycin An **anti-microbial** substance produced by **Streptomyces** and which can now be synthesised. Its spectrum of activity is broad, including **Staphylococci**, **Neisseria**, **Enterobacteriaceae** and some strains of **Streptococcus** and **Pseudomonas**. The drug interferes with **cell wall** synthesis by inhibiting the conversion of N-acetylglucosamine to N-acetylmuramic acid. The drug is little used in the United Kingdom.

Fouchet's test A test to detect bilirubin in urine. Bilirubin is adsorbed on to insoluble barium salts. A blue-green colour appears when Fouchet's reagent, which contains ferric chloride in trichloracetic acid, is added.

Fragility test See **Osmotic fragility**.

Francisella A rod-shaped **bacterium** which does not exhibit **motility**, is **pleomorphic**, negative by **Gram's stain** and grows best on **culture medium** containing cysteine. *F. tularensis* causes a plague-like illness in rodents and the organism is spread by arthropods. Humans contact tularaemia by contact with infected animal tissues or by inhalation. The disease is absent from the United Kingdom, though it occurs throughout northern Europe and north America. After the appearance of an ulcer at the site of inoculation, **bacteraemia** and **pneumonia** develop. Because of laboratory hazards of attempted isolation, serological diagnosis is usually used. While other drugs are somewhat ineffective, **Streptomycin** is the drug of choice.

FRCPath Fellow of the Royal College of Pathologists. See **RCPath**.

Freemartin The female of non-identical bovine twins which share a common placenta and are thus exposed to each others' tissues *in utero*. Each twin will tolerate grafted tissue from the other in later life.

Freeze drying A method of preservation in which water is removed from fast frozen material by sublimation under vacuum. See **Lyophilisation**.

Freeze substitution An alternative to **freeze drying** in which water is removed from the frozen material by **dehydration** at low temperatures ($-60°C$ to $-70°C$). In the case of tissue this is subsequently **embedded**, usually in **paraffin wax**.

French-American-British classification A uniform system of nomenclature for the morphological classification of **acute leukaemia** based on examination of **blood films** which have been **Romanowsky stained**, supplemented where appropriate by **cytochemical** reactions.

Fresh frozen plasma See **Frozen fresh plasma**.

Fresnel fringe Rings formed at the edge of holes in specimens under observation in the **transmission electron microscope**, at either side of the focus position.

Freund's adjuvant A water-in-oil **adjuvant** which is known as incomplete Freund's adjuvant in this form, but is called complete Freund's adjuvant on addition of killed **mycobacteria**.

Frozen fresh plasma A product for **transfusion** obtained by separating the plasma from a donation of **whole blood** and freezing it at $-30°C$ or below within 18 h of collection. Used as a source of **coagulation factors**, especially factors V, VIII and IX and fibrinogen.

Frozen section A **microtome** section cut from fixed or unfixed tissue in the frozen state, thus obviating the need for **processing**. A rapid technique which retains many soluble and labile elements.

FSH See **Follicle stimulating hormone**.

F-test In statistical usage, a method of **hypothesis testing** based on the F-**distribution**. It is widely used in **analysis of variance** to assess the importance of certain **factors** or treatment groups in causing variation in the **variable** of interest.

Fungus A member of a large and extremely varied group of eukaryotes, which usually have rigid **cell walls** of different construction from that of **bacteria**. Phycomycetes such as mucor have no cross walls and thus a continuous multi-nucleate **cytoplasm**, while the higher fungi such as **Aspergillus** have separate hyphae. **Candida**, a yeast-like fungus, **cryptococcus**, the **dermatophytes**, **histoplasma** and a few others can cause disease in otherwise healthy individuals, while a wide range of other fungi cause serious disease in **immunocompromised** individuals.

Furunculosis Recurrent appearances of tense, acutely inflamed and painful **abscesses** in the skin, usually over areas of abrasion or excessive perspiration. The lesions are commonly referred to as boils. Sometimes they progress to become **carbuncles**.

Fusidic acid   An **anti-microbial** substance with a steroid-like structure, produced by Fusidium species. Its main activity is against **staphylococci**, including many **methicillin**-resistant strains. The drug acts by inhibiting the translocation step in **protein** synthesis. It is almost free from side-effects in use, other than mild gastro-intestinal upsets.

Fusiform   Spindle-shaped. A term used to denote rod-shaped **micro-organisms** with tapered ends, as in the **Fusobacterium** species.

Fusobacterium   One of three genera in the family Bacteroidaceae which do not produce **spores**, may or may not exhibit **motility**, are **oxidase** negative and **catalase** negative obligate **anaerobes**, and which are rod-shaped and negative by **Gram's stain**. They are **commensals** of the alimentary tract and cause wound infections, **abscesses** and intrathoracic sepsis.

G

GACRIA   Acronym for IgG Antibody Capture RadioImmunoassay. The general principle of this test is described under **MACRIA**. GACELISA is a similar test employing an **enzyme** label.

Galactosuria   The excretion of galactose in the urine. This sometimes occurs in lactating women but is more significant in infants who have a recessive inherited disorder due to the inability to metabolise galactose, which is formed from lactose in milk.

GALT   See **Gut-associated lymphoid tissue**.

Gamete   A reproductive cell.

Gametocyte   The parental stage from which **gametes** or mature sex cells develop. For example, malaria parasites seen in **Romanowski**-stained preparations of peripheral blood.

Gamma chain   The **heavy chain** of **IgG**.

Gardnerella   Rod-shaped **bacteria** which do not exhibit **motility**, are **oxidase** negative, **catalase** negative and negative by **Gram's** stain. They grow well on **chocolate agar** in an atmosphere of CO_2 or anaerobically, and are considered to be a cause of vaginosis, possibly in association with other **anaerobes**. 'Clue cells' (vaginal **epithelial** cells with adherent *G. vaginalis*) and amine production adding potassium hydroxide to vaginal fluid, are said to be diagnostic.

Gas gangrene   A progressive **necrosis** of skeletal muscle with toxaemia and gas formation in the tissues. The muscle is rapidly destroyed. Predisposing factors include trauma, surgery, **diabetes** and vascular disease. The causative organisms are **Clostridia**, with *Cl. perfringens* predominating. Treatment includes prompt surgical debridement, high-dose **penicillin** dosage and hyperbaric oxygen.

Gas liquid chromatography   A **chromatography** separation technique which depends upon the partition between gaseous and liquid phases. There is one solvent which is coated on a stationary inert phase.

Gastrin   A **hormone** secreted from the antral part of the stomach and the small intestine. It stimulates the secretion of hydrochloric acid from the parietal cells.

Gastritis   Inflammation of the gastric mucosa. Infective causes are rare but include fish worms and *Campylobacter pyloridis*.

Gastroenteritis   Inflammation of the intestine lining, occurring anywhere between the stomach and the rectum. It may be caused by a variety of infectious and non-infectious agents, bacteria, **protozoa**, **viruses**, **toxins** and poisons. The actual inflammation is usually limited to the small (and sometimes large) intestine, and is manifest by **diarrhoea**. The gastric component is inferred by ac-

122

companying vomiting, but this is not necessarily due to gastritis. Many cases of gastroenteritis are caused by **viruses** or have an undiagnosed cause. However, *Campylobacter jejuni*, **Salmonella** species and *Shigella sonnei* are common bacterial causes. The term gastroenteritis is generally held to cover a range of syndromes which include **diarrhoea**, but which might or might not include vomiting. The stools might contain blood and mucus, as with *Sh. sonnei* infection, and this indicates invasion of the mucosa and submucosa of the ileum and colon; or they might be very watery with no blood, indicating the effect of **enterotoxin** on the entero-cytes of the ileal and colonic mucosa, as with enterotoxigenic *Escherichia coli*.

Gel diffusion test A test in which **antibody** and **antigen** are allowed to diffuse and interact to form a precipitate in an **agar** gel.

Gel filtration See **Molecular exclusion chromatography**.

Gel precipitation A technique in which point sources of **antigen** and **antibody** are allowed to diffuse towards one another through a transparent or opalescent **substrate** such as **agar** or **agarose**. The point where reagents meet in optimal proportions is indicated by the development of a white line of precipitation.

Gene The unit of inheritance. Genes occur in linear formation along **chromosomes**.

Gene frequencies The frequency of a **gene** in the population as a whole. (i.e. When calculating the frequency of the **blood group** O gene, people of **genotype** AO and BO must be included as well as those of OO). Gene frequencies are given as a decimal figure per individual (e.g. The gene frequency of O in Britain is 0·6827, therefore the frequency of the genotype OO is $0·6827 \times 0.6827 = 0·47$, or approximately 47%).

Gene probe See **DNA probe**.

Generation of diversity The process by which **B cells** and **T cells** differentiate, during the maturation of the **immune** system, to develop differing specificities for **antigen**.

Generation time The 'instantaneous generation time' of a bacterial cell population is the time taken for a doubling in numbers to take place, if the rate of cell mass synthesis remains constant through-out this period. In practice this is rarely so, and the 'mean generation time' applies. Also called the doubling time, this is therefore shorter than the instantaneous generation time in exponential growth.

Genetic re-assortment Occurring in **viruses** with segmented **genomes**, when each segment represents a single **gene**. Co-cultivation of (e.g.) **influenza viruses** of different types results in exchanged genes in some of the progeny.

Genetic transmission A means by which **viruses**, having invaded host germ cells and integrated with the cell **genome**, can be transmitted to a new individual.

Genome The complete set of **genes** carried on a representative of each of the pairs of **chromosomes** in an individual.

Genotype A statement of the complete genetic constitution of an individual, in respect of any particular factor or **blood group** system. See also **Phenotype**.

Gentamicin An **aminoglycoside** type of **anti-microbial** substance produced by Micromonospora species. The drug is active against a wide range of rod-shaped bacilli which are negative by **Gram's stain**, and Gram positive cocci, but **anaerobes** are usually resistant. **Enterococci** are also relatively resistant, but a combination of **penicillin** or **ampicillin** and **gentamycin** is usually effective clinically. Gentamicin acts by binding to the 30s subunit of the ribosome, thus interfering with protein synthesis. Resistance is mediated by **aminoglycoside-modifying enzymes**.

Geometric optics The approach to light transmission which conceives that light travels in straight lines. See **Wave optics**.

Geotrichium A common **fungus** which is found widely distributed in nature in wood pulp, leaf mould, milk, cow dung and dairy products. It grows as a **yeast** at 37°C but as a filamentous **fungus** at room temperature, but in both phases typical rectangular arthrospores are present which germinate by producing a germ tube from one corner. The fungus is an uncommon cause of human disease but has been known to cause pulmonary infections (including a family outbreak) and **septicaemia**. It is susceptible to **Amphotericin** B and to **fluocytosine**.

Gerhardt's test A test for ketone bodies in urine, which gives a red-brown colour in the presence of ketones or salicylates when 100 g/l ferric chloride is added. Ketones may be differentiated from salicylates by boiling the urine. Ketones are unstable and will boil off; salicylates will remain.

Germinal centre An area within lymphoid tissue which consists of **B cells** and B cell **lymphoblasts**. Germinal centres become enlarged in secondary **antibody** responses and may be regarded as sites of B cell memory.

Germ line theory One theory for the **generation of diversity** in B **cell** surface membrane **immunoglobulin**. Proponents of the theory suggest that all **antibody** genes are present in all B cells, and that during differentiation translocations of **genes** and **chromosome** looping generate the capacity of the B cells to respond to different **antigens**.

124

GGT See **(gamma) Glutamyl transpeptidase**.

GH See **Growth hormone**.

Ghost cell An abnormally shaped non-nucleated cell characteristic of **squamous carcinoma**.

Giant cell An aggregated, elongated **macrophage** which has indistinct interdigitating cell boundaries and thus the appearance of a **giant cell** with multiple nuclei. Found in granulomatous disease, foreign body reactions and as the cell involved in bone resorption **(osteoclast)**.

Giardia A common intestinal **protozoan** with **flagellae**, which is spread largely by ingestion of contaminated drinking water. The life cycle has two forms, the cyst and the trophozoite. Infection with *G. intestinalis*, the only species known, is followed by multiplication of trophozoites in the upper small intestine, and their attachment in large numbers to the enterocytes. This causes **diarrhoea**, flatulence and abdominal cramps with watery stools. A chronic form with malabsorption and steatorrhoea sometimes develops. **Metronidazole** is the treatment of choice.

Giardiasis A clinical condition caused by the **parasite** *Giardia lamblia*, presenting as a range of symptoms from mild abdominal disturbance to fulminating diarrhoea.

Gibson and Harrison standard An aqueous mixture of chromium potassium sulphate, cobaltous sulphate and potassium dichromate, which has a colour equivalent to a 1 in 100 dilution of blood with a **haemoglobin** concentration of 16·0 g/dl.

Giemsa stain See **Romanowsky stains**.

Gigantism A condition in which there is abnormal increase in bone dimensions, and the overall height of the adult exceeds 200 cm (6 feet 7 inches). It is caused by over-secretion of pituitary growth **hormone** in early childhood, as a result of a **benign** eosinophilic **adenoma**.

Gingivitis A **periodontal disease** affecting the gums. The condition, if unchecked, may progress to cause loss of teeth. Plaque is an important factor. The organisms considered to cause gingivitis include **Bacteroides** species, **Capnocytophagia** and oral **streptococci**. An acute necrotising form is caused by *Borrelia vincenti*. Treatment includes debridement, plaque removal, local application of **antiseptics** and the administration of **penicillin** and/or **metronidazole**.

Giving set A device for the intravenous administration of fluids, as in blood **transfusion**.

GLC See **Gas liquid chromatography**.

Glia See **Neuroglia**.

Globin The protein fraction of the **haemoglobin** molecule.

(gamma) Globulin A class of **globulins** defined by its migration on **electrophoresis**, and which includes the **immunoglobulins**.

Globulins A group of proteins, soluble in dilute solutions of mineral salts but not in water, and which are coagulated by heat. **Antibodies** are gamma globulins of the type known as **immunoglobulins**.

Glomerular filtration rate The volume (usually the number of decilitres) of blood cleared of a substance by the renal glomeruli in a specific period of time. It is normally recorded as dl/min. and is calculated by measuring levels of **plasma** and urinary **creatinine**, and the volume of urine passed during a carefully timed period. See **Creatinine clearance test**.

Glomerulonephritis Inflammation of the glomerulus of the kidney. In infective glomerulonephritis, such as that sometimes following infection with *Streptococcus pyogenes*, **endocarditis** and ventriculoatrial shunt infections, the lesion is on the glomerular **basement membrane**, and is associated with deposition of **immune complexes**, **complement** and **immunoglobulins**. The condition, which may be reversible, leads to hypertension, loin pain, haematuria and proteinuria and may progress to renal failure.

Glucagon A **hormone** secreted by the Islets of Langerhans in the pancreas. It promotes **glycogenolysis** and gluconeogenesis, and promotes **insulin** secretion.

Glucocorticoid A **hormone** produced by the adrenals, which affects the **metabolism** of carbohydrates and speeds up the breakdown of **proteins** such as albumin. When present in raised amounts, glucocorticoids inhibit the inflammatory and allergic reactions of steroids. **Cortisol**, and to a lesser extent cortisone and 11-dehydrocorticosterone, have glucocorticoid activity

Glucose oxidase (EC 1.1.3.4) An **enzyme** that catalyses the oxidation of glucose, in the presence of oxygen, to gluconic acid and hydrogen peroxide. In the use of this enzyme for glucose determination the hydrogen peroxide is catalysed to release the oxygen, which forms a colour with a chromogen, and this may be measured. The use of an oxygen electrode obviates the use of the secondary reaction.

Glucose-6-phosphatase (EC 3.1.3.9) An **enzyme** involved in the breakdown of glycogen to glucose. A deficiency in this enzyme, which is found in the kidney, liver and intestine, causes an increase in the amount of glycogen stored in the liver.

Glucose 6-phosphate dehydrogenase A red cell **enzyme** which catalyses the conversion of glucose 6-phosphate to 6-phosphogluconate in the **hexose monophosphate shunt**. Congenital deficiency of this enzyme may be associated with **haemolytic anaemia**. See also **Favism**.

Glucose tolerance test   A test which involves the intake of glucose, either orally or intravenously. This produces a rise in blood glucose levels, and the subsequent rate of fall to a normal concentration is a measure of the secretion of **insulin**. It is a test which is diagnostic of **diabetes**.

Glucuronate   A **conjugate** of glucuronic acid and another substance, often a drug. It enables the material to be excreted in the urine.

(beta) Glucuronidase   (EC 3.1.1.31) An **enzyme** that hydrolyses beta galacturonides. It is widespread in human tissues and is found particularly in liver, adrenal glands, breast and spleen. White blood cells have high concentrations as opposed to red cells, which have little or none of the enzyme.

Glucuronyl transferase   (EC 2.4.1.76) An **enzyme** involved in the reaction in the liver which converts bilirubin to the more-soluble bilirubin glucuronoside, which can be secreted into the bile. The enzyme is generally poorly developed or absent in the **fetus** and the neonate, resulting in jaundice and brain damage in haemolytic disease of the newborn due to accumulation of non-excretable bilirubin. See **Kernicterus**.

Glu-plasminogen   See **Plasminogen**.

Glutaraldehyde   1. A bactericidal, sporicidal and viricidal **disinfectant** widely used in virology. Effective as a 2% aqueous solution at alkaline **pH**, it is less readily inactivated by contaminating **protein** than many other disinfectants. 2. A very efficient agent for cross-linking amino groups of the polypeptide chain of collagen. Used for **fixation**, especially in **electron microscopy**.

Glutathione   A tripeptide which, in its reduced state (GSH) protects **haemoglobin** and other intracellular proteins from oxidative damage, and in the process is converted to its oxidised form (GSSG). Re-conversion into GSH is catalysed by glutathione reductase.

Glutathione peroxidase   An **enzyme** present in **erythrocytes** which plays a major role in protecting cellular components from oxidative damage by peroxide.

Glutathione stability test   A test in which the **glutathione** content of blood is determined before and after incubation with **acetylphenylhydrazine**. Normal blood is relatively unaffected by this procedure, but blood from a **G6PD**-deficient subject shows a marked reduction in **glutathione** content.

Glycerol kinase   (E.C. 2.7.1.30) An **enzyme** that catalyses the transfer of the glutamyl group from glutamyl peptides to another peptide. High concentrations are found in the kidneys, liver and pancreas. Serum concentrations are elevated in all forms of liver disease.

Glycocalicin   A **glycoprotein** found in **platelet** membranes and which is a hydrolytic product of glycoprotein 1b.

Glycocalyx   A general term denoting the loosely attached carbohydrate layer around the outside of many types of cell including mammalian cells such as enterocytes, plants and **bacteria**. The term is not interchangeable with **slime layer**.

Glycoconjugate   Modern alternative description for **mucin**.

Glycogen   A polysaccharide which is the chief carbohydrate storage material in animals.

Glycogen body   Seen in **cysts** of amoeba which act as **parasites** in man. When stained with iodine the glycogen body in *Iodamoeba buetschlii* **cysts** is particularly evident as a large deeply staining discrete mass which distinguishes it from all other amoebic cysts. The *Entamoeba* species may also show a glycogen body which is rather diffuse and only evident in young cysts.

Glycogenesis   The process of utilisation of glycogen to form glucose.

Glycolysis   Also known as fermentation. The degradation of glucose to lactic acid. It occurs in fresh blood, even when taken aseptically. Retardation of glycolysis in blood collected for **transfusion** is essential if the blood is to be stored, and this is achieved by the addition of **adenine** and storage at low temperatures (4°−6°C).

Glycoprotein   A type of protein which contains oligosaccharide moieties.

Glycosaminoglycan   The term given to the carbohydrate moieties of proteoglycans. The latter are proteins containing large amounts of covalently-bound carbohydrate and which function as structural elements of connective tissue. Glycosaminoglycans include substances such as chondroitin sulphate and **heparan sulphate**.

Glycosuria   The excretion of glucose in the urine, which occurs frequently in **diabetes**. It occurs when the renal threshold for glucose (8·9−10·00 mmol/l) is exceeded.

Gm allotype   Genetically determined **antigen** sites on the **heavy chain** of IgG.

Goblet cell   A mucus-secreting **columnar cell** of the bronchial **epithelium**, showing a distortion of the **cytoplasm** by the presence of mucus.

Goitre   Enlargement of the thyroid gland. Often caused by an error of **metabolism**, or by a reduction in the intake of iodine.

Golgi apparatus   Cytoplasmic structure concerned with the processing of cell-synthesised **protein**. Ultrastructurally, a curved organelle with a forming and a maturing face in which **protein** is either packaged or combined with **carbohydrate** (glycolysation) prior to release via the cell membrane.

Golgi complex An **organelle** near the nucleus, composed of spherical **vesicles** and parallel canals. Associated with secretory and excretory functions in the cell.

Gonad A sex gland. An ovary or testis.

Gonadotrophin A **hormone** which regulates the activity of the **gonads** (i.e. the ovaries or the testicles).

Goniometer A type of specimen stage in the **transmission electron microscope** which allows samples to be tilted and rotated during observation.

Gonorrhoea A venereal disease caused by *Neisseria gonorrhoeae*. The infection is usually mild, affecting the mucosa of the male and female urogenital tracts, the pharynx and the rectum. The pharynx becomes infected mainly in females who practise fellatio and the rectum becomes infected in both sexes when anal intercourse is practised. In some females the disease progresses to salpingitis and other forms of pelvic inflammatory disease. In both sexes gonococcal **bacteraemia** may occur and may lead to septic arthritis. Babies born to infected mothers may develop *ophthalmia neonatorum*. The treatment of choice is high dosage of **penicillin**, which is also effective against **syphilis**. However, in areas where **penicillinase**-producing strains are likely, **Spectinomycin** is preferred.

G6PD See **Glucose 6-phosphate dehydrogenase**.

Gradient The mixing together of reagents so that when placed in a column there is a gradual change of **pH** or ionic strength through the length of the column.

Graft-versus-host reaction A reaction in which immunocompetent cells in a graft mount an **immune response** to the recipient's tissues. The abbreviation 'GVH' is often used.

Gram, Hans Christian Joachim (1853–1938) Danish bacteriologist who in 1884 introduced a method of distinguishing bacteria on the basis of their staining reactions. See **Gram's stain**.

Gram's stain A method of staining **bacteria** so that they are more easily seen by **light microscopy**. They can also be divided into Gram positive and Gram negative organisms, based on the final staining reaction and this, together with observation of their morphology, provides valuable data for preliminary identification purposes. The method, developed by Hans Christian **Gram** in 1884, entails staining a fixed preparation of bacteria on a glass slide with crystal violet, followed by treatment with aqueous iodine solution. All bacteria in the preparation will then be stained blue-black. The slide is then treated with ethanol or acetone and the stain is removed from those bacteria which are Gram negative, the Gram positive bacteria retaining the stain. The decolourised bacteria are counter-stained with a suitable stain such as neutral red or safranin. In Gram positive bacteria the **cell wall** prevents **elution** of the crystal violet-iodine complex by the solvent, but the Gram negative cell wall is unable to do this.

Granulation tissue A young **vascular** connective tissue formed during the healing process.

Granulocyte A **leucocyte** of the myeloid series showing cytoplasmic granulation. Granulocytes include **neutrophils, eosinophils** and **basophils**.

Granulocytosis An increase in the number of circulating peripheral blood **granulocytes**.

Granuloma A chronic inflammatory lesion of the **reticulo-endothelial system** in which the main cell type is the **histiocyte** or **macrophage**. These tend to fuse to form **giant cells**. Though inflammatory, the lesion does not exhibit other inflammatory features such as local vascular changes or formation of exudate. One of the factors in granuloma formation is retention of **antigen** within the macrophages, and this occurs classically in **tuberculosis** and **brucellosis**, and in **staphylococcal** infections in patients with chronic granulomatous disease, where the organisms are ingested but cannot be killed due to a defect of the intracellular killing mechanism.

Granulosa cells The solid mass of cells which surround the ovum in a developing graafian **follicle**.

Granulosa cell tumour An ovarian tumour originating in the **granulosa cells**. Associated with excessive **oestrogen** production.

Grave's disease Thyrotoxicosis caused by **auto antibodies** stimulating thyroid cells.

Grey syndrome A serious, often fatal, form of cirulatory collapse in newborn infants, associated with administration of **chloramphenicol**. With normal dosage, blood levels of the drug rise in the newborn due to poor elimination by the liver, and appropriately reduced doses should be used.

Grid 1. A grating or framework. 2. In **electron microscopy**, a very small metal grating used to support specimens in the **transmission electron microscope**.

Grieg's acid hydrolysis A simple substitute for the **Feulgen reaction** which employs **hydrolysis** to demonstrate **DNA**.

Griffith type A serological sub-division of Lancefield group A betahaemolytic **streptococci**, based on M, T and R **proteins**. One or more of these is present at the cell surface. M-proteins are associated with **virulence**.

Griseofulvin An **anti-microbial** substance active against **dermatophytes** but not other **fungi**. The drug is given orally to treat

ringworm of the skin, hair and nails. It becomes concentrated in the keratinised layer and is actively taken up by the fungi. The exact mode of action is not clear. The drug is relatively free from side-effects, sometimes producing transient headaches, **diarrhoea** and asymptomatic disturbances of **porphyrin** metabolism.

Ground section Undecalcified material prepared for microscopy by rubbing against an **abrasive** until thin enough (15−20 **microns**) for transmitted light microscopy. The only satisfactory method of producing sections of **enamel** suitable for microscopy.

Ground state The stable state of an atom or molecule. The state to which atoms and molecules return after excitation.

Ground substance The acellular component of connective tissue, often rich in **acid mucopolysaccharide**.

Groupamatic™ A trade name for a system of automated **centrifugal analysers** for determining **blood groups**.

Group and screen See **Type and screen**.

Growth factor A soluble product (**hormone**) of several cell types (e.g. **platelets**, epidermal cells, **fibroblasts**), the action of which is to stimulate growth in cells with surface receptors. Has a role in cell proliferation and differentiation.

Growth hormone A pituitary **hormone** that increases the growth in bony, connective and epithelial tissues. It is an antagonist to **insulin** and so raises the level of blood glucose. Increases in the level of growth hormone after puberty lead to abnormal skeletal growth and **gigantism**. In contrast, dwarfism is caused by lack of the hormone.

GTT See **Glucose tolerance test**.

Guillan-Barre syndrome Peripheral neuropathy: a paralysing, usually self-limiting, condition of unknown aetiology. Cases usually occur after a viral infection, no particular **virus** being clearly associated, although 'outbreaks' often occur after **epidemics** of **influenza**.

Gumma A **granuloma** found in late **syphilis**, which affects skin, bone, central nervous system, liver and other viscera. **Penicillin** is curative.

Gut-associated lymphoid tissue Lymphoid tissue anatomically associated with the gut (e.g. tonsils, appendix and **Peyer's patches**).

GVH See **Graft-versus-host reaction**.

H

Haem An iron-containing compound that is composed of four pyrol rings in combination with ferrous iron.

Haemadsorption The adherence of **erythrocytes** to the surface of infected cell **monolayers**. The phenomenon is confined to those **viruses** which have **haemagglutinins**, and are released from infected cells by budding (e.g. **orthomyxoviridae** and **paramyxoviridae**). The adherence of cells to the surface of colonies of *Mycoplasma pneumoniae* grown on **agar** has also been termed haemadsorption. See also **Agglutinin**.

Haemagglutination 1. **Agglutination** of **erythrocytes** by a specific **antibody**. 2. Agglutination of erythrocytes by **antigens** – particularly viral antigens – which adhere to specific receptors on the cell surface.

Haemagglutination inhibition A type of **assay** which utilises the phenomenon of **haemagglutination**. An **antibody** is placed in contact with an unknown substance prior to being placed in further contact with an example of its specific **antigen**. Presence of the same antigen in the unknown is indicated if the activity of the antibody against the known antigen is inhibited. The technique may be used to demonstrate the presence either of specific **antibody** in **serum** or of a particular antigen (e.g. on a **virus**) in a suspension.

Haemalum A universal nuclear stain in which **haematein**, the oxidation product of **haematoxylin** (which in itself is a poor dye), becomes active and powerful in the presence of a metallic **mordant**.

Haematin A derivative of **haemoglobin** which has differing **absorption** spectra according to whether it is in acid or alkaline solution. See also **Alkaline haematin**.

Haematocrit The volume of red cells expressed as a percentage of the volume of **whole blood** in a sample.

Haematogenous pigment See **Haem pigment**.

Haematoidin Yellowish granules or masses seen in sections of old haemorrhages, particularly in **infarcts** of spleen and brain.

Haematology The study of blood cells and **haemostasis**. The branch of clinical and laboratory medicine which deals with the diagnosis and treatment of disorders of the blood, and the blood forming (haemopoietic), lymphoreticular and haemostatic systems.

Haematoxylin A natural dye extracted from the logwood tree, used as a nuclear **stain**.

Haemochromatosis A condition in which the body deposits excessive amounts of iron, usually in the skin, liver, heart and pancreas. This leads to tissue damage, manifesting as skin pigmentation, cirrhosis of the liver, heart failure and diabetes.

132

Haemocytoblast The primitive cell which gives rise to **erythropoiesis** during early embryonic development and which later develops into recognisable haemopoietic precursors.

Haemocytometer See **Counting chamber**.

Haemoglobin The respiratory pigment in the red cells of vertebrates, responsible for gas transport and exchange in the circulation. A water-soluble crystalline substance consisting of four polypeptide subunits. It is a globular **protein** consisting of two pairs of polypeptide chains, each chain containing a haem group. The role of the haem groups is to transport oxygen, and the function of the surrounding protein chains (**globin**) is to provide a suitable environment for the haem groups. The tertiary structure of all globin chains found in fetal or adult blood is the same, but these chains (alpha, beta, gamma and delta) differ in the number and sequence of amino acids. The structure of the normal haemoglobins may be written as follows:

Hb A	Adult haemoglobin	$alpha_2$ $beta_2$
Hb A_2		$alpha_2$ $delta_2$
Hb F	Fetal haemoglobin	$alpha_2$ $gamma_2$

Haemoglobinaemia The presence in the **plasma** of free **haemoglobin**, which may occur in some cases of intravascular **haemolysis**.

Haemoglobinopathy A type of congenital disorder which is due to the synthesis of structurally abnormal **haemoglobin** chains. They are usually the result of a single **amino acid** substitution in a **globin** chain, which in some cases may radically alter the function or stability of the haemoglobin molecule. See also **Sickle cell anaemia**.

Haemoglobinuria The finding of **haemoglobin** in the urine, which may occur in some cases of intravascular haemolysis. See also **Paroxysmal cold haemoglobinuria** and **Paroxysmal nocturnal haemoglobinuria**.

Haemolysate A solution of **haemoglobin** extracted from washed, lysed red cells, and commonly used for demonstration or measurement of haemoglobin variants.

Haemolysin A substance which disrupts **erythrocytes**. It might be a blood group **antibody** which reacts with its specific **antigen** in such a manner as to cause haemolysis of the red cell carrying the antigen, in which case the reaction depends upon the presence of **complement**. Haemolysins might also be produced by **microorganisms**, in which case the effect might be observable only under certain conditions, as in the oxygen-labile O lysin of *Streptococcus pyogenes*, or it might only apply to erythrocytes of certain species as in the alpha, beta and delta haemolysins of *Staphylococcus aureus*. Other factors influencing **haemolysis** are temperature, the presence of other **enzymes**, and the sequence in which the erythrocyte is exposed to the various factors.

Haemolysis The disruption of erythrocytes. *In vitro* haemolysis can be brought about by the action of **bacterial** or **fungal** extracellular products, **antibodies**, **complement**, chemicals, or physical means such as freezing the red cells or exposing them to vigorous mechanical trauma. When haemolysis is due to extracellular products of **micro-organisms** growing on **agar** media containing intact erythrocytes, it can be classified according to the completeness or otherwise of the disruption. Beta haemolysis is the complete clearing of the blood, while alpha haemolysis is a zone of greening and partial clearing around the colonies. *In vivo* haemolysis is usually caused by the action of **antibodies** directed against antigens on the patient's red cells, as in auto-immune **haemolytic anaemia**, or the action of a patient's antibodies against incompatible red cells introduced into the circulation in **transfusion**. See also **Haemolytic disease of the newborn**.

Haemolytic anaemia An **anaemia** resulting from abnormal destruction of circulating red cells without a compensating increase in cell production.

Haemolytic disease of the newborn A **syndrome** consisting of a more or less severe **haemolytic anaemia** affecting the **fetus** and the **neonate** as a result of the passage of maternal **IgG antibodies** across the placental barrier into the fetus, where they become attached to fetal red cells. The resulting **anaemia** may be so severe as to be fatal, or may lead to **hyperbilirubinaemia** and thence to **kernicterus**. The most commonly implicated antibody is anti-D of the **Rh blood group system**. Treatment is by **exchange transfusion** or **phototherapy**. See also *Erythroblastosis fetalis* and *Icterus gravis neonatorum*.

Haemolytic-uraemic syndrome A **syndrome** mainly affecting children and characterised by proteinuria, **uraemia**, **thrombocytopaenia** and **haemolytic anaemia**, and having a poor prognosis. Onset is often preceded by bloody **diarrhoea** and the condition has been shown to be due to **vero toxin**-producing strains of *Escherichia coli*.

Haemophilia A The congenital deficiency of blood **coagulation factor** VIII. The disorder is sex-linked, normally affecting only males but transmitted by females.

Haemophilia B See **Christmas disease**.

Haemophilus Rod-shaped **bacteria** which do not exhibit **motility**, are facultative **anaerobes** which are **catalase** positive, **oxidase** negative, and which are negative by **Gram's stain**; they require either haemin (**X factor**) or co-enzyme I (**V factor**) or both for growth. *H. influenzae*, the species of greatest medical importance, is usually capsulated when found in association with disease, while non-capsulated strains are often found in the healthy respiratory tract and only rarely cause disease, except in chronic bronchitics. The organism can be typed serologically according to capsular **antigens**, and type b is often involved in acute infections of the respiratory tract, including **pneumonia** and **epiglottitis, meningitis** and suppurating conditions in other sites. Many strains produce **beta lactamase**, and neither **ampicillin** nor **amoxycillin** is effective in these cases, although **augmentin** is. Most strains are susceptible to **trimethoprim**, and **chloramphenicol** is the drug of choice for meningitis.

Haemopoiesis The term given to the production of haemopoietic cells (i.e. **erythrocytes, leucocytes** and **platelets**) in the **bone marrow** or extra-medullary sites.

Haemorheology See **Rheology**.

Haemorrhagic disease of the newborn A bleeding disorder seen in the first week of life and which is associated with unusually low levels of the **vitamin K**-dependent **coagulation factors**. This disorder is totally preventable by the prophylactic administration of **vitamin K**.

Haemorrhagic fever A severe disease in which the main pathological lesion is vasculitis, resulting from greatly increased vascular permeability. Patients bleed into the skin − often exhibiting a rash − and into the liver, kidneys and central nervous system. The condition is particularly associated with **virus** infections.

Haemosiderin A breakdown product of **haemoglobin**, composed of ferric iron and **protein** and seen as a fine yellow/brown pigment in cells and tissue sections. **Perl's Prussian blue reaction** is the classical method of demonstration.

Haemosiderosis The accumulation of iron in the tissue of the **reticuloendothelial system** following repeated blood **transfusion** over many years. In the absence of blood loss, iron is deposited at the rate of 200−250 mg per unit of blood. After about 100 units the liver, heart muscle and **endocrine glands** may become damaged.

Haemostasis The process by which blood is confined to the circulatory system, and which depends on the contributions and interactions of the vessel wall, **platelets, coagulation factors, fibrinolysis, complement** and **kinins**.

Haemozoin A malarial pigment found in the parasite and in phagocytes and blood-rich organs of infected tissues. Shares many properties with **formalin pigment**.

Haem pigment An **endogenous** material derived from **haemoglobin**. Includes haemoglobin itself, **haemosiderin, haemozoin, haematoidin** and **bilirubin**.

Hageman factor See **Coagulation factors**.

Hairy cell The malignant cell with irregular cytoplasmic villi, giving a 'hairy' appearance, seen in the peripheral blood and **bone marrow** in cases of leukaemic reticulo-endotheliosis.

Half life The time taken for the activity or concentration of a compound to be reduced or to fall by half. Frequently used to refer to the extent of emission of **radioactivity** by a radioisotope.

Halo cell See **Koilocyte**.

Ham's test See **Acid serum test**.

Hand, foot and mouth disease A mild condition caused by **coxsackie A viruses**, in particular type A16. Patients have a mild **pyrexia** and small vascular lesions in the mouth, on the palms of the hands and on the soles of the feet. Virus may be isolated from the lesions and from faeces.

H antigen The flagellar **antigen**(s) of flagellated **bacteria**. **Antibodies** to these are useful for typing purposes in **epidemiology**.

Haploid Having a single set of **chromosomes** – as is normally carried by a **gamete** – or having one complete set of non-**homologous** chromosomes.

Hapten A substance which reacts serologically with a specific **antibody** but which is not itself capable of acting as an **antigen** to stimulate the formation of a specific antibody.

Haptoglobin A plasma **protein** which binds free **haemoglobin**. The haptoglobin-haemoglobin complex is rapidly cleared by the **reticulo-endothelial system**, preventing the loss of haemoglobin (and therefore iron) in the urine.

Hard disc In computing, a non-flexible magnetic-coated disc, permanently sealed in a drive unit and used for storage of data. A hard disc is capable of storing much more data than is a **floppy disc** – typically between 10 and 50 megabytes.

Hartridge reversion spectroscope An instrument used for the differentiation of pigments with similar **absorption** bands, or for the detection of abnormal pigments (e.g. **methaemalbumin**).

HBD See **Hydroxybutarate dehydrogenase**.

HD$_{50}$ **The concentration of complement** capable of lysing 50% of a suspension of sheep **erythrocytes** coated with an optimal dose of sheep erythrocyte **antibody**.

HDL See **High density lipoprotein**.

HDN See **Haemolytic disease of the newborn**.

Heaf test A method of skin testing for hypersensitivity to **tuberculin**, a **protein** extracted from *Mycobacterium tuberculosis*. When positive, the test denotes previous exposure to the organism, including the presence of currently active disease.

'Heart failure' cells **Macrophages** which have ingested **haemosiderin**, and the presence of which indicates haemorrhage.

Heated block incubator A block of metal, drilled with holes to receive closely-fitting test tubes of a standard size, and heated electrically for the incubation of tests.

Heat inactivation The destruction of the biological activity of **complement** or **coagulation factors** by heat. The term is usually applied to the exposure of **serum** to 56°C for 20 min to destroy heat-labile complement components.

Heat labile haemoglobin An unstable form of **haemoglobin** which precipitates when heated to 50°C. See also **Haemoglobinopathy** and **Isopropanol precipitation test**.

Heavy chain A polypeptide present in all **immunoglobulin** molecules. In **IgG** this polypeptide has a molecular weight of approx 50 000 D and is joined to another, identical, heavy chain by at least one **disulphide bond**. Each of the heavy chains is joined to a separate smaller chain (25 000 D) called a **light chain** by another disulphide bond. Other immunoglobulin classes have heavy chains of slightly different structure.

Heiffor knife A small biconcave knife with an integral handle. The original type of knife blade used in the earliest **microtomes**; now largely obsolete.

Heinz body Small red cell **inclusion body**, 1.4×10^{-6} m in diameter, consisting of denatured and precipitated **globin** chains following oxidation of the **haemoglobin** molecule.

Heinz body provocation test A test for deficiencies of **enzymes** of the **hexose monophosphate shunt** in which blood is incubated with **acetylphenylhydrazine** and the number of resultant **Heinz bodies** counted. A positive result is most commonly due to **G6PD** deficiency. See also **Glutathione stability test**.

HeLa cells Hetaroploid cells derived from a **carcinoma** of the cervix, and used in the laboratory in **monolayer cell culture** for the isolation of **viruses**. They have proved useful for growing **enteroviruses**, **adenoviruses**, **herpes simplex** and **respiratory syncytial virus**. They are thought to have contaminated a number of other cell lines in the past.

Helical symmetry A structural form utilised by some **viruses** to allow them to make a large structure from limited genetic information. The animal viruses showing this symmetry all contain **RNA** and the **helix** is coiled inside a cell-derived **envelope**.

Helix aspersa A species of snail, the albumin gland and eggs of which yield an extract which behaves as a specific anti-A **blood group** agglutinin. See **Protectin**.

Helix hortensis A species of snail, the albumin gland and eggs of which yield an extract which behaves as a specific anti-A **blood group** agglutinin. See **Protectin**.

Hellem's test A method of measuring **platelet adhesion** by comparing the **platelet** count of blood before and after passage through a column of glass beads.

Helminth A type of parasitic worm belonging to the **Nematodes** (roundworms, e.g. **Ascaris**), the Trematodes (**Flukes**, e.g. **Schistosoma**) or the **Cestodes** (tapeworms, e.g. Echinococcus). All are visible to the naked eye. They cause enormous numbers of infections annually, and give rise to a wide range of syndromes varying from the sub-clinical to the fatal or severely disabling. (From the Greek, *helmins* = worm).

Helminthology The branch of medical **parasitology** which deals with parasitic worms.

Helper cell A **T cell** whose presence is required for the synthesis of **IgG** by **plasma cells** derived from **B cells**. T helper cells are also required for certain cell-mediated **immune responses**.

Henderson-Hasselbalch equation An equation used to explain the action of **buffers**, and their role in maintaining the **pH** of a solution. It defines the concentration of hydrogen ions liberated by the dissociation of an acid and the relationship to the dissociation constant. It may be expressed as:

$$pH = pK_a + \log\frac{[\text{salt}]}{[\text{acid}]}$$

where pk_a is the negative logarithm of the dissociation (equilibrium) constant of a buffer and the square brackets indicate the molar concentration of the named compounds.

Heparan sulphate A polysaccharide composed of amino sugars and uronic acids with a **heparin**-like action. See also **Glycosaminoglycans**.

Heparin A mucopolysaccharide found in the body, especially in the liver and the lungs, and which inhibits **coagulation**. It is used as a prophylactic and as an **anticoagulant** for blood samples in medical laboratories.

Heparin analogue A partially-synthesised polysulphated polysaccharide which has a **heparin**-like inhibitory effect on blood **coagulation**, but which shows significant differences from natural **heparin**.

Heparin cofactor See **Antithrombin III**.

Heparin fractions Natural **heparin** is a heterogenous compound and may be separated into fractions of differing molecular size which have different biological properties and **anticoagulant** effect.

Heparinoid A **heparin**-like substance which has been prepared by sulphating various polysaccharides and other biological and organic polymers. See also **Heparin analogues** and **Glycosaminoglycans**.

Hepatic Pertaining to the liver.

Hepatitis Strictly, inflammation of the liver, in particular of the **hepatocytes**, often leading to jaundice. A generic term which should be qualified (e.g. viral hepatitis, *q.v.*). The term is often wrongly used in connection with liver disease due to obstruction or poisons.

Hepatitis A Inflammation of the liver due to infection with **hepatitis A virus** (**enterovirus** type 72). Infection is acquired by the **faecal−oral route**, and is frequently asymptomatic − especially in children. The disease is due to viral destruction of **hepatocytes**. The virus is difficult to isolate in the laboratory and diagnosis is usually made by detection of virus-specific **IgM** using **MACRIA** or **MACELISA**.

Hepatitis A virus The cause of **hepatitis A**. It is now classified as **enterovirus** type 72.

Hepatitis B Inflammation of the liver due to infection with **hepatitis B virus**, in conjunction with an immunopathological response. Infection is acquired by the **parenteral** route, or by repeated sexual − in particular, homosexual − contact. In some cases infection is asymptomatic. Approximately 10% of infected individuals fail to clear the infection and become carriers of the virus and this can lead to **chronic** sequelae such as persistant **hepatitis**, **cirrhosis**, and primary hepatocellular **carcinoma**. Laboratory diagnosis is made by detection of viral **antigens** in **serum**. See **Hepatitis B surface antigen**.

Hepatitis B 'e' antigen A degradation product of the **nucleoprotein** core of **hepatitis B virus**. Its presence in the peripheral circulation indicates the presence of large amounts of circulating **infectious** virus, and suggests a high level of infectivity. Presence of **antibody** to 'e' antigen, when found in conjunction with **hepatitis B surface antigen**, suggests low levels of **virus** in the peripheral blood and relatively low infectivity.

Hepatitis B surface antigen An **antigen** of the **hepatitis B virus** which is produced in excess by infected **hepatocytes**, and released into the peripheral circulation. Its natural function is to form the **protein** coat of the virus. The antigen bears the common antigenic determinant 'a', and mutually exclusive determinants 'd' and 'y', and 'r' and 'w'. Thus (with rare exceptions) there are four **serotypes** of surface antigen: adr, adw, ayr and ayw. The presence of the four types has been important in establishing the **epidemiology** of hepatitis B **infection**.

Hepatitis B virus A **hepadna** virus, the cause of **hepatitis B** and its various sequelae, including **carcinoma**. The virus specifically infects **hepatocytes**; replication results in the release of large amounts of the protein coat of the virus, **hepatitis B surface antigen**, which is readily detectable in **serum**. A wide variety of diagnostic tests, and an effective **vaccine**, have been developed without the usual preliminary step of *in vitro* isolation of the virus. The importance of hepatitis B virus in the laboratory lies in its ability to establish **chronic** infection, and the relative ease with which such infection can be acquired by needle-stick injuries or the splashing of infected material onto open wounds or mucous membranes. Historically the virus was an important cause of post-transfusion **hepatitis**, but screening of blood donations has now reduced this risk to a very low level.

Hepatitis non-A, non-B   An unsatisfactory name given to infectious **hepatitis** caused by one or more as yet unidentified **viruses**. The diagnosis is made biochemically, and by the exclusion of other causes of hepatitis.

Hepatocyte   The functional cell of the liver. They have a variety of different roles in storage, nutrient and energy processing, and detoxification.

Hepatotoxicity   Toxic effects on the structure and/or function of the liver. Some **anti-microbial** substances (e.g. **Amphotericin** B, **erythromycin** estolate and **Rifampicin**) are known to be hepatotoxic in certain circumstances.

HEp2 cell   A heteroploid cell derived from a nasopharyngeal **carcinoma**, with similar properties to **HeLa cells**.

Hepnaviridae   A family of non-enveloped DNA **viruses** 42 nm in diameter, and which includes the **hepatitis B virus**.

Herpes   See **Herpes simplex virus** and **Varicella zoster virus**.

Herpes simplex virus   A member of the **Herpetoviridae**, and a cause of vesicular lesions, often recurrent. There are two **serotypes**: type I is found most commonly in facial lesions, while type II is a common cause of genital infection. Both types have been found in a variety of sites. The virus exhibits **latency** and recurrent infections − often associated with physical or mental trauma − are common. Rarely, the virus can cause a severe, often fatal, **encephalitis**. Laboratory diagnosis is by isolation of the virus in **cell culture**, the characteristic **cytopathic effect** being seen within 5 days, and often within 24 hours.

Herpetoviridae   A large family of enveloped cubical **DNA** viruses found throughout the animal kingdom. Four **viruses** are **endemic** in man: **herpes simplex virus**, herpes varicella/zoster virus, **cytomegalovirus** and **Epstein-Barr virus**. **Simian herpes virus** is **zoonotic** in man, causing severe **encephalitis**.

Hess's capillary resistance test   See **Tourniquet test**.

Hetero-   A prefix word. 1. Of a different type (e.g. **Heterozygous**). 2. Pertaining to a different individual or species (e.g. **Heterophile**).

Heteroagglutination The **agglutination** of cells of one species by an **antibody** produced in another species.

Heterochromatin Material in the **chromosome** which remains tightly coiled so that it can be stained and viewed with a light microscope.

Heterogeneic A term used to describe tissue from one species grafted to a host of different species. See **Xenogeneic**.

Heteroglycan An alternative term for **acid mucopolysaccharide**, but now largely in disuse.

Heterograft A graft between individuals of dissimilar species. See **Xenograft**.

Heterophile antibody A non-specific **antibody**, in the sense that it is active against an **antigen** other than that which may be responsible for a given **infection**. For example, the sheep cell **agglutinins** found in cases of **infectious mononucleosis** caused by the **Epstein-Barr virus** are heterophile.

Heterotroph A **micro-organism** which cannot synthesise its requirements of organic nutrients from inorganic sources. Medically important **bacteria** are heterotrophs.

Heterozygous Having two different **allelomorphic** genes on the corresponding loci of a pair of **chromosomes**. See also **Homozygous**.

Hexachlorophane An **antiseptic** substance which is particularly active against **staphylococci** but which has no useful activity against **bacteria** which are negative by **Gram's stain**. This sometimes leads to overgrowth by Gram negative bacteria during the use of hexachlorophane, and in some instances the antiseptic itself has become contaminated. It is used in powders and soaps for skin antisepsis, but is a potential neurotoxin in neonates.

Hexadecimal An arithmetical system using base 16 (rather than base 2 as in **binary**, or 10 as in decimal, systems). Numbers from 1 to 16 are each represented by a single digit, 1 to 9 being the same as in the decimal system while 10 to 15 are represented by the letters A to F. In computing the value of the hexadecimal system is that one **byte** can be represented by only two hexadecimal symbols.

Hexokinase A red cell **enzyme** which converts glucose into glucose 6-phosphate in the first step of the **Embden-Meyerhof** pathway of **glycolysis**.

Hexose monophosphate shunt A metabolic pathway which, in a reaction catalysed by **G6PD**, is the major source of NADPH in **erythrocytes**. The major function of the shunt is to maintain **glutathione** in a reduced state.

H-2 histocompatibility system The **major histocompatibility complex** in mice.

Hickman catheter A silicone catheter for central venous use, inserted into the skin some distance from the target vein, into which it is inserted by tunnelling subcutaneously. The tunnel is intended to reduce **infection** of the system, and this is further reduced by the use of a Dacron cuff around the subcutaneous segment, which allows infiltration by fibroblasts which anchor the catheter and form a barrier to **micro-organisms**. These catheters nevertheless become infected or colonised, most often with **coagulase** negative **staphylococci**. Hickman catheters are used for long-term administration of **cytotoxic** drugs or **parenteral** nutrition fluids.

High density lipoprotein cholesterol The fraction of lipoprotein which has the highest **protein** concentration. It is made up of cholesterol and phospholipid.

High dose tolerance Acquired immune tolerance seen after the administration of large doses of some **antigens**.

High level language In computing, a **language** which approximates to familiar everyday language rather than to **machine code**. A **program** written in a high level language has to be translated into machine code by an **assembler** in order for it to be understood by the computer.

High molecular weight kininogen A **coagulation factor** involved in the **contact activation** phase of **haemostasis**. It binds **coagulation factor XI** and **prekallikrein** to negatively-charged surfaces, allowing optimal activation by surface-activated **coagulation factor XII**. It has also been known as Fitzgerald factor and Flaujeac factor.

High performance liquid chromatography A chromatographic separation technique in which a mobile carrier phase is pumped under high pressure through a static phase of fine particles in a column.

High responder A term used to describe particular animals, or inbred strains of animals, which produce unusually powerful **immune responses** to specified **antigens**.

High risk sample A sample which is known or suspected to contain hazardous constituents (such as **radioisotopes**), or to have come from a person known or suspected to be suffering from an infectious disease (such as **viral hepatitis B**). Such samples need to be handled with appropriate precautions and contained within a laboratory, or an area of the laboratory, designated for the purpose, possibly within a **biological safety cabinet**.

Hill's constant A measurement of the degree of haem-haem interaction during oxygen uptake and release by the **haemoglobin** molecule, calculated by plotting $\log pO_2$ against $1/1-y$, where y is the differential saturation of the molecule at any given pO_2.

Hinge area A region of the **heavy chains** of **immunoglobulin** molecules which is particularly rich in the amino acid proline. These regions are flexible and act as a 'hinge' on which the **Fab fragments** may move to combine with **antigen**.

Hirudin An **anticoagulant** with a powerful and specific antithrombin activity. It is derived from the leach.

Histidine loading test A test for **folic acid** deficiency, in which the intermediate metabolite **formiminoglutamic acid** is measured in the urine after oral administration of histidine.

Histiocyte See **Macrophage**.

Histochemistry The science of applying defined chemical procedures to cells or tissue sections, and visualising the results microscopically.

Histocompatibility antigen An **antigen** carried on many nucleated cells, which is capable of eliciting an **immune response** when present on grafted tissue from a genetically dissimilar individual. These antigens are determined by the **H−2 histocompatibility system** in mice and the **HLA** genes in man. See **MHC**.

Histogram If the number of statistical observations of a **variable** (e.g. an **assay** measurement) in non-overlapping intervals are counted, then a histogram is a diagram where rectangles are drawn on a section of the horizontal axis with each rectangle having as its width the appropriate interval, and having its area proportional to the frequency in that interval. It gives an approximate pictorial representation of the **distribution** of the **variable** being studied.

Histology The microscopic study of the structure and composition of normal cells and tissues. See **Histopathology**.

Histopathology The microscopic investigation of the structure and composition of diseased cells and tissues. See also **Histology**.

Histoplasma *H. capsulatum* is a dimorphic **fungus** which grows as a **yeast** at 37°C but is **filamentous** at lower temperatures. It is found in the soil, particularly where bird droppings have collected, and enters the body by inhalation, causing **histoplasmosis**. *Histoplasma duboisii*, which in Africa gives rise to **histoplasmosis**, frequently spreads to skin and bone.

Histoplasmosis A pulmonary infection − usually self-limiting − with the pathogenic fungus *Histoplasma capsulatum*. Inhalation of organisms from contaminated soil leads to primary lung infection. This organism tends to invade the bloodstream, thus leading to progressive disease. Disseminated, usually fatal, histoplasmosis occurs in those with defective **immunity**. In some central states of the USA the infection is **endemic**.

HIV See **Human Immunodeficiency Virus**.

HLA See **Human Leucocyte Antigen**.

HMK See **High molecular weight kininogen**.

HMP shunt   See **Hexose monophosphate shunt**.

Hockey stick   A piece of glass rod bent at right angles and used to manipulate free-floating tissue sections.

Hodgkin's disease   A **malignant neoplasm** involving lymph nodes, spleen and general lymphoid tissues. Characterised by **Sternberg-Reed cells**.

Hollander test   A test used to assess the completeness of a vagotomy. Hypoglycaemia increases gastric hydrochloric acid secretion. Using **insulin**, hypoglycaemia is induced and if vagotomy is complete there will be no increase in acid secretion.

Homeostasis   The maintenance of a steady state by a physiological process. Physiological systems are held in balance automatically to maintain the homeostatic state.

Homo-   A prefix word. 1. Of the same type. Identical (e.g. **Homozygous**). 2. Pertaining to the same species (e.g. **Homograft**).

Homocytotropic antibody   A term usually used to describe **antibodies** which bind to **mast cells**. When these bound antibodies interact with specific **antigen**, the mast cells degranulate and liberate vaso-active amines such as histamine. The antibodies most usually involved are of the **IgE** class.

Homogeneous immersion   In microscopy, the condition in which the air between an objective lens and the slide is replaced by either oil or water, depending whether an oil immersion or water immersion objective lens is employed. Because the **numerical apperture** (NA) of an objective working in air cannot exceed 1·0 the effect of using immersion materials of a higher **refractive index** is to increase the NA.

Homogentistic acid   See **Alkaptonuria**.

Homoglycan   Sometimes used synonymously with glycogen, but includes also starch, cellulose, **dextran** and **chitin**.

Homograft   A graft of tissue from one individual to another of the same species.

Homologous   Of identical composition.

Homology region   A region of **immunoglobulin** molecules having a similar chemical structure in **antibody** molecules of differing specificity (e.g. C_H1 domains in **IgG**).

Homozygous   Having the same **allelomorphic** genes on the corresponding loci of a pair of **chromosomes**.

Hone   A slab of stone with **abrasive** properties, or a composite slab made from abrasives; or a glass, bronze or copper plate dressed with abrasive. Used to sharpen **microtome** knives or other tools.

Hookworm   Either *Ancylostoma duodenale* or *Necator americanus*; when seen as ova in fresh faeces they are morphologically indistinguishable. Adult worms of both species attach by their mouth parts to the wall of the small intestine and suck blood. Heavy infestations of hookworm frequently give rise to 'hookworm anaemia', seen in immigrants from tropical countries to Europe.

Hormone A chemical substance produced in the living body, which is transported in the blood or other body fluids and exerts a regulatory effect on other target tissues or organs. The term was originally applied to **endocrine** gland secretions, but is now applied also to other substances not produced by glands but having similar activities.

Horror autoxicus An hypothesis that the **immune response** of an individual will not be elicited against the same individual's own tissues. This was first described in 1901 by Paul **Ehrlich**.

Horseradish peroxidase An easily demonstrated **enzyme** frequently used as a **conjugate** to mark **antigen** sites in **immunocytochemistry**, immunochemistry, and **enzyme-linked immunosorbent assays**.

House dust allergy A hypersensitivity **type 1 reaction** to house dust.

Howell-Jolly body A red cell **inclusion body**, approximately 1×10^{-6} m in diameter, appearing purple by **Romanowsky staining**. They represent nuclear remnants and are most prominent in conditions associated with **dyserythropoiesis**.

HPL See **Human placental lactogen**.

HPLC See **High performance liquid chromatography**.

HRP See **Horseradish peroxidase**.

HTLV III Human **T-cell** lymphotropic **virus** type III. See **Human Immunodeficiency Virus**.

Human amnion cell culture Cell cultures obtained by enzymic disruption of human amnion (optimally obtained at caesarian section), which are susceptible to a variety of **viruses**. These **primary cell** cultures can be maintained for long periods *in vitro*.

Human embryo kidney cell culture Mixed **monolayers** of **epithelial** and **fibroblast** cells, obtained by enzymic disruption of the cortex of fetal kidneys. They are used as **primary cells** or **secondary cells**, and are in relatively short supply. They are particularly useful for **rhinoviruses** and **adenoviruses**.

Human embryo lung fibroblast culture A type of **cell culture** consisting of **monolayers** of **fibroblasts**, prepared by enzymic digestion of fetal lung tissue obtained at hysterotomy. The cells may be maintained through 30–60 passages in the laboratory before they become senescent; careful storage of early passage cells can ensure prolonged availability of suitable cells. They are particularly useful for the isolation of the **Herpetoviridae** (excluding **Epstein-Barr virus**), **rhinoviruses**, and some **enteroviruses**. **W138 cells** are a well-known strain of embryo lung cells.

Human foreskin cell culture   **Monolayers** of **fibroblasts** prepared by enzymic disruption of human neonatal foreskin. They provide an alternative source of human **fibroblasts**, but have a limited laboratory life span.

Human Immunodeficiency Virus   A **retrovirus** which is the causative organism of **acquired immune deficiency syndrome** in man. Previously known as **HTLV III** and **LAV**.

Human leucocyte antigen   An **antigen** carried on many human nucleated cells, and most easily detected on **lymphocytes**. Some of these antigens are important in tissue transplantation since they influence the survival of tissue grafts. The antigens are determined by **genes** within the **major histocompatibility complex**. See also **Class I antigen** and **Class II antigen**.

Human placental lactogen   A polypeptide produced in the syncytial layer of the placenta. The **half life** is about 25 min and the polypeptide is found in high concentrations. It can be detected in **plasma** very early in pregnancy and its estimation is used to assess placental function.

Human T lymphotropic virus (HTLV)   HTLV I and HTLV II are **retroviruses**. Type I is the cause of a T cell **leukaemia**, Sezary's **syndrome**. Type II was isolated from a case of **hairy cell** leukaemia, which has not been associated with human disease to date. **Human immunodeficiency virus** was, until recently, called HTLV III, but it is not closely related to HTLV I or HTLV II.

Humoral   Relating to molecules in solution in the body fluids (e.g. **antibodies**).

Huyghenian eyepiece   In microscopy, a lens comprising two plano-convex lenses − an eye lens and a field lens − mounted with their plane surfaces uppermost. Sometimes referred to as a negative eyepiece.

Hyaline   Transparent, glassy.

Hyaline membrane   1. Material which lines alveoli and bronchioles in patients with diffuse alveolar damage. Composed of debris from sloughed cells, mixed with **fibrin**. 2. In a hair **follicle**, the membrane between the outer sheath of the hair root and the inner fibrous layer.

Hyaluronidase   An **enzyme** which hydrolyses hyaluronic acid, which is an important glycosaminoglycan in connective tissue. It is produced by several **bacteria**, including *Staphylococcus aureus* and *Streptococcus pyogenes*, and is considered to assist spread of the infection in the tissues.

Hybrid   An organism produced by crossing parent organisms that are unrelated, or of two different species.

Hybridisation   The formation of double-stranded nucleic acid molecules from single-stranded **polynucleotides** with complementary base sequences. Nucleic acids may be characterised by the measurable percentage of **hybridisation** between known nucleic acid and a test sample. The method may also be used to detect and identify intracellular and extracellular nucleic acid of **pathogens**, and may form the basis of some future diagnostic tests.

Hybridoma A cell culture consisting of a **clone** of cells of different kinds (e.g. mouse **lymphocytes** and rat **myeloma** cells fused together).

Hydatid cyst A **cyst** formed in various organs of the body as a result of infection by the tapeworm *Echinococcus granulosus*. The cysts contain fluid and larvae and should not be aspirated as rupture leads to dissemination of the larvae. Surgical removal is usually indicated.

Hydrocortisone See **Cortisol**.

Hydrogen bonding A weak form of attraction between hydrogen and other atoms carrying a strong electro-negative charge. Plays a part in staining procedures in which alcoholic **dye** solutions are used (e.g. Best's carmine stain).

Hydrogen ion concentration Commonly known as pH. A reflection of the acidity or alkalinity of a substance. A pH level of 7·0 is neutral, figures below this being acid and those above it being alkaline.

Hydrolase A group of **enzymes** which catalyse hydrolytic reactions.

Hydrophobic bonding A mechanism whereby **dyes** in aqueous solution isolate themselves from surrounding water molecules by binding to similarly reactive tissue groups.

Hydrophobicity The property of having poor affinity for water. In **bacteria** this is usually mediated by protein groups on the cell surface. Hydrophobicity (and related properties of the cell surface) are important in **adhesion** of bacteria to each other and to inanimate surfaces, which themselves might exhibit the same properties. Hydrophilic organisms have less tendency to adhere to host cells and to inanimate surfaces.

Hydroxyapatite A lattice of small (20 nm) needle-shaped crystals formed when calcium phosphate acquires hydroxyl ions. The inorganic calcific component of bone and tooth **enamel** in which small crystallites unite to form larger crystals.

Hydroxybutarate dehydrogenase An **isoenzyme** of lactate dehydrogenase which acts on the **substrate** alpha-oxybutyrate.

17-Hydroxy progesterone A **steroid** produced in the adrenal cortex and testes. Levels in serum are raised in congenital adreno hyperplasia, as a result of deficiency of 21-beta-hydroxylase.

5-Hydroxytryptamine A powerful muscle stimulant and vasoconstrictor which can be secreted by abdominal carcinoid **tumours**. It causes tachycardia, diarrhoea and cardiac changes. It is also taken up by the blood **platelets** against a concentration gradient, and stored in the **dense bodies**. Sometimes used as a **platelet aggregation** reagent. Also known as Serotonin.

Hyperbilirubinaemia A condition characterised by levels of serum **bilirubin** raised above those normally to be expected.

Hyperchromasia Exhibiting an increase in nuclear staining intensity.

Hypercoagulability A state in which there is an abnormal tendency for the **blood coagulation** system to be activated within the circulation.

Hyperfibrinogenaemia An increase in the level of plasma **fibrinogen** above the upper limit of the normal range (4·5 g/l).

Hyperfibrinolysis Abnormal activation of the **fibrinolytic system**, leading to increased levels of **fibrin degradation products**, usually in association with **disseminated intravascular coagulation**.

Hyperimmunoglobulin A concentrated preparation of an **immunoglobulin** used prophylactically to produce passive immunity.

Hyperkeratosis Thickening of the corneous layer of the skin.

Hyperplasia An increase in the number of normal cells in normal arrangement in a tissue.

Hypersegmentation A term usually applied to **polymorphonuclear leucocytes** that have more than the normal number of nuclear lobes, and which is often seen in **megaloblastic anaemia**. See also **Shift to the right**.

Hypersensitivity Literally, highly increased sensitivity. In medicine, a high degree of reaction to exposure to specific **allergens**.

Hypertension An increase in arterial blood pressure above the range which is considered normal for the population concerned. Individuals with hypertension are at increased risk of developing cardiovascular and cerebrovascular diseases.

Hypertonic Having an osmotic pressure greater than that normally exerted by blood plasma. See also **hypotonic** and **isotonic**.

Hypervariable region An area within the variable region of a **heavy chain** or **light chain** of an **immunoglobulin**, having an amino acid composition peculiar to that immunoglobulin. See V_H **region (domain)** and V_L **region (domain)**.

Hyperviscosity syndrome A clinical condition in which the blood **viscosity** is greatly increased. This occurs most commonly as a result of a **paraproteinaemia**, or in association with **polycythaemia**.

Hypnozoite Part of the life cycle of the malaria parasite, which passes through the liver. The hypnozoite may remain dormant in liver cells, particularly in infections with **malignant malaria** (*Plasmodium falciparum*), relapsing at some time after parasitological cure has been demonstrated.

Hypochromasia The appearance of **erythrocytes** in **blood films** which have been **Romanowsky stained**, with a greater area of central pallor than normal. This is associated with a reduction in the **mean cell haemoglobin** and is due to deficient haemoglobinisation of the individual red cells.

Hypochromic-microcytic anaemia A form of **anaemia** in which the **erythrocytes** in **blood films** which have been **Romanowsky stained** appear more pale and smaller than normal. This is associated with reduction in the **mean cell haemoglobin** and **mean cell volume**, and is most commonly the result of iron deficiency.

Hypofibrinogenaemia A reduction in the level of plasma **fibrinogen** below the lower limit of the normal range (1·5 g/l).

Hypogammaglobulinaemia A condition in which there are abnormally low levels of circulating **gamma globulins**.

Hypophysis The pituitary gland, which has two main components: (i) the adenohypophysis (anterior pituitary), which is **hormone** producing and part of the **APUD** system; and (ii) the neurohypophysis (posterior pituitary), which is composed of neural cells and fibres.

Hypoplasia A reduction in the number of normal cells in normal arrangement in tissue. See **Di George's syndrome**.

Hypothesis testing In statistical usage, a specified hypothesis concerning certain **parameters** (e.g. the **means** of two **populations** being equal), or concerning the form of the **distribution** (e.g. **independence** in a **contingency table**) is tested by calculating test values and comparing them with tabulated values. Improbable test values lead to rejection of the hypothesis under study. See **Chi-squared test**, **t-test** and **F-test**.

Hypotonic Having an osmotic pressure less than that normally exerted by blood plasma. See also **Hypertonic** and **Isotonic**.

Hypoxia A lack, or deficiency, of oxygen in the tissues.

Hysteresis 1. The failure of two associated phenomena to coincide. 2. In **electron microscopy**, variation in the strength of electromagnetic lenses, depending on whether the current arrives at a given value from a higher or a lower value.

I

Ia antigen An **antigen**, encoded by **IR genes**, which may influence the capacity of an individual to mount an **immune response** against particular antigens.

IAG Indirect **antiglobulin test**. An **antiglobulin test**, applied to cells or serum, in which the reactants are incubated together *in vitro*, washed clear of free protein and then exposed to **antiglobulin** reagent. Also known as the indirect Coombs' test.

IAMLT International Association of Medical Laboratory Technologists. Founded 1958.

Ice crystal artefact A consequence of slow or inadequate freezing of tissue. Water crystals enlarge to distort the tissue, leaving characteristic spaces in **frozen sections** or **cryostat sections**.

Icosahedron A geometric figure having 20 equilateral triangular faces and 12 vertices. The structure of many cubical **viruses** is based on this figure.

ICT Indirect **Coombs' test**. See **IAG**.

Icterus Jaundice. Often a sign of liver disease or of intravascular **haemolysis**. See also **Haemolytic disease of the newborn**.

Icterus gravis neonatorum Literally, severe jaundice of the newborn. The stage of **haemolytic disease of the newborn** in which the infant manifests **hyperbilirubinaemia**. If untreated, the disease may progress to **kernicterus**.

Idiopathic Without known cause.

Idiotype An inherited amino acid variation in a protein (**immunoglobulin**).

IEOP Immune electro-osmophoresis. See **Counter immunoelectrophoresis**.

Ig Abbreviation for **Immunoglobulin**.

IgA See **Immunoglobulin A**.

IgA$_1$ The main sub-class of **immunoglobulin A** (IgA), which comprises about 85% of **serum** IgA.

IgA$_2$ A sub-class of **immunoglobulin A** (IgA) which comprises about 15% of **serum** IgA.

IgD See **Immunoglobulin D**.

IgE See **Immunoglobulin E**.

IgG See **Immunoglobulin G**.

IgG$_1$ The main sub-class of **immunoglobulin G** (IgG), which comprises about 66% of **serum** IgG. This sub-class is able to activate the **classical pathway** of **complement**.

IgG$_2$ A sub-class of **immunoglobulin G** (IgG) comprising about 22% of **serum** IgG. This sub-class, relative to some other IgG sub-classes, is a weak activator of the **classical pathway** of **complement**.

IgG$_3$ A sub-class of **immunoglobulin G** (IgG) comprising about 8%

of **serum** IgG. This sub-class is able to activate the **classical pathway** of **complement**.

IgG₄ A sub-class of **immunoglobulin G** (IgG) comprising about 4% of **serum** IgG. This sub-class does not activate the **classical pathway** of **complement**.

IgM See **Immunoglobulin M**.

Image analysis The technique of examining and reporting upon images, as visualised electronically or photographically, by means of a computer rather than by human observation and interpretation.

Imidazoles A group of related derivative substances having a heterocyclic structure and including **Nitrofurantoin** (a broad spectrum urinary **anti-microbial** substance), **Metronidazole** (which is active against **protozoa** and **anaerobic** bacteria), **Miconazole** (which is an anti-**fungal** drug), and others.

IMLS Institute of Medical Laboratory Sciences. The oldest established professional body for medical laboratory scientists, founded in 1912 as the Pathological and Bacteriological Laboratory Assistants' Association.

Immediate hypersensitivity The immediate response of an individual to an **antigen** to which (s)he has previously been exposed, following often within seconds, and within no more then a few hours, after further exposure. See also **Delayed hypersensitivity**.

Immortalisation A **virus**-induced change in cells which falls short of **transformation**, but which nevertheless confers an ability to replicate *in vitro* far beyond the normal expected span.

Immune A state of protection against specific infection, as a result of previous infection, **vaccine** prophylaxis, the administration of pre-formed **antibody**, or genetic factors. The term may also be applied to any circumstances in which contact with **antigen** leads to a heightened antibody or **cell-mediated immunity** response to subsequent exposure to the same antigen.

Immune adherence Adherence of **antigen/antibody** complexes, or cells coated with **complement** component C3b, to **macrophages**.

Immune antibody Strictly, an **antibody** produced by a process of immunisation. Loosely used in serology to describe an antibody produced in response to an identifiable stimulus, and generally IgG in nature.

Immune complex A complex formed between specific **antibody** and soluble **antigen**. Such complexes may activate the **alternative pathway** of **complement**.

Immune cytolysis The lysis of cells by **complement** activated by **antibody**. The term is usually reserved for the lysis of cells other than **erythrocytes**.

Immune response The response of a body to exposure to a foreign

antigen. The response may comprise **antibody** production, the development of **cell-mediated immunity** or the induction of **immune tolerance**. A primary response takes place after the initial exposure to the antigen and results in formation of an **antibody**, generally **IgM** at first followed by **IgG**. A secondary response may occur after previous exposure to an antigen, a second exposure resulting in more rapid production of antibody.

Immunise　To administer **antigen** or **vaccine** to an individual in order to induce **immunity**.

Immunity　The ability of a host organism to defend itself against foreign **antigens**. Immunity may be **humoral**, involving production of **antibodies**, or cellular, involving the responses of **leucocytes** and **macrophages**. It may also be active, in which the host produces its own response to foreign antigens, or passive, in which pre-formed antibodies are introduced **parenterally** into the host.

Immunoadsorbent　An insoluble material to which **antigen** is linked covalently. The immunoadsorbent may be used to adsorb **antibodies** from a mixture. The antibodies may then be recovered from the immunoadsorbent material by **elution**.

Immunoassay　An assay system making use of the affinity of an **antibody** for an **antigen**.

Immunochemistry　The study of the chemistry and biochemistry of all aspects of the **immune** system and **immune response**.

Immunocompromised　A general term used to describe an individual not able to produce a normal **immune response**. This may be due to genetic factors or it may be an acquired state due to (e.g.) drug therapy or **infection**. See also **Immunodeficiency**.

Immunocytochemistry　The application of immunological methods to cells or tissue sections, the result being visualised by the demonstration of a marker **conjugated** to the final reactant.

Immunodeficiency　Any condition in which one or more elements of the **immune response** is sub-optimal. Such elements include **innate immunity, complement, cell-mediated immunity**, production of **antibody** and **phagocytosis**.

Immunodiffusion　See **Gel diffusion test**.

Immunodominant　That part of the structure of an **antigen** which makes the largest contribution to the binding of that antigen to **antibody**.

Immunoelectron microscopy　The application of **immunocytochemical** methods at the ultrastructural level, using electron-dense markers such as (e.g.) **colloidal gold** or **ferritin**. **Antigens** are made to **agglutinate** by a specific **antibody** prior to preparation for **electron microscopy**. Objects exhibiting **pleomorphism** become more readily recognisable using this method; the **immunoglobulin** molecules attached to the objects may also be visible.

Immunoelectrophoresis A process by which **proteins** are separated by **electrophoresis** in a gel, and then located by allowing specific **antibody** to diffuse through the gel. Areas of **precipitation** develop where the two combine.

Immunoenzyme A type of immunological method which uses **conjugated** enzymes as markers of **antigen/antibody** activity.

Immunoferritin An immunological method employing **conjugated ferritin** as a marker of **antigen/antibody** activity. Can be used in **immuno-electron microscopy**.

Immunofluorescence A type of immunological method employing **conjugated fluorochrome** as a marker of **antigen/antibody** activity. Most commonly applied to cytological preparations or tissue sections.

Immunogen A substance capable of generating an immune response; in contrast to a substance which binds to an **antibody** (i.e. an **antigen**).

Immunogenic The capacity of an **antigen** to elicit an **immune response**. The response may be **antibody** production and/or **cell-mediated immunity**.

Immunoglobulin One of a group of gamma **globulins** which have **antibody** activity. See **Immunoglobulin A**, **Immunoglobulin D**, **Immunoglobulin E**, **Immunoglobulin G** and **Immunoglobulin M**.

Immunoglobulin A (IgA) A class of **antibody** which exists as a monomer in blood, but as a dimer in secretions. Each monomer is composed of two **heavy chains** and two **light chains**. Each heavy chain has four **domains**. The dimer is associated with an extra structure, produced in secretory tissue, called a **secretory piece**. The monomer has a molecular weight of 160 000 D and the dimer a molecular weight of approximately 385 000 D. Two sub-classes of IgA exist, **IgA$_1$** and **IgA$_2$**.

Immunoglobulin D (IgD) A class of **antibody** found in very low concentration in blood. IgD is present on the surface of **B cells**, where it acts as a receptor for **antigen**. Each IgD molecule is composed of two **heavy chains** and two **light chains**. Each heavy chain has four **domains** and the whole IgD molecule has a molecular weight of 184 000 D.

Immunoglobulin E (IgE) A class of **antibody** found in trace amounts in blood, but which is present on the surfaces of **mast cells**. IgE plays a role in **immunity** to some **parasites** and mediates **type I reactions** of **hypersensitivity**. The molecule consists of two **heavy chains** and two **light chains**. Each heavy chain has five **domains** and the whole IgE molecule has a molecular weight of 188 000 D.

Immunoglobulin G (IgG) A class of **antibody** which has the highest concentration of any in the blood. The molecule consists of two

heavy chains and two **light chains** and has a molecular weight of 150 000 D. Four sub-classes exist, **IgG₁**, **IgG₂**, **IgG₃** and **IgG₄**. IgG is actively transported across the placenta.

Immunoglobulin M (IgM) A class of **antibody** which is mainly found intravascularly, where it exists as a pentameric structure. Monomeric IgM may be present on the surfaces of **B cells**, where it serves as an **antigen** receptor. Each monomeric unit consists of two **heavy chains** and two **light chains**. The heavy chains have five **domains**. To form the pentamer, five monomeric units are joined by **disulphide bonds** to form a circular structure with the **Fab** regions on the outside. The pentamer has a molecular weight of 900 000 D and is a potent activator of the **classical pathway** of **complement**, but does not cross the placenta.

Immunoglobulin sub-class Variation of **immunoglobulin** structure within an immunoglobulin class. **IgG** has four sub-classes, IgG₁, IgG₂, IgG₃ and IgG₄, while **IgA** has two sub-classes, IgA₁ and IgA₂.

Immunological memory The capacity of the immune system to respond more quickly and powerfully to second or subsequent exposure to **antigen** than it did on first exposure.

Immunological surveillance A hypothetical mechanism by which the immune system monitors for the appearance of aberrant or **neoplastic** cells. It is suggested that any such cells which develop are destroyed by **antibodies** and/or **cell-mediated immunity**.

Immunology The study and practise of the science relating to the **immune response**, and the properties of agents able to stimulate this.

Immunopathology Pertaining to diseases arising from the reactions of the **immune** system with **antigens** which would themselves not normally cause damage. These diseases are often the result of **infection**, although the term is also applied to **auto-immune** diseases and to problems associated with organ **transplantation**.

Immunoradiometric assay An **immunoasay** method in which the **antibody** is labelled with a **radioisotope** rather than the **antigen**. After the antigen/antibody reaction the bound and unbound fractions are separated and the **radioactivity** of the complex measured, indicating the concentration of the antigen.

Immunosorbent Describes a substance capable of being attached to an **antigen** in such a manner that the antigen can adsorb a **homologous antibody** and then be separated from the remaining solution.

Immunosuppression The diminution of the **immune response** by artificial means (e.g. by irradiation or the administration of drugs).

Immunotherapy The treatment of disease states by the administration of drugs and other agents which are designed to enhance or suppress the **immune response**, or specific elements of it.

Impedance The resistance to alternating electrical current. In **bacteriology** the impedance of a fluid decreases as **bacteria** multiply in it, and the measurement of this phenomenon can be used to monitor bacterial growth for both diagnostic and research purposes. The method detects both viable and non-viable bacteria and certain metabolic products.

Impedance aggregometry A method for the assessment of **platelet aggregation** which measures the change in resistance to an electrical current across two platinum electrodes during platelet aggregation, and is suitable for use with whole blood and **platelet-rich plasma**.

Impedance plethysmography A non-invasive method for measuring changes in the volume of blood in a particular limb. It is based on the principle that blood volume changes in the limb produced by temporary venous obstruction result in proportional changes in electrical resistance (impedance) which may be detected by skin electrodes placed around the limb.

Impenem An **anti-bacterial** derivative of the **beta lactam** thienamycin. It is active against most **enterobacteriaceae**, other Gram negative and Gram positive organisms, **anaerobes**, **Campylobacter**, **Haemophilus** and **Neisseria**. Exceptions are some strains of **enterococci**, **pseudomonas** and **serratia**.

Impetigo A superficial **infection** of the skin caused by *Streptococcus pyogenes*, and sometimes *Staphylococcus aureus*. The lesion begins as vesicles which rupture to form crusts, and the infection is contagious. **Penicillin** is the drug of choice. The strains of *Streptococcus pyogenes* involved have different **M-proteins** from strains causing **pharyngitis**.

Impregnation In **histology** and **histopathology** the stage of tissue **processing** in which the ante-medium is replaced by, and the tissue infiltrated with, the material used for **embedding** prior to **microtomy**.

Inactivation (of serum) Treating to render **complement** inactive, usually by heating, or exposure to an anti-complementary chemical such as **EDTA**. See also **Complement**.

Inborn error of metabolism A fashionable term for an acquired or developmental metabolic abnormality, usually − although not necessarily − expressed during early life.

Inbred strain Laboratory animals produced by mating siblings. If this is performed for several generations the animals gradually become genetically more similar. Inbred strains of animals are required for various (carefully controlled) experimental purposes.

Incident light 1. Light striking an object and being reflected back, as occurs in some forms of **fluorescence microscopy**. 2. Light striking a lens at the **angle of incidence** and leaving at the **angle of refraction**.

Inclusion Extraneous or intrinsic particles contained within cytoplasm or a cell nucleus.

Inclusion body A type of intracellular structure which cannot be classified as a normal cell **organelle**, and which usually occurs in association with a disease state. In **haematology**, these may occur in **erythrocytes** (e.g. **Howell-Jolly bodies**, and **Heinz bodies**) or **leucocytes** (e.g. **Dohle bodies** and **Auer rods**).

Incompatibility Literally − not in harmony, antagonistic. Used in serology to refer to a situation in which an **antibody** and its specific **antigen** are both present in the same environment, as in a **transfusion** when the patient has an **antibody** active against an **antigen** on the **blood donor's** red cells.

Incomplete antibody An obsolete term used to describe antibodies which will not directly **agglutinate** red cells suspended in saline; usually IgG in nature.

Incubate To allow a reaction to procede under particular conditions of time, temperature, gaseous atmosphere and humidity.

Incubator An insulated container for establishing and maintaining standard conditions of temperature and/or humidity, in which tests may be allowed to **incubate**. Special incubators with cooling circuits and carbon dioxide atmospheres are also available.

Independence In statistics, two quantities are said to be independent if whatever value one has does not affect the **distribution** of values of the other quantity.

Indicator system A type of system used in a variety of laboratory tests by which the results of a reaction are visualised − often colorimetrically − for the purpose of observation or recording.

Indices See **Absolute values**.

Indole A substance (2,3-benzopyrole) which (*inter alia*) is responsible, to some extent, for the odour of faeces. It is the product of hydrolysis and deamination of tryptophan, which also yields pyruvic acid. Indole can be detected after growth of certain **microorganisms** in a **culture medium** containing tryptophan by reaction with p-dimethylaminobenzaldehyde to give a red colour. The test is useful for identification of some organisms.

Ineffective erythropoiesis A situation where there is evidence of red cell destruction prior to, or shortly after, release from the **bone marrow**, usually as a result of defective **erythroid** maturation (for example, in **megaloblastic anaemia**).

Inert particle agglutination test   A test which uses inert particles, such as latex, to which soluble **antigen** or **antibody** has been artificially coupled. Such tests may then be used to detect antibody or antigen as appropriate.

Infarct   An area of **necrosis** in tissue, arising as a result of reduced oxygen availability relative to metabolic need (**ischaemia**).

Infection   The presence of viable multiplying **micro-organisms** in the tissues of a host, or in body cavities in which such organisms are not usually found in health. The term implies a host response which is almost always present but is extremely variable in extent. Often the host response component is responsible for many of the unwanted effects of the infection.

Infectious   A term applied to an **infection** or to its causative agent, denoting that it is readily transmitted from the infected person to a healthy one by various means.

Infectious mononucleosis   A febrile condition with severe sore throat and **lymphadenopathy**. The disease is a result of **infection** with **Epstein-Barr virus** or **cytomegalovirus**, together with an immuno-pathological response to the infection. Laboratory diagnosis is by the detection of atypical **mononuclear** cells in **blood films**, and the demonstration of **heterophile antibodies** using the **Paul-Bunnell-Davidsohn test**. The specific cause may be identified by **virus** specific **IgM** tests.

Infective   A term describing an agent which causes an **infection**, but which is not necessarily readily transmissable from the infected person to a healthy one.

Infective dose   The number of **micro-organisms** required to initiate an **infection**, either experimentally or naturally. The term is an expression of the **virulence** of the organisms, the resistance of the host, and the route of inoculation.

Inflammatory cells   Migratory **leucocytes** involved in inflammation.

Infra-red   Electro-magnetic radiation with a wavelength between 700 nm and 12 000 nm.

Influenza   An acute upper respiratory disease featuring sore throat, malaise, aching muscles and **pyrexia**. The elderly, those with chronic chest disease and, occasionally, adults in the prime of life may succumb to an acute viral **pneumonia**. The **orthomyxoviruses** known as **Influenza A** and **Influenza B** are the main causative agents, though many other infectious agents cause illnesses called 'influenza'. The myxovirus-induced disease occurs in **epidemics** affecting whole communities; periodically, influenza A epidemics span the world.

Influenza A virus   An **orthomyxovirus**, the major cause of **epidemic** and **pandemic** forms of **influenza**. Its capacity for major **antigenic** changes (**antigenic shift**) and continuous minor variations (**anti-**

genic drift) mean that this virus will continue to be a major problem for virologists. Genes for 15 haem**agglutinins** and 10 **neuraminidases** are known. The virus may be isolated in fertile hen eggs, and in monkey kidney **primary cells**. Trypsin-modified canine kidney cells have been used as an alternative to monkey kidney. Influenza A viruses occur in a variety of animals and birds; it is known that **genetic re-assortment** occurs naturally in some species of ducks and geese.

Influenza B virus A member of the **Orthomyxoviridae**, infecting only man. The **virus** exists as a single species with a variety of **antigen**ic variants, and shows **antigenic drift**, but no major **antigenic shift**. It is a cause of **epidemic** and **endemic** forms of **influenza**. It may be isolated in the same way as **influenza A**.

Inhibisol^{TM} A proprietary industrial cleaning agent employed in **histology** and **histopathology** for **clearing** tissues.

Inhibition The total or partial prevention of a process from continuing. For example, the prevention of a reaction between an **antibody** and red cells carrying its specific **antigen**, by the addition of the antigen in a soluble form to the serum containing the antibody. Another example is the prevention of further multiplication of **bacteria** around a paper disc placed on the surface of a solid **culture medium**, by **anti-microbial** substances diffusing from the disc, and resulting in a surrounding zone which can be measured. See also **Inhibitors**.

Inhibition test A test in which the agglutinating activity of an **antibody** is blocked by the prior addition of a soluble **antigen**.

Inhibitors A general term given to any substance which interferes with a particular biological process. The action of an inhibitor may be physical, biochemical, pharmacological or immunological. See **Inhibition**.

Innate activity A term for the collective inborn capacities of an individual to resist infection. This is sometimes called non-lymphoid immunity, as activities of **B cells** and **T cells** are usually excluded from the meaning of the term.

Inoculate 1. To introduce **micro-organisms** (or material containing them), or tissue cells, into or onto a **culture medium** for cultivation (i.e. for the purpose of multiplication). 2. Historically, the practice of introducing material containing **micro-organisms** into the body for the purpose of inducing a state of **immunity** which would protect the individual against further exposure to the disease. See also Edward **Jenner** and **Smallpox**.

Inoculator, multipoint See **Multipoint inoculator**.

Inoculum Material used to **inoculate** a **culture medium**, animal or person. The term is commonly used to denote a volume of culture medium containing a known number of viable organisms in a known phase of growth, which is to be introduced into a second culture system, such as a test for **minimum inhibitory concentration** of an **anti-microbial** substance. The term is also used to refer to clinical material which is inoculated into culture medium.

Input Information fed into a computer.

INR See **International normalised ratio**.

In situ **hybridisation** A method of introducing labelled nucleotide sequences (probes) to matching sequences in RNA or denatured DNA in tissue sections or smears, and visualising the results microscopically.

Inspissation The thickening or solidification of a fluid **culture medium** by applying just sufficient heat to coagulate **protein** constituents such as the albumin in serum (Loeffler medium) or egg (**Lowenstein-Jensen medium**). The temperature usually used is 75°C.

Instructive theory An hypothesis which suggests that **B cells** and **T cells** have no pre-existing specificity for **antigen** until they come into contact with it. On contact, antigen instructs these cells to produce a corresponding specific response to that antigen, e.g. **antibody** production. See **Burnett's monoclonal selection theory**.

Insulin A polymer that is secreted by the beta cells of the Islets of Langerhans in the pancreas. The main action of insulin is to speed up the rate of passage of glucose across cell membranes. See **Diabetes**.

Interaction If, when examining statistically the effects of two **factors** on a **variable**, it is found that the effect of one factor depends on the value that a second factor takes, then there is said to be an interaction between them. For example, when looking at the heights of children, one would expect to find an interaction between sex and age group, as the difference between the sexes is not the same for all ages.

Interface An assembly which connects two electronic devices, permitting them to interact with one another (e.g. an external device such as a printer, linked to a computer).

Interference A phenomenon exhibited by a number of unrelated **viruses**, infection by one blocking subsequent attempts to infect cells with another. This effect has been used in the laboratory to demonstrate the presence of **rubella virus** in **cell culture**.

Interference microscopy A system based on the principle of **wave optics**, employing a microscope fitted with polarisers and prisms acting as **birefringent** wedges. It combines the properties of **phase contrast** and **polarising microscopy**, producing finely-detailed coloured three-dimensional images.

Interferon　A class of proteins which inhibit the replication of **viruses** and the growth of some **neoplasms**, and which have a regulatory role in the **immune response**, enhancing cellular **immunity**. Interferons produced in living bodies are species-specific (i.e. they protect against viral infection only the cells of the species in which they were formed). Three types of human interferon are currently recognised, which have been called alpha, beta and gamma interferon respectively. Work is still in progress on the clinical use of interferons both to combat viral infection and to treat **malignant neoplastic** disorders, but there are problems in their large scale production.

Interleukin I　(IL1) A soluble factor released by activated **macrophages**, and which influences the proliferation of **lymphocytes**.

Interleukin II　(IL2) A soluble factor released from activated **T cells**, which non-specifically amplifies the proliferation of other T cells.

Intermediate filament　A cytoplasmic constituent of eukaryotic cells, smaller than microtubules but larger than microfilaments, and consisting of polypeptides of five major types. Intermediate filament linkage is maintained through neoplastic change.

Intermediate lens　An electromagnetic lens in the **transmission electron microscope**, situated between the **objective lens** and the **projector lens**.

Internal quality control　A system operated by the staff of a given service (e.g. a laboratory) for continuously monitoring the **quality** of a product or of results produced within the service, using statistical analysis and usually by examining a representative sample of the items against previously laid down standards and tolerances. The aim is to maintain the accuracy of the processes and to determine whether the results and products are sufficiently reliable and consistent to be released.

Internal standard　A signal produced within an instrument, which can be compared to the signal produced by a compound of unknown concentration. Alternatively the compound, not originally present in the unknown, can be introduced with the unknown. Changes within the instrument (such as the temperature of a flame in flame photometry) will affect the internal standard as well as the unknown, so that the ratio between the two remains unaltered.

International normalised ratio　The **prothrombin time** ratio which would have been obtained if the first primary **WHO** reference **thromboplastin** had been used to perform the test. For a prothrombin time (PT) ratio obtained using a thromboplastin with an **ISI** value of x, the INR is calculated as: INR = (observed PT ratio)^x

International reference preparation A **thromboplastin** preparation intended for use in calibrating other **thromboplastins** to enable **prothrombin time** ratios obtained with those thromboplastins to be converted to a universal scale.

International sensitivity index For any given **thromboplastin** preparation, the International Sensitivity Index is the slope of the calibration line obtained when the logarithms of **prothrombin times** obtained with the first primary international reference preparation are plotted against the logarithms of **prothrombin times** obtained with the **thromboplastin** on the same set of **plasmas** from normal and anticoagulated patients.

Interphase The period during which a cell is not dividing. The interval between the production of a new cell and its **mitosis**.

Interpreter In computing, a **program** which converts each instruction in a **high level language** into **machine code**, and then executes it before converting the next instruction.

Interstitial Situated between the parts (the inter-spaces) of a cell or tissue.

Intestinalisation A process of **metaplasia** in which normal gastric cells are replaced by clear cells which resemble the mucus cells lining the large intestine.

Intraperitoneal Within the peritoneal cavity.

Intrauterine Within the uterus.

Intrauterine infection A variety of **pathogenic** and non-pathogenic agents are capable of infecting the fetus *in utero*. Those known to cause damage are **rubella virus, cytomegalovirus** and *Treponema pallidum*. Herpes varicella/zoster and **vaccinia** viruses are rare causes of severe disease. It seems likely that intrauterine acquisition of **Human Immunodeficiency Virus** will frequently result in **Acquired Immune Deficiency Syndrome** (AIDS) in early life.

Intravital staining Staining of living cells in the body by certain **dyes (vital stains)**. The staining of living cells outside the body is termed **supravital staining**.

Intrinsic blood coagulation system The term given to that part of the coagulation cascade which can be initiated by **contact activation** and involving **BMWK, Prekallikrein** and **coagulation factors** XII, XI, IX, VIII and X.

Intrinsic factor A **glycoprotein** produced in the gastric parietal cells, which binds dietary **vitamin B12** and aids its absorption through the ileum.

Inv allotype An inherited **antigenic** determinant on the **kappa chain** of human **immunoglobulin** molecules.

In vitro Outside a living organism.

In vivo Within a living organism.

5-Iodo—2-deoxyuridine A **nucleotide** analogue which is used (i) in the topical treatment of **herpes simplex virus** infection, and (ii) in **cell cultures** of **McCoy cells**, to arrest their division and to make them more susceptible to **Chlamydia** species.

Iodophore A compound of iodine with an inert vehicle. A common example is povidone-iodine, a complex of iodine with polyvinyl-pyrrolidone, used as an **antiseptic**. The compound retains much of the **anti-microbial** properties of iodine but is more stable and does not have the toxic and irritant effects on tissues and mucous membranes.

Ion An electrically charged atom or molecule. A negatively charged ion is called an **anion**, and a positively charged ion a **cation**.

Ion exchange chromatography A system for the separation of molecules, usually **proteins**, based upon their electrical charge. Mixtures of molecules in solution are applied to charged resins. Molecules which bind to the resin, because of an opposite charge, may be recovered by changing the **pH** or the ionic strength of the medium surrounding the resin.

Ionophore See **Calcium ionophore**.

Ion selective electrode An electrochemical sensor, the potential of which has a linear relationship with the logarithm of the activity of a particular **ion** in solution, despite the presence of other ions.

Ir gene An **immune response** gene. Such **genes** govern the overall capacity of an individual to mount an **immune response** to a particular **antigen**. See **MHC**.

IRMA See **Immunoradiometric assay**.

Iron-binding capacity A measure of the amount of iron that can be transported in the **plasma**. Serum iron is bound to the plasma protein **transferrin**, and the total iron-binding capacity is therefore related to the transferrin level. The transferrin to which iron is not currently bound is known as the unsaturated iron-binding capacity (UIBC). The serum iron levels plus the UIBC gives the total iron-binding capacity (TIBC).

Iron deficiency anaemia An **anaemia** which follows a reduction in the body's **iron stores** from whatever cause, and which is associated with **hypochromasia** and **microcytosis** in the peripheral **blood film**.

Iron ore pigment An exogenous deposit present in the lungs of those following certain occupations. The colour varies from black to blue, green, yellow or red depending upon the composition.

Iron overload A general term applied to situations in which there is an abnormally high amount of body iron. This may occur as a result of excessive dietary absorption of iron (**haemochromatosis**) or through numerous blood **transfusions** over a prolonged period of time (**haemosiderosis**).

Iron stores The reserves of body iron, stored mainly as **haemosiderin** which may be mobilised to meet increased body requirements for the synthesis of **haemoglobin** or iron-containing **enzymes**.

Iron turnover The **plasma** iron turnover is a measure of the total amount of iron leaving the plasma per unit time. It may be calculated following administration of radio-labelled iron, and is a measure of iron taken up by erythroid cells and non-erythroid elements.

Irregular antibody An antibody which is not normally found in a given situation.

ISBT International Society of Blood Transfusion. Founded 1937.

Ischaemia The state of an organ or tissue resulting from reduced oxygen availability due to lowered arterial supply relative to metabolic demands.

ISI See **International sensitivity index**.

Iso- A prefix word. Literally, equal, alike, the same. In **Immunology**, from a genetically-alike individual. See **Allo-**.

Iso-antibody See **Allo-antibody**.

Isoelectric focusing An **electrophoretic** technique used to separate mixtures of molecules (usually **proteins**), according to their electrical charge, in a medium in which a **pH** gradient has been established. Molecules move through the medium until they reach their **isoelectric point**.

Isoelectric point The **pH** value at which molecules (usually **proteins**) have no overall positive or negative charge and therefore do not migrate in a medium under the influence of direct current.

Iso-enzyme A closely related, but slightly different molecular form of an **enzyme**. Iso-enzymes may originate from different organs and can be differentiated by their physical and chemical characteristics.

Isolate Part of a population separated by transfer into an artificial state, as by inoculation of laboratory animals or cultures.

Isoniazid Isonicotinic acid hydrazide (INAH) is a synthetic anti-tubercular **anti-microbial** substance. Like most other anti-tubercular agents it cannot be used alone because of development of resistance. Its precise mode of action is unknown, but it probably inhibits **mycolic acid** production. It is relatively non-toxic, though neurotoxicity (in the form of confusion and psychosis, and peripheral neuropathy) can occur.

Isopropanol precipitation test A method for the detection of unstable **haemoglobins,** in which a freshly prepared **haemolysate** is added to a solution of isopropanol. Unstable haemoglobins precipitate under these conditions whereas normal haemoglobin does not. See also **Haemoglobinopathy** and **Heat-labile haemoglobin**.

Isopyknic gradient centrifugation The form of **density gradient centrifugation** used to determine the **buoyant density** of a molecule or particle. Classically, the **substrate** employed is caesium chloride.

Isotonic Exerting the same osmotic pressure as blood plasma. In humans this implies a freezing point of $-0.56°C$. Solutions of sodium chloride and dextrose are isotonic at (respectively) 8·8 g/l and 51·0 g/l.

Isotope One of a number of species of an element which have the same atomic number but different atomic weights: (e.g. ^{125}I and ^{131}I are different isotopes of iodine).

Isotropic Material which is unaffected by crossed polarizers — (i.e. it appears dark). See **Anisotropic**.

Isoxazolyl penicillin A group of semi-synthetic **anti-microbial** substances based on the **penicillin** nucleus. The two drugs of this group used in Britain are **Cloxacillin** and **Flucloxacillin**. They are resistant to staphylococcal **penicillinase** and can be taken orally, being resistant to gastric acid.

Ivy test See **Bleeding time**.

J

Jacob and Jandl ascorbate cyanide test   A test used mainly for the diagnosis of **G6PD** deficiency, in which sodium cyanide and sodium ascorbate are added to the blood under test. In the absence of G6PD the hydrogen peroxide generated by this mixture will convert **haemoglobin** to **methaemoglobin** and the blood will become brown within 1−2 hours. Positive results are also found in deficiencies of **glutathione** and **glutathione peroxidase**.

Jacuzzi rash   Skin lesions − confined to the trunk, legs and forearms − associated with the use of Jacuzzi whirlpool baths, especially if multiply occupied or over-used. The lesions are due to infection with **pseudomonas**, which grows rapidly in vigorously-aerated water.

J chain   In **Immunology**, a polypeptide chain (MW 36000 D) associated with pentameric **IgM** and dimeric **IgA**. J chains play a role in the formation of the pentamer and the dimer from monomeric forms.

Jenner, Edward (1749−1823)   English physician credited with making the first use of a **vaccine** in 1796. Jenner claimed to have used the organism of cowpox to protect against **smallpox**, the **viruses** of which are very similar. However, the **vaccinia** virus used until recently for smallpox vaccination is not the same as the viruses of either cowpox or smallpox, and it is probable that Jenner's original cowpox material was contaminated either with the related virus of horsepox or with the **variola** virus of smallpox, and that today's vaccinia virus is a hybrid derived from all three organisms.

Jenner's stain   See **Romanowsky stains**.

Jigger flea *(Tunga penetrans)*   Occurs in tropical areas of Africa and South America. Gravid females bury into the skin, usually in the foot and particularly under the toe nails. Eggs are passed through the entry hole. The flea is imported into, but not disseminated in, the United Kingdom.

JK coryneform   Rod-shaped **bacteria** which are positive by **Gram's stain** and which belong to the genus **Corynebacterium**. They are characterised by their lack of biochemical action and by poor growth in the absence of lipids, and by their resistance to a wide range of **anti-microbial** substances other than **Vancomycin**; however, fully susceptible strains also occur for which the name *J. jeikeium* has been proposed. The organisms cause serious infection in immuno-deficient or debilitated patients, or those with implants.

K

K 1. The symbol for the quantity of 2^{10}, or 1024. See also **k** and **Kilobyte**. 2. The chemical symbol for potassium. See also **K antigen**.

k Abbreviation for Kilo-, representing a number raised to the power of 10^3.

KAF Obsolete term for the **enzyme** responsible for the inactivation of **complement** C3b.

Kala Azar Also known as Visceral leishmaniasis, Dum Dum fever, Black sickness, Sahib's disease, Poros, and Mard el Bicha. An infective disease, becoming chronic with irregular fever, leading to enlargement of the spleen − and occasionally the liver − in both of which *Leishmania donovani* (Leishman Donovan bodies) may be demonstrated. The disease is disseminated by sandflies, and has an uneven distribution across the world. It is found particularly in India, Africa and South America, but also in countries surrounding the Mediterranean. Associated parasites (cutaneous leishmaniasis) causing limited eroding lesions are found in many parts of the world and are not infrequently imported by visitors to the United Kingdom. A grossly disfiguring form of visceral leishmaniasis (Espundia), usually only affecting the face, is found exclusively in central and south America.

Kallikrein An **enzyme** derived from the **plasma** precursor **prekallikrein** by the action of activated **coagulation factor** XII. The preferred substrate for plasma kallikrein is **high molecular weight kininogen**, and its main role in **haemostasis** is in **contact activation** of the **intrinsic system**.

Kanamycin An **aminoglycoside** produced by **Streptomyces** species, and similar in structure to **streptomycin**. It is active against a wide range of **aerobic** Gram positive and Gram negative organisms, but **plasmid**-mediated resistance is quite common. **Streptococci**, including *Strep. pneumoniae* and **enterococci**, are resistant, as is **pseudomonas**. The drug is also active against *Mycobacterium tuberculosis*. Irreversible deafness is the main toxic effect and this is more likely to occur than with streptomycin.

K antigen 1. A polysaccharide **antigen** on the surface of *Escherichia coli* and other **Enterobacteriaceae**. The antigens can be detected and characterised using **immune** sera. Many appear to be **virulence** factors and the K1 antigen is found frequently on strains of *Esch. coli* causing **meningitis**, while K13 is associated with **pyelonephritis**. 2. An antigen of the Kell **blood group** system; also known as K1. It is present in about 8% to 10% of Caucasians, and the antibody to this antigen readily causes severe adverse haemolytic reactions to **transfusion**, and also **haemolytic disease of the newborn**.

Kaolin-cephalin clotting time   See **Activated partial thromboplastin time**.

Kaposi's sarcoma   A rare skin tumour associated with **cytomegalovirus** infection; seen more commonly in some **immunodeficient** individuals. See **Acquired Immune Deficiency Syndrome**.

Karyolysis   A form of degeneration in which the nucleus of the cell swells and loses its **chromatin**.

Karyopyknotic Index   See **Cornification Index**.

Karyorrhexis   Degeneration of the nucleus of a cell, resulting in nuclear fragmentation.

Karyosome   See **Caryosome**.

Karyotype   The **chromosome** complement of an individual defined by number, size and form. Demonstrated by a systematised array of photomicrographs of the **metaphase chromosomes** of a single cell.

Kawasaki disease   A disease also known as Mucocutaneous lymph node syndrome, which mainly affects children and is of unknown aetiology. The mortality rate is low and death is due to **endocarditis**. The symptoms include **fever**, desquamation of the skin of palms and soles, **conjunctivitis**, buccal mucosal lesions and **lymphadenopathy**. **Pyuria** is also found. **Anti-microbial** substances are ineffective and salicylate is the drug of choice. Various microbial causes have been suggested, including organisms of the **Propionibacterium** species.

KB cells   An epithelial cell line grown in **monolayers**, and derived from a human buccal epithelioma. They have similar properties and laboratory applications to **HeLa** cells.

KCCT   See **Activated partial thromboplastin time**.

K cell   See **Killer cell**.

Keratin   An insoluble and fibrous protein which is the main constituent of **epidermis**, hair, nails and the organic part of tooth enamel.

Keratinisation   Formation of **keratin** within cells of the **squamous epithelium**.

Keratinised cancer cell   A **malignant squamous epithelial** cell which has excessively **keratinised** the **cytoplasm**.

Keratitis   Corneal inflammation which can be caused by a variety of agents including chemicals and trauma. Many **micro-organisms** have been incriminated including *Staphylococcus aureus*, *Pseudomonas aeruginosa*, *Streptococcus pneumoniae*, *Chlamydia trachomatis* and **fungi** and **parasites**.

Keratohyalin   Strongly haematoxyphil granules seen in the *stratum granulosum* of **epithelium**.

Kernicterus   A condition of **hyperbilirubinaemia** in which the levels of bilirubin rise to a point at which they become attached to brain and central nervous tissue, causing irreversible brain damage. See **Haemolytic disease of the newborn**.

Keto acid A product of the metabolism of fat. They are generally aceto-acetic acid and beta-hydroxybutyric acid.

Ketoacidosis See **Ketosis**.

Ketoconazole An **imidazole** type of **anti-microbial** substance which is active against many **fungi**, although resistant strains of **Candida** and of *Aspergillus niger* do occur. It does not penetrate sufficiently into the cerebrospinal fluid to be useful in the treatment of **meningitis**. Toxic effects include nausea, vomiting, and **hormone** disturbances which may lead to gynaecomastia.

Ketone bodies The products formed as a result of increased fat metabolism, including acetoacetic acid, acetone and beta-hydroxybutyric acid.

17-Ketosteroid One of a group of neutral **steroids** which produce a red colour with *m*-dinitrobenzene in alkaline solution. They are metabolites of adrenal cortical and gonadal steroids, and urinary levels are raised in pregnancy, some **neoplasms** of the adrenals and patients being treated with **ACTH**. Reduced levels are found in Addison's disease, individuals with reduced **androgen** production, and occasionally in **myxoedema** and anorexia nervosa.

Killer (K) cell A cell which may bind to target cells coated with **antibody** and subsequently lyse the target cell. See **Antibody Dependent Cell-mediated Cytotoxicity**.

Killing curve A method of assessing the **bactericidal** effect of a drug or a combination of drugs *in vitro*. A suitable fluid **culture medium** is inoculated with the test culture and the **viable count** is determined. The **anti-microbial** substance is then added and mixed and the culture incubated. The viable count is determined at intervals over 24 or 48 h and plotted. For a bactericidal drug there is an initial fall, or no change, followed by a logarithmic rise. The method is particularly suitable for studying **synergism** and **antagonism**.

Kilobyte In computing, a measurement of **memory** representing the closest power of 2^{10} (i.e. 1024 bytes). In practice, a Kilobyte is regarded as 1000 bytes so that (e.g.) 64 K is considered to represent 64 000 rather than $64 \times 1024 = 65\,536$ bytes.

Kinetic Describes the velocity of a reaction. When measuring **enzyme** activity, kinetic or continuous monitoring methods may be used as opposed to end-point determinations.

Kingella Rod-shaped **bacteria** which do not exhibit **motility**, are **oxidase** positive, **catalase** negative and are negative by **Gram's stain**, and which are **commensals** of mucous membranes. They occasionally cause **septicaemia** and **arthritis**.

Kinin See **Kininogen**.

Kininogen There are two forms of plasma kininogen: a high molecular weight form (HMW kininogen − **HMWK**) and a low molecular weight form (LMW kininogen). The kininogens are cleaved by **kallikrein** to yield kinins, a family of polypeptides with a variety of pharmacological actions including vasodilation, muscle contraction and production of pain.

Kirby-Bauer test A method of testing for **anti-microbial** susceptibility by **disc diffusion**. The standard test uses **Mueller-Hinton agar** medium and the inoculum size is adjusted to the density of a barium sulphate standard, to give confluent growth. The concentrations of **antibiotics** in the discs are generally higher than those used in other methods.

Klebsiella Rod-shaped **bacteria** which do not exhibit **motility**, are facultative **anaerobes** which are **catalase** positive, **oxidase** negative, staining negative by **Gram's stain** and which are usually capable of utilisation of citrate as their sole carbon source. The organisms are responsible mainly for hospital-associated **urinary tract infection**, **septicaemia**, chest infections and **meningitis**. They are capable of developing **plasmid**-mediated resistance to a wide range of **anti-microbial** substances. They are members of the **Enterobacteriaceae**.

Kleihauer test A test devised by Kleihauer and Betke in which a film of blood is stained differentially to demonstrate the presence of **fetal** red cells in a population of predominantly adult cells. The technique depends upon the fact that adult **haemoglobin** is susceptible to **elution** by acids, while fetal haemoglobin is not.

Km See **Michaelis constant**.

Kohler illumination In **light microscopy**, an illuminating system requiring a light source fitted with a **condensing lens** and an iris diaphragm. The condenser is used to focus an enlarged image of the source at the focal plane of the microscope condenser, and the latter is used to focus the image of the lamp condenser into the object plane. This is the illumination system of choice for all microscopy requiring **critical illumination**.

Koilocyte An enlarged superficial or intermediate epithelial **squamous cell**, often showing one or more irregular **nuclei** and surrounded by a perinuclear clearing, peripheral to which the **cytoplasm** is quite dense due to an excess of tonofilaments. Also known as Ballon cells or Halo cells.

Kringle structure A term given to a section of polypeptide chain which contains three disulphide bridges, arranged in such a pattern that in two dimensions it resembles a triple loop structure, not unlike a pretzel or 'kringle'. Such a structure occurs in the **prothrombin** and **plasminogen** molecules.

Krukenberg's tumour   A special type of **carcinoma** of the ovary, **metastatic** from the gastro-intestinal tract.

Kupffer cell   A 'fixed' **macrophage** found in the liver.

Kurthia   Rod-shaped **bacteria** which do not exhibit **motility**, do not form **spores**, and are **aerobes** which are **catalase** positive and **oxidase** negative, staining positive by **Gram's stain**. They do not exhibit **haemolysis** on horse blood **agar** and are asaccharolytic, which helps to distinguish them from **Listeria**. They occasionally cause infection in the immuno-incompetent.

Kuru   A progressive and fatal **spongiform encephalopathy** found in the Fore tribe of Papua New Guinea. It was spread by the ritual cannibalising of recently deceased relatives in the hope of perpetuating their better qualities. The infectious nature of the disease is shown by its slow disappearance since the practice was stopped. The causative agent resembles that inducing **Creutzfeldt-Jakob disease**.

Kviem test   A test for sarcoidosis, in which a sterilised suspension of sarcoid tissue is injected into the dermis. A positive result is determined by the presence of follicular granulomas in a **biopsy** of the site.

L

Labile factor See **Coagulation factors**.

Laboratory strain A strain of micro-organism perpetuated for long periods in the laboratory. These strains may show characteristics – in particular, growth characteristics – not associated with the naturally-occurring agent.

Lac operon The genetic unit of co-ordinated expression of the ability to absorb and ferment lactose, consisting of LAC O (operator), LAC Z (coding for beta galactosidase production) and LAC Y (coding for permease production). The operator locus can be repressed by specific proteins in order to prevent lactose fermentation. In inducible production of **enzyme**, the repressor is inhibited.

(beta)-Lactam A term used for those **anti-microbial** substances, both natural and semi-synthetic, whose molecular structure includes the beta-lactam ring. Such substances include the **penicillins** and **cephalosporins**, and **clavulanic acid**. They exert their anti-bacterial action by binding to **penicillin-binding proteins** in the cytoplasmic **membrane**, thereby preventing these substances from taking part in cell wall synthesis. Resistance to beta-lactams is usually mediated by **beta-lactamases**, which hydrolyse the beta-lactam ring, inactivating the anti-microbial substance. Whilst some organisms (such as *Streptococcus pyogenes*), are typically susceptible to beta-lactams, strains of most others are capable of showing resistance to one or more of these drugs. In use, the beta-lactams have very few toxic side-effects other than hypersensitivity.

(beta)-Lactamase (EC 3.5.2.6) A group of **enzymes** produced by micro-organisms which are capable of hydrolysing the **beta-lactam** ring of anti-microbial substances possessing it. Beta-lactamases have been classified in various ways but a scheme devised by Sykes and Richmond is considered the most useful. The enzymes are divided into five classes according to their **substrate** profiles. Beta-lactamases may be mediated by **chromosomes** or by **plasmids**, and may be inducible or constitutive. Those produced by bacteria positive by **Gram's stain** usually escape into the surrounding cells, whereas those found in Gram-negative bacteria are often retained in the cell wall between the cytoplasmic **membrane** and the **peptidoglycan** layer. Also known as **Penicillinase**.

Lactate dehydrogenase (EC 1.1.1.27) An **enzyme** that catalyses the reversible oxidation of lactate and NAD^+ to pyruvate and NADH. It is widely spread and is found particularly in the heart, kidneys and liver.

Lactobacillus Rod-shaped **bacteria** which do not exhibit **motility**, do not form **spores**, are facultative **anaerobes** which are **catalase** negative, **oxidase** negative, and prefer an acid **pH**. Many are found in foodstuffs and some are found as **commensals** in the mouth, vagina and large intestine.

Lactoferrin   An iron-binding **protein** found in mucous secretions, breast milk and various cells in the body including **neutrophils**, in which it plays an important part in oxygen-independent killing of ingested organisms. By binding free iron, lactoferrin makes it unavailable to **bacteria**, thus preventing their further multiplication and metabolism. Those whose **reticulo-endothelial system** is saturated with iron — as in **thalassaemia** — are at risk from **septicaemia** due to organisms such as **Yersinia**, because all lactoferrin has been saturated.

Lacunae   1. Literally, a gap, as a space in a piece of text where something has been lost; or a missing link in a chain of arguments. 2. In **histopathology**, spaces in bone within which are the bone cells (**osteocytes**).

Lag phase   1. The phase of bacterial growth during which there is little or no increase in the **viable count** after introducing **bacteria** into fresh **culture medium** or into a susceptible host. During this phase the bacteria synthesise **enzymes** to metabolise the components of the fresh medium and prepare for rapid multiplication in the **log phase**. 2. The period in a test during which there is apparently no reaction or activity, despite the fact that all necessary constituents are present and mixed together.

Lake   Result of the combination between a **dye** and a **mordant**. The resultant complex is invariably basic in action.

Lambert's law   See **Beer-Lambert's law**.

LAN   See **Local Area Network**.

Lancefield group   The serological group to which a beta **haemolytic streptococcus** is assigned by virtue of its group carbohydrate. This is generally found in the **cell wall** between the **M-protein** layer and the peptidoglycan, and can be extracted by heating with hydrochloric acid or by other means, including the use of an **enzyme** produced by **Streptomyces**. In *Strep. pyogenes* (group A) the group specific **antigen** consists of rhamnose and N-acetylglucosamine, while those of groups B, C and G are of slightly different composition. The group D-specific antigen found in **enterococci** is a glycerol teichoic acid.

Landsteiner, Karl (1868–1943)   Viennese scientist who, in 1900–1901, was the first to discover the existence of blood groups. In 1930 he was awarded the Nobel prize in medicine for his discovery of the **ABO blood groups** and in 1940 he reported the finding of the **Rh blood groups**.

Landsteiner-Miller technique A method of **elution** in which red cells **sensitised** with an **antibody** are subjected to heat so that the antibody is removed from the cell surface into solution in the supernatant fluid.

Langerhans' cell A **dendritic** cell of the outer layer of the epidermis: a modified type of **macrophage** which possesses **IgA** surface **receptors**.

Langhan's giant cell A multi-nucleated giant **histiocyte** associated with tuberculosis.

Language In computing, a set of instructions used in a **program** to communicate instructions to the computer. See **Assembly language**, **High level language**, **Low level language** and **Machine code**.

Lanthanum hexaboride filament Small tips of lanthanum hexaboride which give greater brightness in the **electron microscope** than the conventional tungsten **filament**.

LAP See **Leucocyte alkaline phosphatase**.

Lassa fever An acute **haemorrhagic fever** caused by a member of the **Arenaviridae**. The **virus** is found in the multimammate rat *Mastomys natalensis* in parts of West Africa. Infection in man is **zoonotic**, man-to-man spread having almost always been achieved by needle-stick. Disease in Caucasians is seen rarely, but seems likely to be severe. The virus is a **risk group 4 pathogen**.

Latency 1. Literally, concealed, dormant. 2. In microbiology, a property of agents capable of establishing a **latent infection**.

Latent image fading In **autoradiography**, high temperature and water present in the emulsion, leading to sensitised specks of non-ionised silver becoming ionised to silver bromide again, destroying the latent image formed during exposure.

Latent infection An **infection** in which the **infectious** agent − usually a **virus** − is not demonstrable until it is activated by some internal or external event such as trauma, pregnancy, physical illness or mental stress. All human **herpetoviridae** establish the state of **latency** after primary infection, although activation does not always result in disease.

Latent period The time between the apparent disappearance of a **virus** once it has infected a cell, and the release of progeny virus.

Latex agglutination A technique utilising latex particles labelled with **antigen** or **antibody**. A sample containing the appropriate reactant will induce visible aggregation of latex particles, often within minutes.

Latex particle test An **inert particle agglutination test** utilising polystyrene latex particles coated with **antigen**. See **Latex agglutination**.

Lattice hypothesis An hypothesis which postulates that maximal

precipitation in an antigen/antibody reaction is only seen when **antibody** and soluble **antigen** are present in **optimal proportions**. The hypothesis may be used to explain why conditions of antibody excess in the presence of optimal concentrations of antigen may lead to an absence of precipitation (i.e. the **prozone phenomenon**).

Laurell test   An **immunoelectrophoretic** technique for the quantitation of protein **antigens**. Proteins are placed into wells towards one end of an **agar** gel containing **anti-serum** to the **protein**. When direct current is applied to the gel the proteins migrate in the electrical field and precipitate with the antibody to form elongated arcs or 'rockets' of **precipitation**. The length of the 'rocket' from the application site to the tip of the precipitation arc is proportional to the concentration of the antigen.

LAV   Lymphadenopathy-Associated Virus. See **Human Immunodeficiency Virus**.

Lazy leucocyte syndrome   A disease in which **neutrophils** show defective **chemotaxis**. Individuals with the condition may suffer from recurrent low-grade infections.

LDL   See **Low density lipoprotein**.

Least significant difference   If several treatment groups are compared statistically by **analysis of variance** and found to differ, then the least significant difference − which can be calculated from the **mean squares** − is the amount by which group **means** have to differ before they are significantly different at the 5% **significance level**. This enables group differences to be investigated. This technique should not normally be used if the treatments have any structure or order (e.g. are combinations of several **factors** or are increasing doses of a drug).

LE cells   A leucocyte. In **Romanowsky-stained** preparations the LE cell appears as a **neutrophil** containing a large, amorphous, purple-staining spherical mass (the LE body). The LE body represents altered nuclear material and the demonstration of LE cells is suggestive, but not diagnostic, of systemic **lupus erythematosus** (SLE).

Lecithin/Sphyngomyelin ratio   A means of assessing the maturity of fetal lung by measuring the concentrations of lecithin and sphyngomyelin in amniotic fluid. In normal development, at about 26 weeks gestation the sphingomyelin concentration is higher than that of lecithin, therefore the ratio is <1: after this period the ratio increases.

Lectin   A haemagglutinin (but *not* an **antibody**) found in extracts of certain plants and fungi; often in the seeds of *leguminosae*. Some lectins have **blood group** specificity. See **Protectins**.

Lee and White clotting time   See **Whole blood clotting time**.

Legionella   Rod-shaped **bacteria** which exhibit **motility**, are **catalase** positive, weakly **oxidase** positive, negative by **Gram's stain** and whose natural habitat is water, either in lakes and streams or in heating, cooling and plumbing systems. The organisms are fastidious and require additional iron and amino acids for growth in culture; they may be isolated on buffered charcoal yeast extract **agar** containing L-cysteine, ferric pyrophosphate and alpha-ketoglutarate, requiring 2–6 days for growth. *L. pneumophila*, the causative organism of Legionnaire's disease, is asaccharolytic. **Antibody** to the organism can be found in the **serum** of those infected, and strains of this and other species can be grouped serologically. Legionnaire's disease is characterised by a severe **pneumonia** affecting particularly the elderly and smokers, and caused mainly by *L. pneumophila*. Pontiac fever is an **influenza**-like illness, often with central nervous system disturbance, caused by certain sero-groups of *L. pneumophila* and *L. feelii*. **Erythromycin** and **Rifampicin** are used in treatment of these Legionelloses.

Leiomyosarcoma   A **malignant neoplasm** of smooth muscle cells.

Leishman Donovan body   See **Amastigote**.

Leishman's stain   See **Romanowsky stain**.

Leishman, William (1865–1926)   Scottish pathologist and military administrator who was an international authority on anti-typhoid inoculation and who introduced the famous blood stain which carries his name. He was the first to associate the so-called **Leishman-Donovan bodies** with trypanosomiasis. See also **Leishman's stain** and **Leishmaniasis**.

Leishmaniasis An **infection** which occurs in two main clinical forms, visceral and cutaneous (**Kala azar**). The causative parasite is disseminated by sand flies and the disease occurs in many parts of the world.

LEP   An abbreviation of Low Egg Passage, a technique used to **attenuate** the **rabies virus** for production of a **vaccine** for dogs.

Leprosy   An infection of the peripheral nerves and skin by *Mycobacterium leprae*. The skin lesions are essentially granulomatous and affected areas are anaesthetised, resulting in injuries and mutilation. The organism cannot be grown in synthetic **culture media** or in **tissue culture** but it has been grown in the footpads of mice and armadilloes. Nasal secretions, rather than direct skin contact, are probably responsible for spread. The drugs used for treatment are **Dapsone**, **Rifampicin**, **Ethionamide** and Clofazimine.

Leptocyte   A term given to abnormally thin **erythrocytes** seen (e.g.) in **iron deficiency anaemia**, in which the red cells stain as rings of **haemoglobin** with large unstained central areas of pallor. See also **Target cell**.

Leptospira A type of **spirochaete** with fine coils, up to 15 micrometres long by 0·1 micrometre wide, and showing hooking at the ends. They exhibit **motility** in either direction and maintain a rigid straight shape for most of the time. They can be grown easily in appropriate artificial **culture media** containing **serum**. Two species are now recognised: *L. biflexa*, representing the saprophytic strains, and *L. interrogans*, of which there are several serotypes such as *var.* canicola and *var.* icterohaemorrhagiae. They are the cause of a **zoonosis** in wild and domestic animals, and of **leptospirosis** in man.

Leptospirosis A disease of wild and domesticated animals, which occasionally affects humans. It may be caused by any of the species of **Leptospira** except *L. biflexa*. The disease takes two forms, a mild anicteric form and a more severe icteric form. The anicteric form often presents in two phases separated by a few days. The first phase is of sudden onset with headache, vomiting, **fever** and **conjunctivitis**, during which the **spirochaetes** distribute themselves throughout all tissues of the body and can be found in blood, **cerebrospinal fluid** and (later) urine. The second phase, which does not always occur, is characterised by aseptic **meningitis**, rash and fever, and is probably of immune origin. The icteric form, known as Weil's disease, begins like the first phase of the mild form but progresses to jaundice, renal failure and cardiovascular collapse with a mortality rate of up to 10%. In both cases spirochaetes can be found in the urine for long periods. Diagnosis can be made by isolation in Tween-80-albumin medium, but this is slow. Leptospires might also be seen by dark-ground microscopy of cerebrospinal fluid, but serology is the usual method. **Tetracycline** is the drug of choice for treatment, but its role is controversial.

Leuckhart mould Two 'L' shaped pieces of brass which, together with a base plate, can be arranged to form a square or rectangular mould for molten **paraffin wax** during histological **embedding**.

Leucocidin An **exotoxin** produced by some pathogenic **Staphylococci** and **Streptococci**, which kills white blood cells either by action on the cell membrane or, more specifically, by inducing discharge of lysosomal **enzymes** into the **cytoplasm** of the cell. The Panton-Valentin leucocidin of *Staph. aureus* is the only one which acts specifically on **neutrophils**.

Leucocyte White blood cells. The body's main defence against infection. There are two main series, **mononuclear** (including **lymphocytes** and **monocytes**) and **polymorphonuclear** (including neutrophil, eosinophil and basophil cells), named for the staining reactions of their intracellular granules.

Leucocyte acid phosphatase An **enzyme** present in the **lysosomes** of many haemopoietic cells. The most important use of the leucocyte acid phosphatase reaction is in the classification of **lymphoproliferative disorders**.

Leucocyte alkaline phosphatase An **enzyme** contained in the secondary or specific granules of **neutrophils**, and which can be demonstrated **cytochemically**. High levels are seen in infections and in **polycythaemia rubra vera**, while low levels are characteristic of **chronic myeloid leukaemia**.

Leuco dye **Chromophore** groups which become colourless on reduction, and re-coloured on oxidation. In use, a colourless **dye** is applied to tissue and the site of oxidation is revealed by colour production (e.g. leuco patent blue applied to **haemoglobin**).

Leuco-erythroblastic anaemia The finding of **anaemia** with a blood picture that appears **leukaemoid** as regards the **leucocytes**, but which also shows large numbers of nucleated red cells. This is most commonly seen in **carcinoma** involving the **bone marrow**, and severe **haemolytic anaemia**.

Leuco-erythrogenic ratio The ratio of immature **leucocytes** to nucleated red cells in the **bone marrow**. It is used as a means of expressing the relative activities of **leucopoiesis** and **erythropoiesis**.

Leucopenia A decrease in the total number of peripheral blood **leucocytes**.

Leucopheresis The procedure of **apheresis** performed with the intention of separating **leucocytes** from the circulation.

Leucoplakia A lesion characterised by a 'whitish plaque' on the **epithelium** of the mucous membrane.

Leucopoiesis The term given to the production of **leucocytes**, either in the **bone marrow** or in other extra-medullary sites. See **Haemopoiesis**.

Leucotrine One of a series of compounds, metabolites of **arachadonic acid**, produced by **leucocytes** and which exert a variety of pharmacological effects.

Leukaemia A generic term for a series of neoplastic diseases. A **malignant** proliferation of **leucocytes**, usually – but not always – associated with an increase in the number of circulating white cells, and the presence of immature **leucocytes** in the peripheral blood and **bone marrow**. The malignant cells may be of myeloid, lymphoid or monocytic origin, and the clinical course may be **acute** or **chronic** in nature. A variety of similar diseases in animals are induced by **retroviruses**.

Leukaemoid The finding of marked **leucocytosis**. Immature or abnormal **leucocytes** in the peripheral blood, suggesting a diagnosis of **leukaemia**, but which is actually reactive and non-malignant in nature.

Leukotrienes A group of substances which are biochemically related to **prostaglandins**. The **slow reacting substance A**, which is released from **mast cells** during **type I hypersensitivity reactions**, is a mixture of leukotrienes C4 and D4.

Leyell's disease A condition characterised by exfoliation, leaving large areas of denuded dermis. The terminology is confused but can be simplified by using the term staphylococcal scalded skin syndrome for Ritter's disease − which is identical to one of the two types of Lyell's disease − and toxic epidermal necrolysis for the second type of Lyell's disease, which is not due to infection. Staphylococcal scalded skin syndrome almost exclusively affects infants and is due to the production of exfoliative toxin by *Staphylococcus aureus*. If excessive fluid loss and secondary infection are avoided, recovery is usually complete. **Flucloxacillin** should be given parenterally.

Ligand See **Hapten**.

Light chain A polypeptide (MW 22 000 D) which is present in all **immunoglobulin** molecules. Each immunoglobulin monomer contains two **lambda** or two **kappa** light chains, each joined to a **heavy chain** by a **disulphide bond**.

Light pen A device for reading **bar codes** and passing the information thereon to a computer.

Limulus assay A very sensitive test for **endotoxin** which relies upon the finding that an extract of amoebocytes of the horse-shoe crab, *Limulus polyphemus*, will form a gel in its presence. The test has been used to diagnose infection with members of the **enterobacteriaceae**.

Line Continuous passage of a parasite in culture. Not necessarily a **clone**, but a strain showing particular characteristics.

Linearity An expression of proportional relationship between response and concentration over a defined range.

Lipaemia The turbidity or milky appearance of **serum** due to an increased amount of lipid (triglyceride).

Lipase (EC 3.1.1.3) An **enzyme** that hydrolyses fats and oils. It is secreted by the pancreas and levels are raised in acute pancreatitis, although less so than occurs with **amylase**.

Lipid A naturally occurring substance which is related either actually or potentially to fatty acid esters, and which is capable of being utilised by the animal organism. Usually, but not invariably, insoluble in water but soluble in 'fat solvents' (e.g. chloroform, acetone, ether). (NB Fat is a lipid which is soluble at room temperature, whereas oil is a lipid which is liquid at room temperature.)

Lipid pigment An oxidation product of a **lipid** seen in tissue sections. The colour darkens with increasing oxidation. See also

Ceroid, Lipofuscin, Dubin-Johnson pigment, Carotenoid, *Pseudo-melanosis coli.*

Lipochrome See **Carotenoid.**

Lipofuscin A yellow-brown or brown pigment in tissue sections, most commonly seen in heart, liver, adrenal, testis and **neurones.** It gives a variable staining reaction depending upon the degree of oxidation of the **lipid** component. Synonyms are **Brown atrophy pigment** and **Wear and tear pigment.**

Lipolysis The breakdown of triglyceride to fatty acid and glycerol.

Lipopolysaccharide One of the main constituents of the **cell wall** of **bacteria** which are negative by **Gram's stain.** It is responsible for somatic **antigen** expression and it also functions as an **endotoxin.** It consists of three segments: lipid, a common core polysaccharide, and side chains of polysaccharide which confer antigenic specificity.

Lipoprotein A combination of lipid and **protein** found in all mammalian plasma, in a structure that enables lipid to become soluble in water and be transported in the blood.

(beta)-Lipoprotein See **Low density lipoprotein.**

Lipoteichoic acid A substance found in the **cell wall** of *Staphylococcus aureus* and *Streptococcus pyogenes.* It contributes to the hydrophobicity of the cell surface and is instrumental in **adhesion** of the organisms to mammalian cells and host proteins.

Lipoxygenase An **enzyme** involved in the metabolism of **arachadonic acid** and which produces the hydroxy-fatty acid 12-hydroxyeicosatetranoic acid (HETE) via its hydroperoxy precursor HPETE.

Liquid nitrogen Nitrogen under increased pressure, with a temperature of −196°C. Used for rapid freezing and low-temperature storage of many biological substances.

LISS Low ionic strength saline. A solution of sodium chloride with an ionic strength of 0·03. Some **blood grouping** reactions can be enhanced under these conditions. See also **Normal saline.**

Lissamine rhodamine isothiocyanate A fluorochrome **dye** which can be used to label **immunoglobulins** for **immunofluorescence** techniques.

Listeria Rod-shaped **bacteria** which do not form **spores,** are facultative **anaerobes,** are **catalase** positive, **oxidase** negative and are positive by **Gram's stain.** They exhibit **motility** at 20−25°C. They are capable of growth at +4°C as well as at 37°C and produce beta **haemolysis** on horse blood **agar.** They can be divided into O and H **antigenic** types. They are found in the intestinal tracts of many animals as well as in decaying vegetation and manure.

Live vaccine A **vaccine** containing live micro-organisms (e.g. **BCG** vaccine).

Local anaphylaxis A localised **type I hypersensitivity reaction** such as hay fever. Sometimes called **atopic allergy**.

Local area network A **network** of several computers linked together by hard wiring.

Locus The position on a **chromosome** occupied by a **gene** (plural = loci).

Loeffler, Friedrich (1852–1915) German bacteriologist, a pupil of Robert **Koch**. A joint discoverer (with Edwin Klebs) of the diphtheria bacillus and an early pioneer virologist, being the first to recognise the filter-passing properties of the foot and mouth disease virus. Author of the first published history of **bacteriology**.

Log phase The phase of rapid cell division of **bacteria**, during which a plot of the logarithm (to any base) of the **viable count** against time results in a straight line. During this phase the optical density is proportional to the viable count, as very few bacteria are dead.

Loop In computing, the repeated execution of a series of instructions in a **program**.

Louse Three species infect man: the head louse, *Pediculus humanus, var. capitis*; the body louse, *P. humanus, var. corporis*; and the pubic or 'crab' louse, *Phthirus pubis*. Infestation with lice is called pediculosis. Lice are the **vectors** of typhus (*Rickettsia prowazekii*) which is cosmopolitan in distribution, and also other 'louse-borne' fevers found particularly in parts of the world where crowding, famine and malnutrition occur.

Low density lipoprotein A **lipoprotein** in which the lipid portion contains cholesterol esters, phospholipid and triglyceride. On **electrophoresis** the lipoprotein migrates with the **beta Globulin** fraction. These lipoproteins are involved in the formation of atheromatous lesions and accumulations. Removal of low density lipoproteins from **serum** prior to assay of **antibody** to **rubella** and **measles** is essential.

Low dose tolerance Acquired immune tolerance seen after repeated administration of very small doses of some **antigens**.

Lowenstein-Jensen medium A **culture medium** for cultivation of **Mycobacterium** species, and consisting of mineral salts, asparagine, glycerol, malachite green and hens' eggs. The medium is treated by **inspissation** to solidify it. The malachite green makes it inhibitory to most other **micro-organisms**.

Low level language In computing, a **language** approximating to **machine code** rather than to everyday language. A **program** written in a low level language needs less interpretation for the computer than one written in a **high level language**, and so runs faster.

Low responder A term used to describe **inbred strains** of laboratory animals which show weak **immune responses** to some **antigens**.

L/S ratio See **Lecithin/Sphyngomyelin ratio**.

Lupus anticoagulant A relatively common inhibitor of blood coagulation found in approximately 10% of patients with systemic
lupus erythematosus, as well as a variety of other clinical conditions. A characteristic feature of lupus anticoagulants is their
ability to prolong **phospholipid**-dependent clotting tests, for example the **activated partial thromboplastin time**.

Lupus erythematosus A skin disease characterised by a scaly rash
on the nose and cheeks, called a 'butterfly rash'. This may be a
sign of **Systemic lupus erythematosus**.

Luteinising hormone A **hormone** of the anterior pituitary which
acts with the **follicle-stimulating hormone** to cause ovulation of
mature **follicles**, and secretion of **oestrogen**.

Lyme disease A disease caused by *Borrelia burgdorferi*, which is
carried by a **tick**, *Ixodes dammini*, which normally feeds on mice
and deer; other related ticks have also been incriminated. Most
cases have been reported from the USA but some have also been
recorded in Europe. The site of the tick bite is marked by a large
erythematous lesion and this is accompanied by an **influenza**-like
illness. Many patients develop **arthritis** and occasionally cardiac
involvement at a later stage. **Penicillin** or **Tetracycline** are the
drugs of choice for treatment.

Lymphadenopathy Strictly, any disease of any lymph node. The
term is often applied to the local or generalised swelling of lymph
nodes which is frequently associated with **infection**.

Lymph node Small organs, widely distributed in the body, made
up virtually entirely of **lymphocytes** and **macrophages**. Lymph
nodes are drained by lymphatic vessels which eventually join to
the blood stream. They are important sites at which **antigen** may
come into contact with lymphocytes and macrophages, thus insti-
gating an **immune response**.

Lymphoblast The characteristic cell seen in the peripheral blood
and **bone marrow** of patients with **acute** lymphoblastic **leukaemia**.
The cell contains a round or oval **nucleus** with one or two **nucleoli**,
and scant agranular basophilic **cytoplasm**.

Lymphocyte A single celled **leucocyte**, the main function of which
is concerned with the immune response.

Lymphocyte transformation A term used to describe the change in
lymphocyte morphology seen when lymphocytes are stimulated *in
vitro* with **mitogens**, or exposed to other immunologically incompatible lymphocytes.

Lymphocytic choriomeningitis virus A micro-organism which is a
pathogen of the mouse and which can cause a **zoonotic** infection of
man. A self-limiting **meningitis** is the usual result of infection;
rare cases develop a severe **encephalitis**. The **virus** is a member of

the **Areniviridae**. Human infection has been very rare in recent years.

Lymphocytopenia A reduction in the number of circulating peripheral blood **lymphocytes** below the lower normal limit of $1 \cdot 5 \times 10^9/l$.

Lymphocytosis An increase in the number of circulating peripheral blood **lymphocytes** above the upper normal limit of $4 \cdot 5 \times 10^9/l$. A 'relative' lymphocytosis is said to occur when the relative proportions of other peripheral blood **leucocytes** is decreased, even though the absolute number of **lymphocytes** is normal.

Lymphocytotoxicity A term used to describe a test for the presence of **HLA** antigens on **lymphocytes**. Because of the expense and difficulty in obtaining some of the reagents used in the test it is usually performed on small volumes of material. See **Microcytotoxicity test**.

Lymphogranuloma venereum A sexually transmitted disease caused by *Chlamydia trachomatis* of **serotypes** L1, L2 and L3. The main feature is of swollen and ulcerating inguinal lymph glands (buboes). Untreated disease can lead to rectal fistulas, infectious **arthritis**, **osteomyelitis** and **peritonitis**.

Lymphography The visualisation of the lymphatic system by X-ray following injection of a radio-opaque **dye** into a lymphatic vessel.

Lymphoid cell A general term for any cell of the **lymphocyte** series.

Lymphokine Part of the **immune response**, lymphokines are soluble factors released during cell-mediated **immunity**, and indicate **lymphocyte** activation. Lymphokines are proteins, glycoproteins or peptides and are neither **immunoglobulins** nor fragments of them. They react with particular target cells and, although they do not have specific antigen binding sites, they appear to affect their targets by reacting with specific membrane receptors.

Lymphoma A general term applied to any **neoplasm** of the lymphoid tissue.

Lymphopoiesis The term given to the specific production of **lymphocytes** by the **bone marrow** and lymphatic system. See also **Haemopoiesis** and **Leucopoiesis**.

Lymphoproliferative disorder A general term given to any condition which is characterised by a malignant proliferation of lymphoid cells.

Lyon hypothesis An explanation for the variable expression of X-linked **gene** products in females heterozygous for X-linked genes. The hypothesis suggests that either the maternally- or paternally-derived X chromosome is inactivated in early embryonic life, and that the descendents of that cell therefore do not express the particular gene product. In **haematology** the Lyon hypothesis is particularly relevant to the detection of carriers of **G-6-PD** deficiency and of **haemophilia**.

Lyophilisation Freeze-drying of (e.g.) **serum**, cultures of **micro-organisms**, or other aqueous fluids. The fluid is first frozen then the water removed in a vacuum drawn over a dessicant such as phosphorus pentoxide. This causes the ice to sublime, thus dehydrating the fluid to leave its non-aqueous constituents which can then be stored indefinitely in sterile evacuated ampoules. The method is particularly useful for **serum** containing rare or delicate **antibodies**, and for cultures of **bacteria**, which do not lose viability over long periods and are not subject to the risks of contamination and emergence of variants inherent in cultural methods of preservation.

Lysis The breakdown of a cell. Haemolysis is lysis of red blood cells.

Lysochrome A disputed term applied to fat stains.

Lysogeny The state in which a **bacterium** is infected by a **bacteriophage** but is apparently unaffected by it, though subsequent generations may undergo **lysis**. The bacteria infected in this way contain prophage which multiplies at the same rate as the rest of the cell and is transmitted to progeny. Lysogeny is associated with toxigenicity in some organisms such as *Corynebacterium diphtheriae*.

Lysosome An **organelle** found within the **cytoplasm** of cells. Lysosomes contain various hydrolytic **enzymes** and **bactericidal** substances capable of hydrolysing the cell wall of certain **bacteria**. In **macrophages** the lysosome contents are responsible for killing micro-organisms taken into the cell by **phagocytosis**.

Lysozyme A hydrolytic **enzyme** with a molecular weight of 14 400 D. It is present in many body fluids and secretions, in lysosomal **vacuoles** of **phagocytes**, in egg white and other biological materials, and is capable of hydrolysing the **peptidoglycan** component of the **cell wall** of **bacteria** by cleaving the beta 1−4 linkage between muramic acid and N-acetyl glucosamine. Lysozyme has high concentrations in tears and nasal secretions, where it is believed to play an important role in the protection of mucous membranes from infection, against **bacteria** which give a positive reaction by **Gram's stain**. **Lysosomes** also contain high concentrations of the **enzyme**.

Lys-plasminogen See **Plasminogen**.

Lyssavirus The generic name of the genus of **Rhabdoviridae** which includes **rabies virus**.

Lytic infection In **virology**, an infection in which viral replication results in cell death.

M

MACELISA An acronym derived from IgM Antibody Capture Enzyme Linked ImmunoSorbent Assay: a method used for the detection of a specific **IgM**. See also **Enzyme immunoassay** and **MACRIA**.

MA 109 cell A monkey cell which, in continuous **cell culture**, is capable of supporting the complete replication cycle of some types of **rotavirus**.

Machine code In computing, a code in which the instructions to the computer are represented by binary numerical values. Any **program** written in **high level language** needs to be translated into machine code by an **assembler** before it can be executed.

MACRIA An acronym derived from IgM Antibody Capture Radio-ImmunoAssay. A **radio-isotope** label is used for the detection of a specific **IgM**. See also **MACELISA** and **Radioimmunoassay**.

Macroamylase **Amylase** which is complexed with **protein** and, as a result, becomes too large to be excreted by the kidney.

Macroautoradiography Whole body **autoradiography** of small animals − mice, rats, rabbits, etc.

Macroconidium See **Macrospore**.

Macrocytic anaemia A term given to the finding of **anaemia**, from whatever cause, associated with the presence of abnormally large **erythrocytes** in the peripheral blood. See also **Macrocytosis** and **Mean cell volume**.

Macrocytosis The presence in the peripheral blood of **erythrocytes** having a **mean cell volume** greater than 96 fl. See **Macrocytic anaemia**.

(alpha₂) Macroglobulin A large **glycoprotein** which can form complexes with a variety of **serine protease** type of **enzyme**. Its main physiological role appears to be that of neutralising **plasmin** formed in excess of the capacity of plasma **anti-plasmin**.

Macroglobulinaemia The presence in the peripheral blood of high concentrations of high molecular weight (**IgM**) forms of **immunoglobulin**, caused by a **malignant** proliferation of lymphocytoid cells. Also known as Waldenstrom's macroglobulinaemia.

Macrolide A group of **anti-microbial** substances with a macrocyclic lactone ring structure, produced by **Streptomyces** species. **Erythromycin**, **Spiromycin**, Oleandomycin and others are included in the group. Although there are similarities, **Clindamycin** and **Lincomycin** are not structurally related to the macrolides.

Macromolecular medium A solution of a chemical which has a high molecular weight (>50 000). Used in some blood grouping techniques (e.g. bovine serum **albumin**).

Macrophage A large motile cell of **interstitial** origin, part of the reticulo-endothelial system, and acting as a **phagocyte**.

Macropolycyte A term sometimes used to describe large **neutrophils** containing a higher than normal number of nuclear lobes. Such cells are most commonly seen in deficiencies of **folic acid** or **vitamin B12**. See **Hypersegmentation** and **Shift to the right**.

Macrospore A type of large, multi-cellular asexual **spore** produced by some **fungi**. They are useful for identification of the **dermatophytes**, each genus of which has macrospores of typical structure and shape.

Macrothrombocytosis The presence in the peripheral blood of abnormally large **platelets**, with or without an abnormal platelet count.

Madura foot A condition in which the aetiological agents vary from **bacteria** to **fungi** which exist freely in soil or plants, so that infection is usually in the feet or lower limbs. While a global disease, it is found more commonly where footwear is not worn. In mycetoma found in Canada and the USA the most common agent is *Petriellidium boydii*.

Magnification In microscopy, denotes this property of eyepieces and **objective lenses**, and is usually indicated on these components by the manufacturer. Total magnification can be calculated by the simple addition of the indicated factors.

Major histocompatibility complex (MHC) A genetic region carried on an **autosomal** pair which codes for **histocompatibility antigens** and some **complement** components. The MHC in mice is known as the H−2 system and in humans as the **HLA** system.

Malabsorption The process of **absorption**, or taking up of compounds from the gut, by diffusion. There are two types of absorption: one requires energy and the other is passive, occuring by diffusion only, depending on differences in concentration.

Malakoplakia A rare disorder of the bladder, associated with **chronic** infection with **bacteria**. Most of the inflammatory cells which accumulate are **macrophages**.

Malaria A febrile illness caused by **protozoa** of the class Sporozoa, genus **Plasmodium**. Four species infect man: *P. falciparum*, also known as malignant tertian (MT), subtertian (ST), malignant or cerebral malaria; *P. vivax*, also known as benign tertian (BT) malaria; *P. ovale*, also known as ovale tertian malaria; and *P. malariae*, also known as quartan malaria. The **vector** of malaria from man to man, or animals to man, is the female mosquito of the genus *Anopheles*, of which there are hundreds of species. Sexual reproduction in the mosquito results in **sporozoites** being injected into the bloodstream of the human victim when the mosquito bites to feed. After multiplication in the liver large numbers of **merozoites** are released which invade the **erythrocytes**, where they can be detected by **Giemsa stain**. They multiply in the erythrocytes, which rupture, releasing large numbers of merozoites which then infect more erythrocytes. The onset and duration of **pyrexia**, which varies depending on the infecting species, is directly related to these events. Infection with *P. Falciparum* is often fatal if untreated. Malaria is widespread, being distributed throughout most tropical and sub-tropical areas of the world, also extending into temperate zones and accounting for about 10^6 deaths annually. **Transfusion** with infected blood may give rise to malarial infection. Numerous species of *Plasmodium* occur amongst the higher primates other than man, and some of these are rarely transmitted to humans. There are also species of *Plasmodium* found in rodents and birds. Treatment involves the use of chloroquine, but *P. falciparum* might be resistant, in which case other drugs such as pyrimethamine are used.

Malaria pigment   See **Haemozoin**.

Malignant   1. Of **tumours**, involved cells invade surrounding tissue and may spread to distant sites. 2. Of cells, showing increased **mitosis**, altered **morphology** (especially size and shape), incomplete **differentiation**, increased nuclear size and staining. The term is also applied to particularly serious forms of other diseases such as malignant hypertension.

Mallory bleach   An oxidising procedure for decolourising **melanin pigment**. Also used as a preliminary to certain **trichrome** staining procedures. The method involves oxidising sections with potassium permanganate and decolourising with oxalic acid.

Mallory body   See **Alcoholic hyaline**.

Malonyldialdehyde   An end product of **prostaglandin** and **thromboxane** synthesis, which can be measured by using the **thiobarbituric acid** assay. Malonyldialdehyde production can be blocked by aspirin, and this forms the basis of a non-isotopic method of measuring **platelet** survival.

Maltase   An **enzyme** that splits maltose into glucose. It is found in the small intestine.

Mancini test   A quantitative **gel diffusion test** in which **antigen** or **antibody** is allowed to diffuse radially into a gel medium incorporating antigen or antibody, as appropriate. Circles of **precipitation** develop, the diameter of which is proportional to the concentration of the diffusing agent.

Mann Whitney U-test   In statistical usage this is a **non-parametric test** which is used to compare the **medians** of two **independent** groups. It assumes that the groups have the same **distributional** shape, and thus the same **variance**, but that the **medians** may differ. It is analogous to an **independent** groups **t-test**, but does not assume that the data are in a **normal distribution**.

Mantoux test   A test for **hypersensitivity** to a **protein** derived from *Mycobacterium tuberculosis*. If positive the test indicates previous or current infection. The purified protein derivative is injected intradermally in a carefully measured dose and the degree of reaction, in the form of induration, is measured at 48–72 h.

Marburg agent   A member of the **Filoviridae**, first isolated from patients with **haemorrhagic fever** and from African green monkeys. The natural host of this **risk group 4 pathogen** has proved elusive and seems unlikely to be the monkey species associated with the original **outbreak**.

March haemoglobinuria   A condition in which red cell **haemolysis** and **haemoglobinuria** occurs following certain forms of exercise; seen mainly in marching soldiers and long distance runners. The phenomenon is due to physical damage to **erythrocytes**, usually in the soles of the feet, and is cured by cushioning the footwear.

Marginating neutrophil   Peripheral blood **neutrophils** which have temporarily adhered to the walls of capillaries and venules and which are then no longer circulating. These 'marginated' cells are in continual exchange with the circulating neutrophil pool and may be mobilised by administration of **epinephrine**.

Masked basophilia   Acid hydrolysis treatment to reveal masked carboxyl groups which stain with **basic dyes**. The reaction simultaneously removes nucleotide phosphates which would otherwise also react.

Mast cell   Cells found in the tissue, which are similar to peripheral blood **basophils** but which differ slightly from basophils in their granule contents and their method of degranulation.

Mastomys natalensis   The species of multimammate rat notorious for being the natural host of the **virus** of **lassa fever**.

Maturation index   A differential count of **parabasal**, intermediate and superficial cells in a vaginal smear, reflecting **hormone** activity.

Maurer's dots   Coarse, purple-staining dots which may appear in parasitised red cells during heavy infestation of falciparum (malignant tertian) **malaria**.

Maximum Surgical Blood Ordering Schedule   A 'menu' stipulating the normal amount of blood which is provided for **transfusion** in a given hospital or group of hospitals for particular surgical procedures. See also **Menu** (2).

May-Grunwald-Giemsa stain   See **Romanowsky stain**.

May-Hegglin anomaly   A rare autosomal dominant condition associated with giant **platelets** and the presence of **Dohle bodies** in **granulocytes**.

MBC   See **Minimum Bactericidal Concentration**.

McCoy cells   A line of mouse heteroploid cells used in the isolation of *Chlamydia trachomatis*. They should be treated with cycloheximide or irradiated before inoculation, to ensure that they will become infected when exposed to the organism.

MCD   See **Mean Cell Diameter**.

MCF   See **Mean Cell Fragility**.

MCH   See **Mean Cell Haemoglobin**.

MCHC   See **Mean Cell Haemoglobin Concentration**.

MCV   See **Mean Cell Volume**.

Mean   In statistical usage this is the most commonly used average value. The true (**population**) mean can be **estimated** using the **sample** mean, which is the arithmetic average of the observation taken.

Mean cell diameter   (MCD) A means of expressing the red cell diameter observed in dry **blood films** and which normally lies between 6·7 and 7·7 × 10^{-6}m, with a mean of 7·2 × 10^{-6}m.

Mean cell fragility   (MCF) A means of expressing the results of an **osmotic fragility** test as a single figure, and is the concentration of sodium chloride at which 50% **haemolysis** occurs. The normal range is 4−4·45 g/l NaCl.

Mean cell haemoglobin   (MCH) An expression of the average amount of **haemoglobin** contained in the red cells, expressed as **picograms**. The normal range is 27−32 pg. The MCH is diminished in **hypochromic microcytic anaemia** and increased in **macrocytic anaemia**. See also **Absolute values**.

Mean cell haemoglobin concentration   (MCHC) An expression of the average **haemoglobin** concentration in the red cells, given in g/dl. The normal range is 30−35 g/dl. The MCHC may be reduced in **hypochromic microcytic anaemia**. See also **Absolute values**.

Mean cell volume   (MCV) An expression of the average red cell volume expressed in **femtolitres**. The normal range is 76−96 fl. Red cells with an MCV below this range are termed **microcytic**, while a raised MCV results in **macrocytosis**. See also **Absolute values**.

Mean squares   Statistical calculations occurring in an **analysis of variance** table, used to **estimate** the **variance** of observations due to certain **factors**, **blocks** or treatment groupings. The residual mean square is a pooled error variance, measuring the average variability of observations receiving the same treatment and situated in the same **block**, if blocking is used.

Measles   A common **acute** disease of childhood caused by **measles virus**. Patients develop **pyrexia**, cough, suffused eyes, and malaise, followed by a typical rash, and 10% of patients suffer sequelae such as *otitis media*, **pneumonia**, **meningitis** and **encephalitis**. Measles in the first two years of life is associated with the (fortunately rare) **sub-acute sclerosing panencephalitis**, which develops 5–10 years after the initial infection. A **vaccine** has been available for some years.

Measles virus A member of the **Morbillivirus** genus of the **Paramyxoviridae**; the cause of **measles** and most cases of **sub-acute sclerosing panencephalitis**. Laboratory diagnosis is by virus isolation in **cell culture**, or by serological methods. The disease in the immunologically competent individual is readily diagnosed clinically; laboratory services may be required in the case of measles in the **immunocompromised** individual.

Mecillinam A semi-synthetic **anti-microbial** substance of the **beta Lactam** type, derived from **penicillin** and active mainly against **bacteria** which are negative by **Gram's stain**. **Haemophilus** and **Pseudomonas** are resistant. Apart from occasional gastro-intestinal disturbances there are few toxic side-effects. The drug is used mainly in urinary tract infection, but has also been used for systemic infections and bronchitis.

Median In statistical usage, the median is an alternative measure of the average value of a **distribution** to the **mean**. The true, or **population**, median is the mid-point of the **distribution** (i.e. half of the distribution will be smaller than the median and half will be larger. The **estimation** of the median from a **sample** is made by taking the middle value when observations are ordered from the smallest to the largest. When there is an even number of observations it is the average of the two middle observations. For asymmetric distributions it is a better measure of the average value than is the **mean**, as it is less affected by occasional unusually large or unusually small observations.

Medical Laboratory Scientific Officer A class of employment in the British National Health Service for individuals skilled in the theory and practise of the procedures of the medical laboratory. Entry to this professional class is normally by possession of a degree in one or more of the biological sciences followed by in-service training prior to statutory registration with the Council for Professions Supplementary to Medicine (**CPSM**). Alternatively, in some areas entry is still open to those in possession of a Higher National Certificate in medical laboratory sciences. Progression to more senior professional grades requires acquisition of a higher professional qualification, normally Fellowship of the Institute of Medical Laboratory Sciences (**FIMLS**).

Megakaryoblast The earliest recognisable precursor cell of the **megakaryocyte**, which arises from the same pluripotential stem cell as the **erythrocyte** and **granulocyte** series.

Megakaryocyte A large cell (35–160 × 10^{-6} m in diameter) with multi-lobed nuclei, found in the **bone marrow**, lung and spleen, and which gives rise to the formation of platelets.

Megaloblastic anaemia An **anaemia**, usually **normochromic** and **macrocytic**, associated with the appearance of **megaloblastic** changes in the **bone marrow**. Megaloblastic red cell precursors are larger than their **normoblastic** counterparts and are additionally distinguished by the more open pattern of the nuclear chromatin. Megaloblastic anaemia is also associated with **hypersegmentation** of the **neutrophils** and is most commonly the result of **folic acid** or **vitamin B12** deficiency.

Meiosis The process by which the **chromosomes** are separated during formation of the sex cells and their number reduced from the **diploid**.

Melanin A yellow-brown to black pigment occuring normally in hair, skin and eyes. Also present in pathological conditions, both **benign** and **malignant**. Synthesised from tyrosine and stored in the melanosomes of melanocytes.

Melioidosis An infection due to *Pseudomonas pseudomallei*, which can occur as a localised infection of the subcutaneous tissues with lymphangitis, or as a generalised infection with **pneumonia**, **septicaemia** and **abscess** formation. The organisms are usually introduced from soil and water into abrasions, and many years may elapse before infection becomes apparent. The disease is **endemic** in south-east Asia, and military personnel and other travellers from western countries sometimes become infected. The causative organism is usually susceptible to several **anti-microbial** substances including **Trimethoprim** and **Chloramphenicol**.

Membrane 1. The thin continuous sheet-like structure which surrounds cells. 2. A thin layer of specialised tissue which divides a space or an organ, lines a cavity or covers a surface.

Memory In computing, a device or series of devices in which information can be stored and retrieved. Memory may be internal, as in the **Read Only Memory** of the **Central Processing Unit**, or external as in a **file** stored on a **floppy disc**.

Memory cell In the body, a long-lived **T cell** or **B cell** which is responsible for **immunological memory**.

Meningitis Inflammation of the meninges, characterised by headache, photophobia, stiff neck, **pyrexia** and vomiting. It can be caused by **bacteria**, **viruses**, **fungi**, **protozoa**, chemicals and **malignant** and auto-immune mechanisms. Bacterial meningitis is frequently septic, severe, and rapidly fatal if untreated. In the laboratory the diagnosis is made by the finding of excess **neutrophils** in the **cerebrospinal fluid**, and the finding of morphologically definable organisms in a **Gram stained** film is invaluable. In the presence of a suggestive clinical history, but the absence of organisms in Gram film or culture, **antigen** can be detected in the cerebrospinal fluid using **latex agglutination** tests. Viral meningitis is usually aseptic and **benign**, but may proceed to **encephalitis**.

Meningo-encephalitis Infection of the meninges (**meningitis**) along with infection of the substance of the brain. The inflammation, microvascular damage and cellular infiltration of the white or grey matter of the brain tissue gives rise to typical neurological signs. The infection is most often caused by a **virus** but can be due to *Listeria monocytogenes*, *Cryptococcus neoformans*, *Naegleria fowleri*, *Toxoplasma gondii* and other organisms.

Menu 1. In computing, a displayed list of options offered in a **program**, for the operator to select an action which will enable the program to proceed in a selected direction. 2. In transfusion medicine, a list stipulating the normal amount of blood which is provided for **transfusion** in a given hospital or group of hospitals for particular surgical procedures. See **Maximum Surgical Blood Ordering Schedule**.

2-Mercaptoethanol A sulphadryl compound used in **serology** to reduce human **IgM** molecules so as to abolish the ability of the **antibody** to behave as an **agglutinin**, thus distinguishing IgM from **IgG** antibodies. Due to its unpleasant odour it is not as much used for this purpose as is **dithiothreitol**.

Mercury pigment Dark brown, grey or black irregular masses of **artefact** in tissue, caused by **fixation** in mercuric solutions. It may be removed by sequential treatment with iodine and sodium thiosulphate.

Merozoite The 'young ring' form in the life cycle of the **parasite** of **malaria**, seen in peripheral blood and usually marking the onset of **febrile** episodes throughout malarial infections. Merozoites also occur in liver cells, from where they are released into the blood stream. See also **Schizont, Hypnozoite, Malaria**.

Mesenteric adenitis A condition characterised by abdominal pain and **pyrexia**, often mistaken for appendicitis. The mesenteric lymph nodes are enlarged and inflamed at laparotomy. The commonest causative organism is *Yersinia enterocolitica*.

Mesonephroma A **tumour** arising from the mesonephros, or primitive kidney.

Mesothelioma A **tumour** derived from mesothelial tissue.

Messenger RNA In normal cells this is transcribed from **DNA**, and carries the message to ribosomes, from which **proteins** are produced. The **genomes** of some RNA **viruses** act as their own messengers, and enable the virus to replicate without the involvement of cellular DNA.

Metabolism The process of altering and converting compounds into structures, followed by breakdown and excretion, by which all living organisms grow and maintain themselves..

Metachromasia The property of certain **dyes** to change colour without change of chemical structure. It is brought about by physical changes involving **Van der Waal's forces**, to form dimers, trimers and polymers.

Metacyclic A term used to describe the infective stage of a **parasite**, usually when it changes in its life cycle from a resting phase to an actively dividing stage.

Metamyelocyte One of the **granulocyte** precursor cells, characterised by a clearly indented or horseshoe-shaped nucleus. The **cytoplasmic** granules classify the cell into **neutrophilic**, **eosinophilic** or **basophilic** type.

Metaphase The middle stage of **mitosis**, during which the lengthwise separation of the **chromosomes** occurs.

Metaplasia The replacement of one mature cell type by mature cells of another cell type.

Metastasis The process by which **malignant** cells are disseminated from a **tumour** to form a new growth at a distant site.

Metathrombin The functionally inactive complex formed when **thrombin** is bound by another protein (for example, **albumin**).

Methacarn A modern formulation for tissue **fixation**. A mixture of methanol and **Carnoy's fluid** used especially in **immunocytochemistry**.

Methaemalbumin A complex of **haem** and **albumin** formed following the liberation of **haemoglobin** into the **plasma** during predominantly intravascular **haemolysis**. It is only found following the saturation of the **haptoglobin** and haemopexin systems for trapping free haemoglobin.

Methaemoglobin A form of **haemoglobin** in which the iron has become oxidised and therefore cannot transport oxygen. Methaemoglobin is continually being formed in normal **erythrocytes**, but is reconverted to normal haemoglobin by NADH diaphorase. Methaemoglobinaemia may develop if the red cells are deficient in this **enzyme** or are exposed to high concentrations of oxidant drugs or chemicals.

Methylation Treatment of **acid mucopolysaccharides** with hydrochloric acid in methanol. Treatment at 37°C for 4 h abolishes **basophilia** of most carboxyl groups (mild methylation) and at 60°C, of all acid mucopolysaccharides (active methylation). Reactivity may be restored by **saponification**.

Metricillin A semi-synthetic **penicillin** which is resistant to staphylococcal **penicillinase**. It is active against both **coagulase**-positive and negative **staphylococci**, and while it is also active against some other organisms positive by **Gram's stain** it is not recommended for treatment of infections due to these. As with other **beta lactam** type of **anti-microbial** substances it acts by interfering with **peptidoglycan** synthesis. Resistant strains of both *Staphylococcus aureus* and coagulase-negative staphylococci occur, in which the resistance is not due to inactivation of the drug by **beta lactamase**. Resistance to **methicillin** (and to **flucloxacillin**) can reliably be detected only by testing on osmotically enhanced **culture media** and/or at 30°C.

Metronidazole A synthetic **nitroimidazole** type of **anti-microbial** substance which is active against **anaerobic** organisms including **Bacteroides** species, **Clostridium** species, **Spirochaetes**, and **protozoa** including *Trichomonas vaginalis*. Though the drug is taken up by both **aerobes** and **anaerobes**, only the latter are susceptible. The drug must be reduced in order to be active, and a very low **redox potential** is required inside the cell. Once reduced, the drug stimulates the formation of toxic-free radicles which directly damage DNA, thus halting protein synthesis. Development of resistance is rare. Toxicity is uncommon, but on high or prolonged dosage peripheral neuropathy has been observed. The drug induces an adverse reaction if alcohol is also consumed.

Mezlocillin A semi-synthetic ureido **penicillin** with activity against **bacteria** which are negative by **Gram's stain**, including **pseudomonas**. Strains of *Staphylococcus aureus* which produce **penicillinase** are resistant, as are **enterococci**.

MHC See **Major Histocompatibility Complex**.

MIC See **Minimum Inhibitory Concentration**.

Michaelis constant The concentration of a **substrate** at which the **enzyme** activity is progressing at half the maximum speed. It is a measure of enzyme-substrate affinity.

Miconazole A synthetic **imidazole** type of **anti-microbial** substance with wide anti-**fungal** activity which includes **yeasts** and **dermatophytes**. Resistant strains of *Candida albicans* and *Aspergillus fumigatus* occur. The drug acts by damaging the fungal cell **membrane**, causing leakage of essential cytoplasmic constituents. Miconazole is relatively free from toxic side-effects, but **haematological** and gastro-intestinal problems are sometimes encountered. Thrombophlebitis may complicate intravenous use.

Microaerophilic (Of **micro-organisms**): requiring an atmosphere depleted in oxygen, but not devoid of it, for growth. Some organisms in this group grow better in the presence of carbon dioxide.

Microangiopathic haemolytic anaemia A haemolytic **anaemia** caused by mechanical damage to **erythrocytes** in the arteriolar circulation, as a result of **endothelial** damage or **fibrin** deposition within the vessel. This process results in red cell fragmentation and the presence of **schistocytes** in the peripheral blood.

Microbiology The study of living organisms which are too small to be seen by the naked eye, including **bacteria**, many **parasites**, **viruses** and many **fungi**. The definition is relaxed to include larger parasites such as **helminths** and filamentous fungi. Medical microbiology is the study only of those organisms of medical importance, but in modern infectious diseases practice the distinction is difficult to maintain.

Microcalorimetry The quantitative measurement of heat emitted by a culture of **micro-organisms** during metabolism. The main use of the technique is in the testing of **anti-microbial** substances, when results become available within 1 or 2 h. In batch microcalorimetry the culture vessel is surrounded by the heat detection system, whereas in flow calorimetry the culture fluid is pumped through the detector and returned to the culture vessel.

Micrococcaceae A family of **micro-organisms** consisting of the genera **Micrococcus**, **Staphylococcus** and Planococcus. The organisms are **cocci** which are positive by **Gram's stain** and which divide in more than one plane to produce packet or cluster shapes. They are **catalase** positive, grow in the presence of 50 g/l sodium chloride, and may be obligate **aerobes** or facultative **anaerobes**. Most strains do not exhibit **motility**.

Micrococcus A group of **micro-organisms** which are **catalase** positive **cocci**, obligate **aerobes** which are positive by **Gram's stain**. Their taxonomy is unclear but it is suggested that there are three species: *M. luteus*, *M. varians* and *M. roseus*. Some strains of the latter are said to exhibit **motility**. They are susceptible to **lysozyme** but resistant to lysostaphin. They grow on ordinary **culture media** to produce colonies which are often pigmented. Various methods for distinguishing micrococci from **staphylococci** are available, but all require care. Micrococci rarely cause disease in humans.

Microcomputer A small computer, the **central processing unit** of which is contained within a **microprocessor**.

Microcytic anaemia Any **anaemia** in which the **mean cell volume** is less than 76 fl. The most common cause is **iron deficiency**, when the peripheral blood picture is usually − but not always − **hypochromic** and **microcytic**.

Microcytosis The term given to red cells which appear smaller than normal in the peripheral **blood film**. This is usually reflected in a reduction in the **mean cell volume**.

Microcytotoxicity test A test used for detecting **antigens** of the **HLA** series on **lymphocytes**, by serological means. Lymphocytes are exposed to **antibody** in the presence of **complement**. Specific reactions between the antibody and an HLA antigen lead to

complement fixation and lymphocyte **membrane** damage. These positive reactions are detected by the failure of damaged cells to exclude dyes.

Microdensitometry **Spectrophotometry** carried out through a microscope. Non-uniform distribution of **dye** in areas of stained sections is overcome by scanning and integrating measurements.

Microembolus A very small blood clot, of microscopic size.

Microfilaria Larvae of filarial worms (e.g. *Loa loa, Wucheria bancrofti*, etc.), which can be demonstrated in blood and other body fluids. The adults block the lymphatics, particularly of the pendulous parts of the body, eventually producing grossly distorted disfigurement. See **Chyle** and **Filariasis**.

(beta) Microglobulin A non-glycosylated peptide of 12 000 D which is associated with the structure of **class I antigens** of the major histocompatibility complex (**MHC antigens**). It also occurs free in **serum** or urine as a globular peptide having a structure similar to that of an immunoglobulin **constant region domain**.

Microhaematocrit A method of measuring the **packed cell volume** by centrifuging a capillary tube filled with blood in a specially designed **centrifuge**.

Micro-incineration Heating of tissue sections to high temperature (e.g. 650°C) and examining the residue in oblique light or by **polarisation** microscopy to determine mineral content.

Micrometry The technique used for determining the size of microscopic objects, employing a **stage micrometer** and an **eyepiece graticule**. In the simplest form, an eyepiece micrometer with an arbitrary scale is employed together with an accurately engraved stage micrometer with a millimetre scale divided into 100 gradations.

Micron A unit of length. The thousandth part of one millimetre. In SI usage it is termed a micrometre.

Micro-organism A small, microscopic living organism. Those of interest in the biomedical sciences include **bacteria**, **fungi**, **protozoa**, **rickettsia** and **viruses**.

Microphage A **polymorphonuclear neutrophil**.

Microprocessor A **central processing unit** contained on a single **chip**.

Microradiography A method used to determine the presence and study the distribution of **radioisotopes** in tissue sections.

Microscopy, electron The microscopical examination of samples, using an electron beam instead of visible or ultra-violet light. The samples have to be prepared in advance by **dehydration**, sectioning, **staining** or coating with metallic compounds before examination. The electron beam is produced in a high vacuum by a hot filament and focused and magnified by electromagnets. Because of the very short wavelength of electrons, high **magnification** and high **resolution** can be achieved. **Scanning electron microscopy** uses electrons which are reflected from the surface of the sample, while in **transmission electron microscopy** the electrons pass through the sample. See **Scanning electron microscope** and **Transmission electron microscope**.

Microscopy, light The microscopical examination of samples using visible or ultraviolet light. The light is focused and the image magnified by conventional glass lenses. The sample must be transparent except where incident light reaches it from above, and it can be stained to distinguish various components by colour. Ultraviolet light is usually employed in order to excite a sample with a fluorescent **dye** which emits light when in contact with ultra-violet light. The dyes are often combined with **antibody** specific for a component of the sample, such as a **capsule** or **cell wall**, so that fluorescence is selective. Because of the relatively long wavelength of light the resolving power is approximately 250 millimicrons compared to less than 0·5 millimicrons for electron microscopy.

Microsome A term originally applied to a cell fraction containing rough surfaced membranous vesicles of **cytoplasm**. Probably represents **ribosomes** and the **membrane** of the **endoplasmic reticulum**.

Microspore Small, usually uni-cellular asexual **spores** produced by filamentous **fungi**, including the **dermatophytes**. They are important in identification of fungi.

Microsporum A genus in the **dermatophyte** group of **fungi**, responsible for ringworm.

Microtitre plate A tray used for serological reactions, made of rigid polystyrene and containing a matrix of wells each of about 500 microlitre capacity. The usual format is of 96 wells in 12 columns and eight rows. The wells may have a round, flat or conical base and resemble a block of small capacity test tubes.

Microtome An instrument used to cut thin sections (from 2 to 20 **microns**) of (e.g.) tissue. Types of microtome include rocking, sliding and base-sledge designs. A freezing microtome is used to produce sections from frozen tissue. See also **Cryostat** and **Ultramicrotome**.

Microtomy The preparation of thin sections or slices of tissue for microscopy using a special cutting instrument, the **microtome**

Minimum Bactericidal Concentration (MBC) The lowest concentration of an **anti-microbial** substance which is lethal to the inoculum *in vitro*. Attention must be paid to inoculum size, type of test medium, growth phase of the organism and time and temperature of incubation. A large difference between MBC and **MIC** indicates **tolerance**.

Minimum Inhibitory Concentration (MIC) The lowest concentration of an **anti-microbial** substance which prevents visible growth of organisms *in vitro*. Attention must be paid to inoculum size, type of test medium, growth phase of the organism and time and temperature of incubation.

Minocycline A member of the **tetracycline** group of **anti-microbial** substances, which has higher activity against susceptible strains than has tetracycline itself. It is also active against some tetracycline-resistant organisms.

Miracidium A stage in the life cycle of the **flukes**. A free-swimming ciliated form which penetrates the **membranes** of an intermediate host (a snail) where it develops before being shed as **cercaria**, which are infective to man.

Miscarriage See **Abortion**.

Mite Many species infect domestic animals but only one − *Sarcoptes scabiei*, the scabies mite − causes disease in man. The burrows made by the scabies mite, around the hairy areas of the body and between the fingers, produce intense itching. Dissemination of the mite is commonly through contact with infested persons, their clothing, towels and bed linen.

Mitochondrion A self-contained cytoplasmic structure responsible for cell respiration. Easily recognised in tissue sections by **electron microscopy** as round or oval shaped cross-banded cell **organelles**.

Mitogen An agent capable of stimulating **mitosis**. In **immunology** this usually refers to substances such as **Con-A** or **phytohaemagglutinin**, which stimulate mitosis in human **T cells**.

Mitogenic factor A soluble factor (**lymphokine**) liberated by activated **T cells**, which stimulates **mitosis** in other **lymphocytes**.

Mitosis The process of cell division, giving rise to two daughter cells, each of which exactly duplicates the **chromosome** content of the parent cell.

Mitotic index The number of cells in any given pool currently undergoing **mitosis**, divided by the total number of cells in the pool. In **bone marrow** the mitotic index is approximately 1−2%.

Mixed field agglutination A reaction in which some of the red cells in a sample are **agglutinated** by a particular anti-serum while others are not.

Mixed lymphocyte reaction or culture A **compatibility test** between **lymphocytes**. Two populations of lymphocytes are cultured together for several days and then examined for the presence of **blast cells**. The number of blast cells present is related to the degree of **histocompatibility** between the lymphocytes.

Mixed vaccine A **vaccine** containing **antigens** derived from two or more different species of **pathogen**.

MLSO   See **Medical Laboratory Scientific Officer**.

Mode   A quantity in distribution that appears more frequently than any other.

Modem   A MOdulator/DEModulator. In computing, a device for converting data from **digital** to **analogue** form and *vice versa*, and either transmitting the modulated signal along a telephone line, or receiving such a signal and re-converting it to digital form. Used to allow computers to communicate with each other through the telephone system.

Modified Thayer-Martin medium   A **culture medium** consisting of heated **blood agar** containing **Vancomycin** 3 mg/l, **colistin** 7·5 mg/l and **Nystatin** 12 500 u/l. It is used as a **selective medium** for *Neisseria gonorrhoaea* and *N. meningitidis*. Strains of *Branhamella catarrhalis* will also grow on it.

Molar absorption coefficient   The absorption of light by a solution of a compound at a concentration of 1 mol/l, with a light path of 1 cm.

Molecular exclusion chromatography   A technique for separating macro-molecules such as **proteins**. Molecules for investigation are applied to a column of beads of gel with known pore size. Smaller molecules enter the beads of gel and are delayed in the column, whereas large molecules are excluded from the gel beads and pass through the column more quickly.

Mollicute   A class of **bacteria**, the cells of which are bounded by a cell **membrane** but no **cell wall**. They vary considerably in size and shape. Enriched **culture media** are usually essential for growth. The class contains two families, Mycoplasmataceae and Acholeplasmataceae. *Mycoplasma pneumoniae* is a common cause of respiratory infections, and other species cause disease in animals. Cell wall-active **anti-microbial** substances are ineffective.

Molluscum contagiosum   One of the **Poxviridae**, causing warty lesions of the skin. Laboratory diagnosis is by **electron microscopy** of a crushed excised lesion. The virus has not been grown *in vitro*.

Monkey kidney cell culture   Derived from the **enzyma**tically digested cortex of excised kidneys and widely used in **monolayers** as **primary cell** or **secondary cell** cultures for the isolation of a variety of **viruses**, particularly **enteroviruses**, **influenza A virus**, **influenza B virus** and the **Paramyxoviridae**. A number of monkey viruses, notably SV5 and **foamy viruses**, interfere with their sensitivity. The cultures are expensive, requiring a constant supply of animals, and a more or less continuous search is in progress for alternatives.

Monkey pox   An **orthopoxvirus** of monkeys, closely resembling **variola** virus. It is **zoonotic** in man, causing a relatively mild **smallpox**-like illness.

Monobactam   A **beta Lactam** type of **anti-microbial** substance which lacks the usual thalizolidine ring found in **cephalosporins** and **penicillins**.

Monochromator   A device used to isolate a selected portion of the electromagnetic spectrum.

Monoclonal   Describing a population of identical cells derived from a single precursor. From a single **clone**.

Monoclonal antibody   An **immunoglobulin** derived from a **monoclonal hybridoma**. Each immunoglobulin molecule is identical in terms of chemical structure and specificity.

Monoclonal selection theory   See **Burnett's monoclonal selection theory**.

Monocyte   A non-granular form of **leucocyte**, comprising 2−10% of the peripheral blood leucocytes. The cell is approximately 16−22 × 10^{-6} m in diameter, with abundant **cytoplasm**, appearing light blue with **Romanowsky stains** and containing a kidney or horseshoe-shaped nucleus.

Monocytosis   An increase in the number of peripheral blood **monocytes** above the upper normal limit of $0.8 \times 10^9/l$.

Monokine   A soluble product released from **macrophages** (e.g. **Interleukin 1**).

Monolayer cell culture   A **cell culture** grown as a single layer of cells attached to a surface − usually clear glass or plastic.

Mononuclear   Having one nucleus.

Mononuclear phagocytic system   See **Reticulo-endothelial system**.

Monospecific anti-serum   A **serum** containing **antibody** directed against a single **antigenic** determinant.

Monospot test™   A rapid and specific test for the **heterophil** antibody of infectious mononucleosis, based on the ability of the **antibody** to cause **agglutination** of formalinised horse red cells.

Montenegro test   A test used to assist the diagnosis of **Leishmaniasis**. **Antigen** prepared from cultures of *Leishmania promastigotes* is injected intradermally, stimulating a response in most cases of cutaneous disease. See **Kala-azar** and **Leishmaniasis**.

Moraxella   Rod-shaped members of the *Neisseriaceae* family of **bacteria** which do not exhibit **motility**, are obligate **aerobes**, both **catalase** and **oxidase** positive, asaccharolytic and negative by **Gram's stain**. Some strains will grow on **blood agar** while others, such as *M. lacunata* − which is associated with **conjunctivitis** − require enrichment with **serum**.

Morbillivirus   A genus of the **Paramyxoviridae** which includes **measles virus**.

Mordant   A substance which acts as an intermediary between a **dye** and tissue, to enhance staining by forming a **lake** with the dye.

Morganella   Rod-shaped **bacteria** which exhibit **motility**, are facultative **anaerobes**, **catalase** positive, **oxidase** negative, urease positive, capable of deaminating phenylalanine, and negative by **Gram's stain**. Unlike **Proteus** species, citrate is not utilised as a sole source of carbon. As with many other members of the **Enterobacteriaceae**, Morganella species cause infections of surgical wounds and the urinary tract.

Morphology   Study of the shapes of cells and organisms.

Morula cell   A **plasma cell** producing **IgM**, occurring typically in the area of perivascular cuffing seen in brain sections (and sometimes in **cerebrospinal fluid**) in cases of Trypanosomiasis.

Mosaicism   Multiple **chromosome** constitution of different cell lines resulting in different numbers of chromosomes in the same person. See **Chimera**.

Mosquito, Anopheline   The **vector** and definitive host of the **plasmodium** (i.e. the **parasite**) of **malaria**. Numerous species occur around the world. Only the female sucks blood and, if infected, inoculates **sporozoites** into the victim.

Motility   The movement of an organism through a fluid medium. Propulsion may be due to the action of **flagella** or, less commonly, by axial filaments as with **Spirochaetes**. A few **bacteria**, such as **Capnocytophagia**, exhibit gliding motility while having no known means of propulsion. Motility is usually in random patterns, but in the presence of a positive or negative stimulus the motility becomes directed towards or away from the stimulus. Motility can be detected microscopically or by using semi-solid **culture media**.

Motor end plate   Nerve ending, especially in muscle.

Mountant   A material used to affix a cover-slip to a microscopical preparation such as a tissue section. Should have a high **refractive index** to improve **resolution**.

Moxalactam   An oxacephem type of **anti-microbial** substance which has a **beta Lactam** ring but in whose accompanying ring the sulphur is replaced with oxygen. The drug is active against a range of rod-shaped **bacteria** which are facultative **anaerobes** and negative by **Gram's stain**, and also *Bacteroides fragilis*, but is poorly active against Gram positive bacteria. While generally free from side effects, development of a haemorrhagic state sometimes occurs.

M-protein   One of three major protein **antigens** situated in the outer **cell wall** of *Streptococcus pyogenes*. M-proteins are associated with **virulence** and, with **lipoteichoic acids**, with attachment to mammalian cells. The various antigenic types are associated more commonly with infection in certain sites and with sequelae such as **nephritis** or rheumatic fever.

MRC Medical Research Council.

MRCPath Member of the Royal College of Pathologists. See **RCPath**.

MSBOS See **Maximum Surgical Blood Ordering Schedule**.

MS.DOS™ MicroSoft Disc Operating System. A proprietory **operating system** in widespread use on **16 bit computers**.

Mucin A common term for describing **mucopolysaccharide**, mucosubstance or **glycoconjugate**. A polysaccharide containing hexosamine and bound to variable amounts of **protein**.

Mucopolysaccharide See **Mucin**.

Mucoprotein Also known as **glycoprotein**. A polysaccharide bound to protein, found mainly in epithelial secretions. See also **mucin**.

Mucormycosis See **Zygomycosis**.

Mueller-Hinton agar A **culture medium** recommended for testing for **anti-microbial** susceptibility. The medium supports growth of most fastidious organisms when supplemented with horse blood. The **pH** of the medium changes little during growth of the organisms and gives reproducible results in **disc diffusion** tests.

Multigravida A woman who has been pregnant more than once, although has not necessarily delivered any live-born children.

Multi-nucleated giant cell A large **macrophage** containing from 2 to 30 nuclei in finely **vacuolated cytoplasm**.

Multipara A woman during or subsequent to her second pregnancy. A woman who has born one previous child is para 1, etc. A woman pregnant for the first time (see **Primigravida**) is para 0.

Multiple myeloma A **malignant tumour** of the bone marrow, marked by circumscribed or diffuse tumour-like **hyperplasia** of the marrow.

Multipoint inoculator A device for simultaneous inoculation of approximately 20 samples onto the surfaces of a large number of **agar** plates. The device is used to identify large numbers of **bacteria** by their inoculation onto agar **culture media** containing various **substrates** and detector systems, or in **bacteriophage** typing. See also **Phage type**.

Multivariate analysis Any statistical method which enables several different **variables** measured on each individual to be analysed together. Two commonly used methods are: discriminant analysis, which is used when individuals belong to predetermined groups and it is desired to find a simple method, based on the variables measured, of determining to which group a new individual belongs; and cluster analysis which is used to group individuals on the basis of the variables observed so that individuals in each group are as like each other as possible, and as unlike those in other groups as possible.

Mumps A common childhood disease characterised by inflammation and swelling of the parotid glands, caused by the **mumps
virus**. A proportion of cases are complicated by **meningitis** and,
rarely, **encephalitis**. Adult males may develop orchitis, though
sterility does not seem to result from this. A **vaccine** has been
available for some years.

Mumps virus A member of the paramyxovirus genus of the **Paramyxoviridae**, which causes **mumps**. It may also be the single most
common cause of **aseptic** forms of **meningitis**. Laboratory diagnosis is by virus isolation in **cell culture**, or by demonstrating
seroconversion using **complement fixation tests** or **haemagglutination inhibition tests**.

Muramidase See **Lysozyme**.

Mutation A change in the characteristics of a gene in the offspring,
as compared with the parent.

Mycetoma See **Madura foot**.

Mycobacterium Rod-shaped **bacteria** which do not exhibit **motility**,
do not form **spores**, are obligate **aerobes** and which retain carbol
fuchsin **dye** during attempted de-colourisation with acid and alcohol, and which generally stain poorly by **Gram's stain**. All grow
relatively slowly and some very slowly, taking several weeks to
form a visible colony. Enriched **culture media** are often necessary
for growth. The **cell wall** is very rich in lipids (**mycolic acids**). *M.
tuberculosis* causes tuberculosis in man, while other species cause
disease in animals but can also infect man, especially individuals
who are **immunosuppressed**.

Mycobactin A lipid-soluble substance produced by *Mycobacterium
tuberculosis*, concerned with capture of iron and its transport into
the cell. Mycobactins are the probable targets for the action of
para-aminosalicylic acid.

Mycolic acids Alpha-branched beta-hydroxy acids found in the **cell
walls** of members of the genera **Mycobacterium**, **Nocardia** and
Corynebacterium. The acids vary in the number of carbon atoms
between the genera and between species, and their characterisation is useful in taxonomy.

Mycology The study of **fungi**. Medical mycology is the study of
those fungi − almost all microscopic − which cause human disease.

Mycoplasma The smallest free-living organisms. A genus of **bacteria** which lacks the ability to synthesise **peptidoglycan**, and therefore does not have **cell walls**, the cell being enclosed in a typical
three-layered cell **membrane** and varying greatly in size and shape.
All members of the genus − of which there are over 30 − require
cholesterol or related sterols for growth, along with fatty acids.
They can be isolated on complex **culture media** enriched with

serum, on which they appear as colonies of 'fried egg' appearance, with a central portion which penetrates into the **agar.** *M. pneumoniae* — the only proven **pathogen** in the group — is the causative organism of 'atypical' **pneumonia** and other respiratory tract infections. Sometimes other (probably non-infective) sequelae occur at distant sites. The organisms are resistant to the **beta Lactam** type of **anti-microbial** substance, but are susceptible to **erythromycin** and **tetracycline.**

Mycoplasma pneumoniae An important cause of primary atypical **pneumonia.** Laboratory investigation is usually serological, using **complement fixation tests** or **passive haemagglutination tests.** The organism will grow in heavily enriched media, although it may be some days before recognisable growth occurs.

Mycosis Infection by a **fungus.** Dermatomycosis is infection of the skin, usually by **dermatophytes.**

Myelin A specialised compound **lipid** of the nervous system, found as a sheath around certain nerve **axons.**

Myeloblast The earliest recognisable **bone marrow** precursor of the granulocyte series of blood cells. The myeloblast is a spherical cell, approximately $11-18 \times 10^{-6}$ m in diameter, containing a relatively large nucleus with several **nucleoli.**

Myelocyte One of the **granulocyte** precursors in the **bone marrow.** By this stage of maturation the **nucleoli** have disappeared and the cell contains the specific granules which characterise neutrophilic, eosinophilic and basophilic lineage.

Myelofibrosis A **malignant** proliferation of **bone marrow** fibroblasts leading to fibrosis of the marrow space, osteosclerosis and extra-medullary **haemopoiesis.**

Myelogram A differential count of all the nucleated cells in the **bone marrow.**

Myelokathexis A synonym for **chronic** idiopathic granulocytopenia resulting from intramedullary (i.e. within the **bone marrow**) retention and death of **neutrophils.**

Myeloma cell A type of cell occurring in the **bone marrow** of patients with **multiple myeloma** (myelomatosis) and which is responsible for the **malignant** production of **immunoglobulin (myeloma protein)** characteristic of this condition.

Myeloma protein An homogenous **(monoclonal) immunoglobulin** produced by neoplastic **plasma cells** in the **bone marrow** of individuals with **myelomatosis.** Myeloma protein is also called **paraprotein.**

Myelomatosis A disease in which **plasma cells** proliferate in the **bone marrow.** The plasma cells are derived from a single neoplastic precursor and produce a **monoclonal** form of **myeloma protein** which appears in the **plasma.** See **Paraprotein.**

Myeloperoxidase An **enzyme** present in high concentration in the primary granules of the **neutrophil** and which generates a powerful **bactericidal** activity in conjunction with hydrogen peroxide and halide ions.

Myelophthistic anaemia A relatively non-specific term given to the appearance of nucleated red cells and myeloid precursors in the peripheral blood film. See also **Leuco-erythroblastic anaemia**.

Myeloproliferative disorder A disorder involving **malignant** proliferation of the myeloid cells including **acute** and **chronic** myeloid **leukaemias, myelofibrosis, erythroleukaemia, polycythaemia rubra vera** and essential **thrombocythaemia**.

Myiasis A condition produced when fly larvae of particular species, found only in Africa and South America, invade living tissue. Occasionally imported into Europe and temperate zones as infections which resemble a boil from which, if not removed, a larva emerges.

Myocarditis Inflammation of the heart muscle. It may have a variety of infectious and non-infectious causes.

Myoglobin A respiratory pigment, similar to **haemoglobin**, but containing only one haem group. Its function is to store oxygen in muscle tissue.

Myoglobinuria The appearance of **myoglobin** in the peripheral blood as the result of massive muscle injury (e.g. by severe trauma or electric shock).

Myoma A **benign tumour** composed of muscular elements.

Myxoedema A swelling of the tongue and face, associated with a reduction in the level of thyroid **hormones**. There is frequently an increase in the level of thyroid-stimulating hormone (TSH) in the serum.

N

N.A. Abbreviation for **Numerical Aperture**.

N.A.D. An abbreviation which is widely and loosely used to indicate, *inter alia*: 1. Nicotinamide Adenine Dinucleotide; 2. No Appreciable Disease; or 3. any combination of the following words.

Nil	Abnormal	Demonstrated
Nothing		
No	Acetone	Detectable/Detected
	Agglutination	Discovered
	Antibodies	

Naegleria Free-living amoeba with a flagellate stage, which live in fresh water. They are able to cause disease in humans who swim in lakes which contain large numbers of the organisms. They enter the nasal cavity and invade by way of the cribiform plate to reach the central nervous system. Here they cause haemorrhagic necrosis to the olfactory bulbs and other structures, resulting in death in a few days. The cerebrospinal fluid is turbid, having a high **neutrophil** count, and sluggishly mobile amoebae can be seen in preparations of warm fluid. They can be isolated on simple **culture media** if heated *Escherichia coli* are first applied to the surface. There is no effective treatment for the **meningoencephalitis**. The related Acanthamoeba causes kerato **conjunctivitis**.

Nalidixic acid A synthetic **quinolone** type of **anti-microbial** substance which is active mainly against **Enterobacteriaceae**, and which is used principally to treat urinary tract infections. Gram positive **cocci**, including **enterococci**, are resistant. The drug exerts its anti-microbial action by inhibiting **DNA** gyrase, thus halting DNA synthesis. Resistant mutants arise with high frequency. Toxic effects include gastro-intestinal and central nervous system disturbances.

NANB hepatitis See **Hepatitis non-A, non-B**.

Nanometre A unit of measurement that is used to describe the frequency intervals of the wave cycles in light radiation (10^{-9} m).

Natural dye Extract of plant or animal used as a **dye**. Carmine and, particularly, **haematoxylin** are examples.

Natural killer cell A **leucocyte** capable of 'recognising' and killing **tumour** cells and cells infected by **viruses**, independently of any specific **antibody**. Natural killer (NK) cells also play a role in the regulation of the **immune response**.

'Naturally occurring' antibody An **antibody** for which the stimulus is not readily apparent and which, in contradiction to the definition of antibody, appears to occur in the plasma of an individual without a specific stimulus. Such antibodies (which are generally IgM in nature) are often **hetero**-immune and may be the result of bacterial (etc.) stimuli.

Navicular cells Cells with a 'boat-like' shape, carrying yellow deposits of **glycogen** in their **cytoplasm**. Found especially in vaginal smears during pregnancy.

NBTS The National Blood Transfusion Service of England and Wales. Contrary to its name, there is no national structure and the NBTS consists of a series of services provided independently by regional health authorities.

NBT test See **Nitroblue tetrazolium test**.

NCCLS National Committee for Clinical Laboratory Standards (both in the UK and the USA).

Nearest neighbour sequence analysis A method of characterising and identifying **DNA** molecules using radio-labelled **nucleotides**.

NEC See **Necrotising enterocolitis**.

Necoloidine An ether-based supporting medium used instead of **paraffin wax** in some procedures in **histopathology**. It has proved useful in making permanent preparations of **monolayers** in **cell cultures**.

Necrosis Death of a tissue, as individual cells, groups of cells or in small localised areas. It may be due either to infective processes and the host response to them, or to non-infective causes such as ischaemia. Some bacterial toxins – especially those of **clostridia** – cause **necrosis**, which is also a feature of necrotising **fasciitis** caused by mixtures of **anaerobes**.

Necrotising enterocolitis A **syndrome** affecting mainly newborn infants (particularly those born prematurely) and consisting of failure to feed, abdominal distension, apnoeic attacks and blood in the **faeces**. Typically, gas bubbles are seen in the bowel wall on radiographs. At laparotomy the mucosa, submucosa and sometimes the muscularis and serosa are necrotic, leading in severe cases to perforation and **peritonitis**. The cause of the condition is unknown and the precipitating event may not be an **infection**, as transient ischaemia can precipitate the lesions in animals. However, the nature of the lesions suggests the involvement of **clostridia**. Treatment consists of parenteral nutrition, resuscitation, **antimicrobial** substances and, if necessary, surgical resection of necrotic segments. The mortality rate is high.

Negative staining A technique used in **light microscopy** and **electron microscopy**, in which objects are seen as light or electron transmitting areas in a dense field. Objects are not stained in the true sense, not being chemically attached to the **dye**. Nigrosin and various inks are popular in light microscopy, while heavy metal salts are used in electron microscopy.

Negative strand   In a nucleic acid, a strand that can only copy its **complementary strand**.

Negri body   An **inclusion body** found in brain cells infected with **rabies virus** and staining with **eosin**.

Neisseria   **Bacteria** which do not exhibit **motility**, are obligate **aerobes**, both **oxidase** and **catalase** positive, and negative by **Gram's stain**. They are very susceptible to drying, and to some extent to rapid change in temperature. *N. gonorrhoeae* is the causative organism of **gonorrhoea**, and *N. meningitidis* is a common cause of **meningitis** and **septicaemia**. For growth in the laboratory both these species require enriched **culture medium** and an atmosphere with high humidity and enhanced carbon dioxide concentration on first isolation. They are usually susceptible to **penicillin**, but **beta Lactamase**-producing strains of *N. gonorrhoeae* occur. Other species are rarely implicated in disease and grow on ordinary media. They are members of the normal flora of the human nasopharynx.

Nelsonian illumination   See **Critical illumination**.

Nematode   In medical **parasitology**, accepted as the true roundworm. Many species of nematodes are parasites of invertebrate and vertebrate animals. They form the largest number of **helminth** parasites of man.

Neomycin   An **aminoglycoside** type of **anti-microbial** substance, which is used only topically due to its toxicity. Most **staphylococci** and rod-shaped **bacteria** which are negative by **Gram's stain** (except **pseudomonas**) are susceptible. **Anaerobes** and **streptococci** are resistant.

Neonatal   During the period of 4 weeks following birth.

Neonatal conjunctivitis   Inflammation of the conjunctiva occurring in the first 4 weeks of life, and often caused by *Neisseria gonorrhoea* or *Chlamydia trachomatis*. Infection is acquired from the cervix or the vagina of the mother at delivery.

Neoplasm   A new growth of cells which may be either **benign** or **malignant**.

Nephelometry   Measurement of the number and size of particles in a suspension by determination of the intensity of light scatter, using a detector placed at right angles to the incident light path but of the same wavelength as the incident light. The procedure is particularly useful in measuring complexes of **antigen** and **antibody** produced by immunoprecipitation.

Nephrosis   A syndrome in which there is proteinuria, hypoalbuminuria, hyperlipidaemia and **oedema**. The patients may have normal renal function, or there may be renal insufficiency indicating severe renal disease.

Nephrotoxicity   Toxicity affecting the kidneys. It may be caused by

anti-microbial substances such as **aminoglycosides, Vancomycin**, certain **cephalosporins, Amphotericin B** and **polymyxins**, and it can be enhanced by combining any of these with each other, or with some other drugs such as frusamide. The toxic effect can be reversible, irreversible or progressive. If drug-induced nephrotoxicity occurs the major route of excretion of the drug is no longer available, and if dosage is not adjusted, further toxicity to other organ systems can occur.

Netilmicin A semi-synthetic **aminoglycoside** type of **anti-microbial** substance with a similar spectrum of activity to **gentamicin**, though it is not susceptible to some of the **aminoglycoside-modifying enzymes** affecting gentamicin. There is some evidence suggesting that it might be less toxic than gentamicin.

Network In computing, a system whereby a number of **microcomputers** are set up to interact with one another so that an operator at any one **terminal** may input data, and have access to the data stored in a central mini or mainframe computer, and to each of the other terminals.

Neubauer counting chamber See **Counting chamber**.

Neuraminidase Syn. Sialidase. An **enzyme** which is specific for **sialic acid** (e.g. in **mucins** and on the surface of red blood cells); however, not all sialic acids are susceptible to neuraminidase digestion. Neuraminidase also cleaves neuraminic acid from certain saccharides, **glycoproteins** and glycolipids. It is the most efficient of all enzymes in reducing the surface electrical charge of **erythrocytes**, removing most of the sialic acid and thus enhancing the ability of the cells to be **agglutinated** by certain **IgG** types of **antibody**. It also removes N-acetylneuraminic acid from the cell surface and in doing so diminishes the **blood group** reactions given with anti-M and anti-N reagents, but has no effect on most other blood group reactions. In **histochemistry** it is used to remove **mucins** from bronchial and intestinal preparations. Neuraminidase is present on the surface of the **Orthomyxoviridae** and some of the **Paramyxoviridae**, having a role in the release of progeny **virus** from the cell. In **virology** it is used to remove neuraminic acids from **serum** prior to testing for influenza antibodies. The enzyme is produced in large amounts by *Vibrio cholerae*.

Neuroglia Specialised connective tissue of the nervous system, including the specialised nerve cells of this tissue.

Neurone Non-connective cells of the nervous system, responsible for transmitting impulses.

Neurone-specific enolase An **enzyme** believed to be common to all components of, and therefore a marker of, the **diffuse neuroendocrine system**.

Neurotoxin A **toxin** which is solely or particularly active on the central and/or peripheral nervous systems. The action can consist of direct damage to nerves causing **necrosis**, de-myelination, or interference with nerve function without physical damage. Examples of organisms producing a **neurotoxin** are *Clostridium tetani*, *Cl. botulinum*, *Corynebacterium diphtheriae*, *Shigella dysenteriae* type I, and some enteropathogenic strains of *Staphylococcus aureus*.

Neutralisation test A general name for any test in which **antibody** neutralises the biological activity of an **antigen** or a microorganism.

Neutropenia A reduction in the number of circulating peripheral blood **neutrophils** below the normal limit of $2 \cdot 5 \times 10^9$/l.

Neutrophil A **leucocyte**, or white blood cell, approximately $10-12 \times 10^{-6}$ m in diameter, and containing a **nucleus** divided into two to five lobes connected by fine chromatin filaments. The **cytoplasm** contains numerous granules, staining pink by **Romanowsky stains**, and which distinguish the neutrophil from the **eosinophil** and **basophil**.

New Oxford unit A means of expressing **coagulation factor** VIII **inhibitor** levels based on the ability of the test **plasma** to inhibit a known amount of added factor VIII. The unit is defined as the amount of inhibitor which destroys $0 \cdot 5$ units of factor VIII:C in 4 hours. See also **Bethesda unit**.

New York City Medium A selective **culture medium** for the cultivation of *Neisseria gonorrhoeae*. The medium does not contain blood and is translucent. The selective agents are **Vancomycin**, **Colistin**, **Trimethoprim** and **Nystatin**. Certain auxotypes are susceptible to Vancomycin and will not be detected by use of this medium.

New Zealand black mice An **inbred strain** of experimental mouse which spontaneously develops **auto-immune haemolytic anaemia**.

Nezelof syndrome A **congenital** state of **immunodeficiency**, characterised by an absence of **T cells** and, therefore, **cell-mediated immunity**.

Niemann-Pick cell Lipid-containing **macrophages** and reticulum cells seen in **bone marrow** and other tissues in patients suffering from the Niemann-Pick lipid storage disease.

Ninhydrin Triketohydrindene hydrate. A compound which, when heated with an amino acid, gives a purple colour. It is an important locating agent, used for detecting amino acids after **chromatographic** separation.

NISS Normal Ionic Strength Saline. See **Normal saline**. 2.

Nissl substance In tissue sections, granular material in the **cyto-**

plasm and **dendrites** of **neurones**, consisting largely of **ribonucleic acid**.

Nitroblue tetrazolium test The reduction of nitroblue tetrazolium (NBT) **dye** to insoluble formazan is stimulated by normal **phagocytosis** of **bacteria** by **neutrophils**. This process is markedly reduced in patients with **chronic granulomatous disease**. Increased NBT reduction is often associated with untreated bacterial **infection**.

Nitrocellulose As low viscosity nitrocellulose (LVN), used as an **embedding** medium for hard (e.g. bone) or dense (e.g. brain) tissues. Has a similar composition, though slightly different properties, to **celloidin**.

Nitro dyes Those **dyes** which contain the acidic **chromophore** group $- NO_2$.

Nitrofurantoin A nitrofuran **anti-microbial** substance used only for urinary tract infections. It is active against most rod-shaped organisms which are negative by **Gram's stain**, though **pseudomonas** and many strains of **proteus** are resistant. **Enterococci** are also susceptible. The drug causes nausea and vomiting, and occasionally peripheral neuritis.

Nitrogen, liquid See **Liquid nitrogen**.

Nitromidazoles A group of synthetic **anti-microbial** substances consisting of **metronidazole**, tindazole, and a few others which are not commonly used.

NK cell See **Natural killer cell**.

NMR See **Nuclear Magnetic Resonance**.

Nocardia Filamentous rod-shaped **bacteria** which do not produce **spores**, do not exhibit **motility**, are **catalase** positive, positive by **Gram's stain** and weakly acid-fast. Aerial hyphae are produced. The organisms are obligate **aerobes** and growth can often be enhanced by carbon dioxide. *N. asteroides*, which is most commonly involved in human disease, grows slowly on ordinary **culture media** to produce leathery colonies which are often pigmented. Infection may be in the form of **abscesses** in the brain or other organs. The organisms are resistant to **penicillin**. The most successful agents have been **sulphonamides**, though **erythromycin**, **chloramphenicol** and **tetracycline** show *in vitro* activity.

Non-A, non-B hepatitis See **Hepatitis non-A, non-B**.

Non-Newtonian fluid Simple fluids generate twice the counter-force (**shear stress**) when flowing at twice the **shear rate** and are said to be 'Newtonian' in nature. Complex fluids like blood, however, respond differently to varying amounts of applied force, and are therefore non-Newtonian.

Non-parametric test In statistical usage this is a **hypothesis test** where the observations are not assumed to have a particular **distribution**. Tests based on the **normal distribution** (e.g. **t-tests**

and **F-tests**) are more accurate when the observations are approximately normally distributed. See **Mann-Whitney U-test**, **Sign test** and **Wilcoxon signed-rank test**.

Non-permissive cell A cell which will not permit complete replication, in spite of the presence of all the genomes. See also **Permissive cell line**.

'Non-specific' antibody An **antibody** for which the specificity is not readily apparent and which appears to react with (e.g.) red cells of all types regardless of their antigenic structure.

Non-specific immunity A collective term for non-specific factors which contribute to **immunity** (e.g. **lysozome**, **phagocytosis**). The activities of **B cells** and **T cells** are specifically excluded from the definition and consequently non-specific immunity is sometimes called non-lymphoid immunity.

Non-specific urethritis An inflammation of the urethra for which there is no apparent specific cause and no evidence of **infection**. It is a common chronic condition amongst women, and in men it is often accompanied by a discharge from the urethra.

Norfloxacin A **quinolone** type of **anti-microbial** substance active against most rod-shaped **bacteria** which are negative by **Gram's stain** (including **pseudomonas**), and Gram positive **cocci**, including most strains of **enterococci**. Its main use is in the treatment of urinary tract infections.

Normal distribution In statistical usage, the most commonly used **distribution**, characterised by a symmetrical bell-shaped **histogram**. Many **variables** (e.g. male adult height, error measurements) have an approximately normal distribution, and sample **means** from any distribution have an approximately normal distribution for large **sample** sizes.

Normal probability paper A type of graph paper used for a simple graphical method for statistical testing of whether data have an approximately **normal distribution**. The data points are plotted on special graph paper, and if the data are normally distributed the observations should lie approximately on a straight line.

'Normal' saline 1. A solution of sodium chloride which is physiologically normal (i.e. one which exerts the same osmotic pressure as human plasma). Theoretically this would be represented by a solution of 8·8 g/l, although in practice a solution of 9·0 g/l is generally used. 2. A solution of sodium chloride which is of normal ionic strength, as distinct from low ionic strength saline (**LISS**); often referred to as NISS (normal ionic strength saline). 3. An obsolete chemical term for a solution (in this case, of sodium chloride), containing the equivalent weight of the solute in grams dissolved in 1 litre of solvent.

Normoblast A general term given to the nucleated **erythrocyte**

precursor cells, normally seen in the **bone marrow**, but which may also appear in the peripheral blood in some disease states. The early (basophilic) **normoblast** has a relatively large **nucleus** and non-**haemoglobin**ised, blue-staining **cytoplasm**. The intermediate (polychromatic) and late (pyknotic) normoblasts become progressively smaller and their cytoplasm contains increasingly larger amounts of haemoglobin, as evidenced by their increasingly pink appearance in **Romanowsky-stained** preparations.

Normochromia The appearance, in **blood films** stained with **Romanowsky stains**, of **erythrocytes** which are normally haemoglobinised and which have a normal area of central pallor. See **Anisochromasia** and **Hypochromasia**.

Normocytic The peripheral **blood film** appearances in which each red cell is of normal size. This is associated with a **mean cell volume** between 76 and 96 fl. See also **Macrocytosis** and **Microcytosis**.

Normotest™ A commercially-available method for screening the **extrinsic blood coagulation system**. The reagent consists of rabbit brain **thromboplastin** and modified bovine **plasma**, and is sensitive to deficiencies of **coagulation factors** II, VII and X.

Norwalk virus A small, round-structured **virus**, as yet unclassified, causing **gastroenteritis**. Laboratory detection is by **electron microscopy** or **enzyme immunoassay**.

Nosocomial Hospital-acquired. The term usually refers to infections contracted during the treatment for a different, initial illness, and often due to organisms **endemic** in the institution.

Novobiocin An **anti-microbial** substance isolated from **Streptomyces** species and active against **Staphylococci**, **Haemophilus**, **Neisseria**, and rod-shaped **bacteria** which are positive by **Gram's stain**. Most other Gram negative rods are resistant. The drug acts by inhibiting protein synthesis, but it also damages the **cell membrane**, and therefore suppresses **cell wall** synthesis. The drug causes a range of side effects and is not now used therapeutically.

NSE See **Neurone-specific enolase**.

5'-NT See **5'-Nucleotidase**.

Nuclear magnetic resonance A phenomenon exhibited by all atomic nuclei which have a magnetic moment. Under the influence of a constant magnetic field the nuclei absorb electromagnetic radiation at characteristic frequencies. Each chemically different form of the nucleus of a given atomic species (such as hydrogen) has a different NMR frequency, so that the structure of an unknown compound can often be determined from knowledge of its molecular formula and NMR spectrum. In medicine, nuclear magnetic resonance has so far been applied mostly to **tomography** and to the study of **virus** infected cells. See also **Nuclear Magnetic Resonance imaging**.

Nuclear magnetic resonance (NMR) imaging A form of **tomography** in which the whole body (or a tissue) is placed within the field of a large electromagnet. The atomic nuclei of the tissues align themselves along the axis of the magnetic field and are subjected to pulsed radio frequency signals. When these signals cease the nuclei return to their original positions, emitting radio signals as they do so. By analysing these latter signals it is possible to produce an image of the distribution of the particular atomic species.

Nuclease One of a group of **enzymes** that disrupt nucleic acids. They include the large number of bacterial enzymes collectively termed **restriction endonucleases**.

Nucleocapsid The core of a **virus**, comprising the nucleic acid and its protective **protein**.

Nucleolus A normally round or oval **eosinophilic** structure in the **nucleus** of a cell. Composed chiefly of **RNA**.

Nucleoprotein A basic **protein** of the **nucleus** which is attached, via salt linkage, to nucleic acids.

5′-Nucleotidase (EC 3.1.3.5) An **enzyme** that hydrolyses nucleotides on the fifth ribose carbon atom. It is widely distributed in tissue but is not found in the intestine.

Nucleotide The pentose sugar and phosphate molecule in combination with either a **purine** or a pyrimadine base, which in molecular chains forms nucleic acids.

Nucleus A membrane-limited body within the cell, containing the **chromosomal** material of the cell and directing its metabolic processes.

Nude mouse A strain of experimental mouse with a **congenital** absence of the **thymus**, and no hair.

Null cell A cell of uncertain lineage which has different characteristics to those of **B cells**, **T cells** or **macrophages**. Null cells are sometimes called 'third population cells'.

Nullipara A woman who has never been pregnant.

Numerical aperture The property which governs the resolving and defining power of an objective or a condensing lens, both properties varying directly with numerical aperture while image brightness varies inversely with its square. It may be expressed as the ratio of the lens diameter to its focal length, but more usually by the formula n *sin* U, where n = the **refractive index** (RI) of the medium in which the lens is working and U = half the angle of acceptance of the lens. In general terms, the higher the numerical aperture, the better the resolution and definition achieved.

Nutrition The processes of intake, digestion, absorption and assimilation of food; involved in the supply of nourishment to tissues.

Nystatin A **polyene** type of **anti-microbial** substance active against **yeasts**, and yeast-like and filamentous **fungi**. It acts by binding to sterols in the **cell membrane**, thus causing lethal leaks. The drug is too toxic for parenteral use and is not absorbed when taken orally, so it is used to treat **candida** infections of the skin and mucous membranes.

O

O antigen A type of **antigen** which forms part of the **cell wall** of **micro-organisms** which are negative by **Gram's stain**, and which consists of lipopolysaccharide which is synonymous with **endotoxin**. The polysaccharide chains confer antigenic specificity on the O antigens, and they are used in serological schemes of identification. They are heat-stable.

Oat cell carcinoma A **malignant** bronchogenic **tumour** composed of small, poorly **differentiated** spindly or round cells.

Objective lens In the microscope, a lens which forms the primary image.

Odontoblast A cell of mesenchymal origin responsible for the production of **dentine**. Found lining the pulp chamber of teeth.

Oedema Excessive accumulation of fluid in tissue spaces.

Oestrogen A **hormone** secreted by the ovaries. Used as a generic term for compounds which induce morphological changes in the **endometrium** and affect the growth and maturation of the vaginal **epithelium**.

Ofloxacin A **quinolone** type of **anti-microbial** substance, which generally has less activity than **ciprofloxacin**.

Oil-in-water emulsion A dispersion of oil in water. The emulsion is stabilised by the addition of surfactant such as Tween 80ⓉⓂ. Oil-in-water emulsions may be used as **adjuvants**.

OKT serumⓉⓂ The brand name of certain **monoclonal** antibodies directed against **T cell** antigens.

Oleandomycin A **macrolide** type of **anti-microbial** substance produced by **Streptomyces** species. The mode of action and spectrum of activity are the same as for **erythromycin**. Clinically it appears to be less active than erythromycin, and is no longer in common use.

Oliguria Reduction in the volume of urine excreted to a level which, if maintained, is incompatible with life.

Onchomycosis Infection of the nails by a **fungus**; often due to **Candida** and sometimes to **dermatophytes**.

Oncofetal antigen An **antigen** which is present on fetal tissues, absent from normal adult tissue, but may be expressed by **tumour** cells. See **carcinoembryonic antigen**.

Oncology The study of **tumours**.

One-stage clotting assay A method for the determination of individual **coagulation factors** based on the ability of a test **plasma** to correct the clotting time of a plasma completely deficient in the factor under test. One stage clotting assays are usually based on the **prothrombin time** or **activated partial thromboplastin time**.

See **Two-stage clotting assay**.

One-stage prothrombin time   See **Prothrombin time**.

Oocyst   A **cyst** containing the **zygote**, or fertilised egg, and in **protozoa** the stage in the life history regarded as its homologue. For example, in **malaria** the oocyst is found in the gut of the mosquito, or in many laboratory animals in the coccidia, where it is excreted with the faeces.

Operating system   1. A set of written specifications for the performance of a task or series of tasks. 2. In computing, a collection of **programs** which control the overall operation of a computer, including the operation and sequencing of other programs.

Ophthalmia   Inflammation of the eye, usually consisting of **conjunctivitis**. A large number of agents can be implicated including **viruses**, **bacteria**, **fungi** and **parasites**. *Ophthalmia neonatorum* is conjunctivitis in the newborn, caused by *Neisseria gonorrhoeae* and/or *Chlamydia trachomatis*.

Opportunistic infection   An **infection** in which the infecting agent is frequently or normally present in the host without causing harm, but it will cause lesions in unusual circumstances. Common precipitants of opportunistic infections are acquired immune incompetence and removal of a substantial part of the natural bacterial flora by **antibiotic** therapy.

Opsonin   A **serum** factor which binds to the surface of a **microorganism** and facilitates its ingestion by **phagocytes**. The main opsonins are **IgG** or **IgM** classes of **immunoglobulin**, and the C3 fraction of **complement**. Other factors, such as **C-reactive protein** and **fibronectin**, may also have a role.

Opsonisation   The coating of **antigenic** material by **opsonins**, such as certain classes of **immunoglobulin G** types of **antibody**, so facilitating **phagocytosis**.

Optical density   See **Absorbance**.

Optimal additive solution   A preservative solution designed to be added to **concentrated red cells** which have been prepared for **transfusion** by removing the whole of the supernatant **plasma**, so restoring the **haematocrit** level to around 70%. This enables removal of larger volumes of **plasma** for production of **blood fractions**. The most commonly used solution of this type is one of **Saline**, **Adenine**, Glucose and Mannitol, known as 'SAG-M'.

Optimal proportions   The ratio of **antibody** to **antigen** which leads to maximal **precipitation**. See **Lattice hypothesis**.

Optochin   Ethyl hydrocuprein hydrochloride. The substance is used in **bacteriology** in the form of impregnated discs to test for susceptibility for identification purposes. *Streptococcus pneumoniae* is susceptible, while the colonially similar *Strep. viridans* is resistant.

Ordinate   The vertical (y) axis on a graph or chart.

Orf virus   A para**poxvirus** of sheep and goats, which causes a **zoonotic** infection in man, resulting in a localised solid lesion of alarming appearance. The lesion is painless and harmless, resolving spontaneously without scarring, in 2–3 weeks. Laboratory diagnosis is by **electron microscopy** of the contents of the lesion.

Organelle   A particular particle of organised living matter present in the **cytoplasm** of practically all cells.

Ornithosis   A **zoonosis** affecting birds. It is usually caused by *Chlamydia psittaci* and is otherwise known as **psittacosis**. The organism is spread to humans from direct contact with infected birds, but more usually by inhalation of dust, feathers and dried droppings. The human disease is systemic, but primarily affects the lungs. There is fever, with chills and malaise developing gradually over several days, and headache. Laboratory diagnosis depends on demonstration by a **complement fixation** technique of a raised or rising **titre** of **antibody**. The drug of choice for treatment is **tetracycline**, given for extended periods in order to avoid relapse.

Orthomyxoviridae   A family of **enveloped** helical **RNA** viruses 100–200 nm in diameter, which includes **Influenza A virus** and **Influenza B virus**. The nucleic acid is segmented in eight pieces, each piece representing a **gene**. **Genetic re-assortment** of the various genes of influenza A is a common natural event. The virus **envelope** consists of cell **membrane** modified by the addition of viral **proteins** such as haem**agglutinins** and **neuraminidase**, which can be seen by **electron microscopy** as short spikes on the membrane.

Orthopoxvirus   A genus of the **Poxviridae** which includes **cowpox**, **ectromelia**, **vaccinia**, **variola** and **'Wild white'** viruses.

Osmolality   The concentration of a solution expressed in osmoles of solute *per* kilogram of solvent. See also **Osmolarity**.

Osmolarity   The concentration of a solution expressed in osmoles of solute per litre of solution. A measure of the osmotic pressure of a fluid in which ionic and non-ionic compounds are dissolved. If molar concentrations are used (mmol/l), the sum gives the molality of the fluid. See **Osmolality**.

Osmosis   The movement of fluid across a semi-permeable membrane separating solutions of different molecular concentration, from the weaker to the stronger solution.

Osmotic fragility   A test of the ability of **erythrocytes** to withstand varying degrees of **hypotonic** shock. Red cells are suspended in solutions of sodium chloride of varying concentration, and the degree of **haemolysis** plotted against the salt concentration. The results are largely dependent on the surface area:volume ratio, being increased in **spherocytosis** and decreased in the presence of **leptocytes**. See **Mean cell fragility**.

Ossification Developmental bone growth; when replacing cartilage, referred to as endochondral, and in the absence of cartilage as intramembranous.

Osteitis Inflammation of the bone, without marrow involvement. Usually the marrow eventually becomes involved, leading to **osteomyelitis**.

Osteoblast A specialised connective tissue cell concerned with bone formation.

Osteoclast A specialised cell, commonly multinucleate, concerned with bone resorption. Of undetermined origin, although probably related to **macrophage**.

Osteocyte A cell concerned with the maintenance of bone as a living tissue. Derived from **osteoblasts**.

Osteoid Non-mineralised bone, most commonly found on the outer surfaces of trabecular bone. This material is increased in certain diseases, most notably **osteomalacia**.

Osteomalacia A bone condition in which there is a decrease in calcified bone due to poor mineralisation. Commonly known as Rickets.

Osteomyelitis Inflammation of the bone marrow, but usually including the bone as well. The infection can present as local pain and inflammation with acute onset, and it also has a tendency to become **chronic**. Causative organisms include *Staphylococcus aureus*, *Mycobacterium tuberculosis*, *Treponema pallidum*, *Brucella abortus* and certain species of **salmonella**. Treatment is by surgical debridement and drainage, and long-term antibiotics.

Osteoporosis A bone condition associated with a decrease in bone mass. There is normal mineralisation of bone mass.

Otitis externa An **infection** of the external auditory meatus and canal, which may be **acute** or **chronic**. Causative organisms include *Streptococcus pyogenes*, *Pseudomonas aeruginosa* and *Aspergillus niger*.

Otitis media An **infection** of the middle ear, commonest in the pre-school age group. Symptoms are severe pain, often with fever and discharge of pus or serous fluid. The commonest causative organisms are *Streptococcus pneumoniae*, *Haemophilus influenzae* and *Streptococcus pyogenes*, as well as **viruses** and occasionally *Mycoplasma pneumoniae*. Amoxycillin is the drug of choice for treatment, but trimethoprim is also useful.

Ototoxicity Toxic damage to the functions of the ear by drugs. **Anti-microbial** substances which may cause ototoxicity include **aminoglycosides**, **vancomycin**, **minocycline** and sometimes **ery-**

thromycin. The damage may affect hearing or balance, or both, and is primarily due to destruction of the hair cells of the cochlea or the vestibule. These cells cannot regenerate, though some compensation usually takes place in milder cases. Afterwards, atrophy of parts of the eighth cranial nerve takes place. Those affected by cochlear damage will suffer partial hearing loss, and those having vestibular damage will experience vertigo, dizziness, tinnitus and sometimes nausea. Toxicity is usually related to **plasma** drug levels and rarely occurs if these do not exceed acceptable limits for that drug, though prolonged administration with normal plasma levels has been implicated.

Ouchterlony test A **double diffusion test** performed in an **agar** gel. Wells are cut in the agar gel and filled with **antigen** or **antibody**, which is then allowed to diffuse in the medium. Where antigen and antibody meet in **optimal proportions** lines of **precipitation** develop.

Outbreak A term usually applied to a small **epidemic** of **infection**, often confined to an enclosed community.

Outlier In statistical usage, an observation which is very different from most of the rest of the **sample**. This may be caused, for example, by incorrect measurement or by faulty equipment. Tests are available to detect significant outliers. Inclusion of such aberrant observations in calculations can lead to misleading conclusions being reached.

Output In computing, data which have been processed by a computer and which are fed to an external device such as a printer.

Overlay 1. In microbiology, the liquid phase of a culture system which usually consists of a solid slope to which an 'overlay' of nutrients is added. In parasitology, material is inoculated into the overlay, where **parasites** develop. 2. In computing, a type of **file** used by other **programs** that require storage of data for overlaying on that program. The file type has the extension .OVR.

Ovum The female **gamete**, including fertilised cells for the first 3 weeks of pregnancy.

Owren's buffer The popular name for barbitone-buffered saline, **pH** 7·35, commonly used in blood **coagulation** testing.

Oxidant drug A general term applied to certain drugs (e.g. phenacetin), which may cause oxidation of **erythrocyte** membrane **proteins** and **haemoglobin**. Such drugs are particularly liable to cause oxidative damage in **enzyme** deficiencies of the **hexose monophosphate shunt**.

Oxidase A type of intracellular **enzyme** which catalyses removal of hydrogen from a substance, using oxygen as the hydrogen acceptor to produce hydrogen peroxide. Generally only those **micro-**

219

organisms which are **aerobes** produce oxidases of the cytochrome system. Tests for oxidase utilise tetramethyl phenylene diamine, or a similar substance, which in the presence of oxidase, oxygen and cytochrome C produces a blue pigment, indophenol.

Oxidation The chemical process resulting in an ion losing electrons to become oxidised.

Oxidation-reduction potential The electrode potential, or tendency to donate or accept electrons, of a substance compared to the potential of the hydrogen electrode. It is assigned the symbol Eh and is measured in millivolts. The more oxidised a system is, the higher its Eh. Those **bacteria** which are **anaerobes** require a negative Eh of several hundred millivolts. **Metronidazole** has an Eh of -560 mV.

17-Oxogenic steroid See **17-Oxosteroid**.

17-Oxosteroid A metabolite of androgens (adrenal and gonadal) and also of **cortisol** and its precursor. Urinary excretion is unreliable and estimation has been replaced by more reliable assays of individual **hormones** in blood.

Oxygen dissociation curve The sigmoid curve obtained when the partial pressure of oxygen is plotted against the percentage of blood **oxyhaemoglobin** content at each pressure. The relative position of the curve is affected by **pH**, temperature and **2,3-diphosphoglycerate** concentration, and is conveniently expressed as the oxygen tension at which the **haemoglobin** is 50% oxygenated (P_{50}).

Oxyhaemoglobin The name used to describe **haemoglobin** in its fully oxygenated – as opposed to de-oxygenated – state.

Oxyntic cell See **Parietal cell**.

Oxytalan fibre Specialised connective tissue fibre of blood vessels, skin appendages, tendon, cornea and periodontium. Probably related to elastic fibres, with which it shares staining reactions – although only following per-acid oxidation.

Oxytetracycline A **tetracycline** produced by **Streptomyces** species. It can be given orally or **parenterally**, and has a slightly lower activity than tetracycline itself.

Oxytocin A **hormone** which is an octapeptide and is secreted by the posterior pituitary. It causes uterine contractions in parturition.

Oxytocinase See **Cystine aminopeptidase**.

Oyster cell An intermediate **squamous cell** of the **epithelium**, with **glycogen**-rich **cytoplasm**.

P

Packed cell volume (PCV) The volume of **erythrocytes** per ml of whole blood, which in normal adults lies between 0·36 and 0·54. The PCV may be measured directly after centrifugation in a specially designed **microhaematocrit** centrifuge, or by calculation from **mean cell volume** and red cell count.

PAF See **Platelet activating factor**.

PAGE See **Polyacrylamide gel electrophoresis**.

Paget's disease **Adenocarcinoma** originating in the underlying ductal **epithelium** of the breast and involving the stratified **squamous** epithelium of the nipple.

Palmitic acid Hexadecanoic acid. The most common fatty acid in the human body.

Panagglutination **Agglutination** of red cells, regardless of their antigenic structure, by all sera. Generally due to bacterial contamination of the cells or of the serum.

Pancytopenia A reduction in all the formed elements of the peripheral blood (i.e. a combination of **anaemia**, **leucopenia** and **thrombocytopenia**).

Pandemic An **epidemic** of **infection** with nation-wide or world-wide spread.

P antigen 1. An **antigen** of the P **blood group** system, which contains antigens known as P_1, P_2, p and P^k. Reference simply to 'P' is usually taken to mean the common antigen P_1, which is present in the blood of 78% of Caucasians and over 95% of West African negroes. The antigen is of variable strength and weak forms may be difficult to detect. (**Anti-P_1** is usually a **cold agglutinin**, and is of no clinical significance.) 2. In **bacteriology**, a class of mannose-resistant **fimbriae** found on uropathogenic strains of *Escherichia coli*, which enable them to adhere to urinary tract **epithelium**. They are so called because they agglutinate **erythrocytes** which bear the **antigen** of the common P **blood group**. (See 1, above.)

PAP Abbreviation for either 1. **Papanicolaou's stain** or 2. **Peroxidase/anti-peroxidase**.

Papain A proteolytic **enzyme** sometimes used in serological reactions. Obtained from the paw-paw.

Papanicolaou, George Nicholas (1883–1962) A pioneer in the study of vaginal smears. He introduced a smear test for oestrus in 1917 and a smear diagnostic test for cancer of the cervix in 1928, although this was not accepted at the time and he re-published his method in 1941. Cervical **cytology** screening is often referred to as a 'Pap smear'. See **Papanicolaou stain**.

Papanicolaou stain A **trichrome** staining procedure which indicates epithelial cell maturation and consequently is used extensively in exfoliative **cytology**.

'Pap' cells Small **squamous** cells with dark, round or oval single nuclei, seen in sputum from patients with upper respiratory tract infections. They are considered to be degenerative cells of the pharyngeal **epithelium**.

Papilloma A branching or lobed **benign tumour** derived from the **epithelium**.

Pappenheimer bodies Iron-containing red cell **inclusion bodies** seen in peripheral **blood films** in some cases of **haemolytic anaemia** or following splenectomy. They appear as minute basophilic dots by **Romanowsky stains** and may also be demonstrated by staining with **brilliant cresyl blue** and **Prussian blue**.

Para- A prefix word meaning alongside; related to; accessory to.

Paracetamol N-acetyl-p-amino-phenol. An analgesic with similar properties to aspirin, but producing less side effects.

Paracoagulation test See **Ethanol gelation test**.

Paracrine cell A cell producing hormone to act locally on neighbouring cells, in contrast to **endocrine cells** which release peptide directly into the blood stream.

Paraffin wax A straight-chain hydrocarbon product of crude oil used for **impregnation** and **embedding** of tissue prior to **microtomy**. Usually a mixture of hydrocarbons varying from C_{17} to C_{35} and characterised by melting point.

Parallel Literally, side by side. In computing, a system in which electrical patterns of **bits** travel simultaneously along parallel wires. See also **Serial**.

Parameter Statistically this is a quantity (usually unknown) which is needed to describe a **distribution** (e.g. the **mean** or **variance**), or to describe an assumed model (e.g. slope or intercept of a linear relationship between two **variables**). Parameters can be **estimated** using the observations in a **sample**.

Paramyxoviridae A family of **enveloped** helical **RNA** viruses 250–400 nm in diameter. There are three genera, **Paramyxovirus**, **Morbillivirus** and Pneumovirus. The RNA **genome** is a single molecule. The viral envelope comprises cell **membrane** with viral **proteins** inserted through it. Members of the family include **measles virus**, **mumps virus** and **respiratory syncytial virus**.

Paramyxovirus A genus of the **Paramyxoviridae**, characterised by possession of both haem**agglutinin** and **neuraminidase**. Members include parainfluenza virus types 1–4, which cause upper respiratory tract infections, and **mumps virus**. Newcastle disease virus has considerable economic significance. The viruses grow in **monkey kidney cell culture**, inducing **haemadsorption** but little **cytopathic effect**.

Paraprotein   Homogenous **immunoglobulin** produced by neoplastic **plasma cells** in individuals with **myelomatosis**. See **Myeloma protein**.

Pararosaniline   A diphenylmethane **dye** found to be the most active component of basic fuchsin, which it may replace in most staining methods, especially in the preparation of **Schiff's reagent**.

Parasite   A **micro-organism** which lives in non-mutualistic **symbiosis** at the expense of its host, which is usually a larger organism providing nourishment and physical protection, and being adversely affected by the relationship. A bacterial **infection** is an example of this, in contrast to the normal intestinal flora, which show mutualistic symbiosis, both they and the host deriving benefit. In colloquial medical microbiological terminology, a parasite is a eukaryotic organism such as **Entamoeba, Plasmodium** or **Ascaris**.

Parasitic light   The light lost by reflection from the surface of a lens. Such light makes no contribution to image formation and lens surfaces are coated to reduce loss of light by reflection.

Parasitology   A biological science embracing the study of the phenomena of dependance of one living organism upon another. In medical parasitology this is usually measured by observation of the abnormal physiology of the host.

Parathormone   See **Parathyroid hormone**.

Parathyroid hormone   A **hormone** secreted by the parathyroid gland, whose main function − in association with vitamin D and **calcitonin** − is to maintain normal serum calcium levels.

Parcentral   The facility of each objective lens on a microscope to cover the same field when the nosepiece is rotated.

Parenchyma   A general term used to designate the functional elements of an organ, as distinct from its framework or stroma.

Parenteral   Administered other than by mouth − generally by injection or infusion.

Parfocal   The facility that ensures that each objective lens of a microscope will remain in focus when changing powers of magnification.

Park nucleotide   An intermediate in the synthesis of **peptidoglycan**, consisting of muramic acid bearing a chain of five peptides. The nucleotide is assembled in the hydrophilic **cytoplasm**, attached to uridine diphosphate and then linked to **bactoprenol** to enable subsequent synthesis to take place in the hydrophobic **cell membrane**.

Paromycin   An **aminoglycoside** type of **anti-microbial** substance with a spectrum of activity similar to that of **Kanamycin**.

Paronychia   An **infection** of the nail bed, often caused by **candida** organisms.

Paroxysmal cold haemoglobinuria   (PCH) An increasingly rare type of immune **haemolytic anaemia** often associated with syphilis or infections with **viruses**, and which is precipitated by exposure to cold, whether local or general. The **antibody** responsible, known as the **Donath-Landsteiner antibody** fixes to red cells in the cold and causes **complement**-mediated haemolysis on warming to 37°C. PCH may be diagnosed simply by means of the **Donath-Landsteiner test**.

Partial thromboplastin time A screening test for abnormalities of the **intrinsic blood coagulation** system, involving re-calcification of the test **plasma** in the presence of a partial **thromboplastin** (e.g. cephalin). Due to its extreme sensitivity to factors affecting **contact activation** it has largely been replaced by the **activated partial thromboplastin time**.

Parvoviridae A family of small cubical **viruses** which are not **enveloped** and are 20−28 nm in diameter. The DNA **genome** is unique among animal viruses in being single stranded. The family includes two genera of significance in laboratory practice, **parvovirus** and adeno-associated virus.

Parvovirus A genus of the **Parvoviridae** which includes type B19, the cause of an erythematous rash called 'fifth disease' or 'slapped cheek syndrome'. It is also a cause of aplastic crisis in patients with **sickle cell anaemia**. Virus for laboratory tests is only available from **acutely** infected volunteers; the virus has yet to be cultivated *in vitro*. Laboratory diagnosis of infection is usually serological, using **MACRIA**.

PAS See **Periodic acid/Schiff**.

Pascal In computing, a **high level language** widely used for writing general **programs**.

Pascal, Blaise (1623−1662) French mathematician and physicist. Inventor of the first mechanical calculator, the forerunner of the computer.

Passage A sub-culture or series of sub-cultures. In **cell culture** the term applies to the transfer of cells from one vessel to one or more further containers.

Passive agglutination test A test in which soluble **antigen** is first attached to an insoluble carrier particle such as polystyrene latex. **Antibody** to the soluble antigen will then **agglutinate** the coated particles. See **Latex agglutination test**.

Passive cutaneous anaphylaxis An *in vivo* method for detecting **IgE** responsible for **type I reactions** of hypersensitivity. Following intradermal administration of **antibody**, an **antigen** mixed with Evans blue **dye** is injected intravenously. Combination between IgE bound to **mast cells** and specific antigen leads to degranulation of the mast cells, histamine release, increased vascular permeability and leakage of Evans blue from the vascular system. Blue spots develop near the site of antibody injection.

Passive immunity Humoral **immunity** conferred by the **parenteral** administration of pre-formed **antibodies** or the transfer of **lymphocytes** to one individual from another (e.g. the transfer of **IgG** across the placenta from a mother to her fetus). The effect is temporary and lasts until the antibody **titre** falls below the protective level, usually a few months later.

Pasteur, Louis (1822−1895) French scientist who was the founder of microbiology. Amongst other work he discovered (and coined the expression for) the organisms now known as **anaerobes**, and was responsible for the development of sterilisation by the process known after him − pasteurisation. He also carried out fundamental research into the organisms of anthrax and rabies, as well as into fermentation.

Pasteurella Rod-shaped **bacteria** which do not exhibit **motility**, do not form **spores**, are **catalase** positive and **oxidase** positive, facultative **anaerobes** and negative by **Gram's stain**. They cause disease in a wide range of animal hosts, including man. Four species are recognised, *P. multocida*, *P. pneumotropica*, *P. haemolytica* and *P. ureae*, and several serotypes and biotypes are recognised within this classification. The types of **infections** caused include **septicaemia, meningitis, sinusitis, pneumonia, osteomyelitis** and **abscesses**. They are a common cause of infection following dog bites.

Pasteur pipette A **pipette** consisting of a length of glass tubing drawn out at one end into a capillary, and controlled at the other end by a rubber bulb, or teat.

Patch In computing, coded instructions fed into a **program** to alter it.

Pathogen A **micro-organism** causing, or capable of causing, disease. The term requires considerable qualification, as organisms previously considered to be non-pathogens are capable of causing serious or fatal infections in patients with underlying immunoincompetence, or in those with implanted **prostheses**.

Pathogenesis The process or mode of causation of disease.

Pathogenicity The ability to cause disease. This is a sum of the **virulence** factors of the organism, introduction of the organism into the host tissues, and the host response, and it depends greatly on circumstances and the immune status of the host.

Pathognomic Distinctively characteristic of a particular disease or pathological condition.

Pathologist One who practises **pathology**. Usually a medical practitioner.

Pathology The study of the underlying processes of disease; especially the changes in structure and function of organs and tissues causing, or which are caused by, disease.

Paul-Bunnell-Davidsohn test A test for demonstrating the **heterophile** sheep cell **antibody** occurring in **infectious mononucleosis**, and differentiating it from the **Forssman antibody** and the antibody found in **serum sickness**. It is often called the Paul-Bunnell test, although strictly the Paul-Bunnell test demonstrates the presence of sheep cell agglutinins while Davidsohn's **absorption** modification helps to identify their possible cause. The test depends on the ability of the infectious mononucleosis antibody to **agglutinate** sheep red cells following absorption of the test serum by guinea pig kidney cells or ox **erythrocytes**. Antibodies induced by **Epstein-Barr virus** infection are removed by treatment of **serum** with guinea pig kidney cells, and not by bovine **erythrocytes**. Commercial tests are now available. See also **Monospot test**.

PCH See **Paroxysmal Cold Haemoglobinuria**.

PCI See **Prothrombin Consumption Index**.

PCV See **Packed Cell Volume**.

PDGF See **Platelet-Derived Growth Factor**.

Peak level The highest concentration of an **anti-microbial** substance in **plasma**, or other body fluids, measured following its administration. The concentration thereafter begins to decline due to excretion or inactivation, until the **trough level** is reached just before the next dose.

'Pearl' formation A group of intermediate **squamous cells** of the **epithelium**, forming a 'pearl-like' formation.

Peek In computing, an instruction used in **BASIC** to give the programmer access to any location in **Random Access Memory**.

Pefloxacin A **quinolone** type of **anti-microbial** substance with less activity than **norfloxacin** and **ciprofloxacin**.

Pelger-Huet anomaly A **congenital** condition of the blood in which the affected subject's **neutrophils** appear almost entirely bi-lobed. It is of no clinical significance.

Peltier effect The result of placing two dissimilar metals (commonly bismuth telluride and copper) in apposition and passing a direct current through them. Depending on the direction of the current, heat is generated on one surface and lost from the other. Used to freeze tissue, with running water conducting heat away from the warm surface.

Penicillin A **beta Lactam** type of **anti-microbial** substance produced by *Penicillium* species. Penicillin G (or **benzylpenicillin**) is used **parenterally** as it is destroyed in the stomach by acid, whereas the acid-stable Penicillin V (or **phenoxymethyl penicillin**) can be given orally. Penicillin is active against Gram positive **cocci**, rod-shaped **bacteria** and **Neisseria**, except for enterococci. Rod-shaped organisms which are negative by **Gram's stain** and facultative **anaerobes**

are resistant, as are **haemophilus** organisms. However, many strains of **staphylococci** and some neisseria and **streptococci** are now resistant to **beta Lactamase** production. Some organisms (such as *Strep. pyogenes*, almost all *Strep. pneumoniae* and all *Treponema pallidum*) can still be relied upon to be susceptible. The drug inactivates **enzymes** concerned with **peptidoglycan** synthesis, so rendering the cell liable to **lysis**. Penicillin is excreted in the urine, and has few side effects except hypersensitivity.

Penicillinase A beta Lactamase which inactivates **penicillin**, but not **cephalosporins**.

Penicillin-binding protein A type of **enzyme** – usually a transpeptidase or a carboxypeptidase – which is involved in **peptidoglycan** synthesis, and to which **beta Lactam** types of **anti-microbial** substances bind. Many have been isolated and characterised. In *Escherichia coli*, for example, penicillin-binding protein (PBP) 2 binds **mecillinam**, **clavulanic acid** and **imipenem**, while PBP 4 binds **benzylpenicillin**, **ampicillin** and imipenem, and PBP 5 binds **cefoxitin**.

Penning gauge A gauge to measure high vacuum. It depends on the ionisation of gas molecules in a high electrostatic field. See also **Pirani gauge**.

Pentagastrin A synthetic gastrin having the same effect as gastrin but being less potent.

Pentosan polysulphate A **heparin analogue** useful as an anti-thrombotic and anti-lipid drug. It has a weak anticoagulant activity as measured by the **activated partial thromboplastin time**, but has a powerful antithrombin and anti-factor Xa activity when measured by **antithrombin III**-dependent methods.

Peptide See **Polypeptide**.

C-Peptide A product formed after the cleavage of endogenous proinsulin when **insulin** is formed. Exogenous insulin does not contain C-peptide.

Peptidase A generic name for a group of **enzymes** secreted by the pancreas and which include endopeptidase trypsin (EC 3.4.21.4) and chymotrypsin (EC 3.4.21.1).

Peptidoglycan The mucopeptide which gives the **cell wall** of **bacteria** its strength and rigidity. It is present as a continuous macromolecule which, in bacteria which are positive by **Gram's stain**, is cross-linked in two planes by peptide bonds, and forms a thick mesh. In Gram negative bacteria the molecule is cross-linked in one plane only and is much thinner. The molecule consists of repeated alternating units of N-acetylmuramic acid and N-acetylglucosamine, each with short peptide chains attached.

Peptococcus A genus of the **bacterial** family of Peptococcaceae, which also includes the genera **Peptostreptococcus**, Ruminococcus and Sarcina. Peptococci are **cocci** which do not exhibit **motility**, are **catalase** negative, weakly or non-saccharolytic **anaerobes** which are positive by **Gram's stain** and are capable of metabolising amino acids and purines to produce acetate, propionate, butyrate, formate, succinate, lactate, ammonia and carbon dioxide. They are rarely implicated in human disease, though they are commonly found in the intestine, vagina, mouth and respiratory tract.

Peptone The heterogeneous products of digestion of animal or vegetable **proteins** by **trypsin**, pepsin or **papain**, used as nutrients in **culture media**. Various types and grades are available depending on the source, method of production and purification. Hydrolysis of casein produces a peptone which has a more constant composition than those derived from beef muscle and similar sources.

Peptostreptococcus **Bacteria** which form chains of **cocci** and which do not exhibit **motility**, are **catalase** negative, saccharolytic, **aerobic** and stain positive by **Gram's stain**. A variety of fatty acids are produced from fermentation, but not lactate. They are rarely associated with human disease and are found in the intestine, vagina, mouth and respiratory tract.

Perfluorocarbon A cyclic or straight chain hydrocarbon in which hydrogen atoms have been replaced with fluorine. In clinical medicine, due to their affinity for gases, perfluorocarbons have been used as substitutes for red cells in **transfusion**. They have also been used as anaesthetic agents. In industry they are used as refrigerants and aerosol propellants.

Pericarditis Inflammation of the **membranous** covering of the heart.

Perinatal An imprecise term for the period shortly before and after birth. From about 29 weeks gestation to about 4 weeks after birth.

Perinuclear halo Cytoplasmic vacuolation, giving the **nucleus** of a cell a 'halo' appearance.

Periodic acid/Schiff A widely used staining technique in which the stains react with any substance containing a 1:2 glucol grouping, thus it stains many structures with a carbohydrate component. Results may be varied by using oxidants other than periodic acid.

Periodontal disease **Infection** of the gingiva (**gingivitis**) and supporting tissues of the teeth. The untreated condition is **chronic** and progressive, leading eventually to permanent loss of teeth. **Abscesses** occasionally form in the soft tissue spaces of the neck and jaw but infection is usually localised within the mouth. Treatment involves topical application of **antiseptics**, surgical drainage and debridement and a course of systemic **anti-microbial** drugs. Vincent's gingivitis is an acute necrotising form due to *Borrelia vincenti* and other **anaerobes**.

Peripheral In computing, a device which is external to the **central processing unit's** main **memory**, and is connected to it (e.g. a printer).

Peritonitis **Infection** of the peritoneal membrane which lines the peritoneal cavity and forms the outer surface of the intestine. Peritonitis may result from perforation of the intestine or appendix, with release of **faeces** and large numbers of intestinal **bacteria**, or it may have no apparent primary cause. In the latter case the causative organisms are predominantly *Streptococcus pneumoniae*, but intestinal **anaerobes** and occasionally *Mycobacterium tuberculosis* are also involved. In females, one possible route of infection is from the vagina via the fallopian tubes. Peritonitis also complicates peritoneal dialysis, when a variety of organisms – including **pseudomonas**, **candida** and **coagulase**-negative **staphylococci** – are involved.

Permeability increasing factor A **lymphokine**, which increases vascular permeability, released from an activated **T cell**.

Permissive cell line A cell line which will allow the complete replication and release of (e.g.) a **virus**. See **Non-permissive cell**.

Pernicious anaemia A form of **megaloblastic anaemia** resulting from defective secretion of **intrinsic factor** and consequent failure of **vitamin B12** absorption.

Peroxidase/anti-peroxidase A stable complex comprising three molecules of horseradish peroxidase and two molecules of antibody (anti-peroxidase), used in **immunocytochemistry**. (Note. Often abbreviated to PAP. Do not confuse with the same abbreviation used for **Papanicolaou's stain**.)

Peroxidase reaction A cytochemical test for the demonstration of **myeloperoxidase**, most useful in the differentiation of early **myelocytes** and late **myeloblasts** from **lymphocytes** and **lymphoblasts** in patients with **leukaemia**. It may also distinguish **monocytes** from **lymphocytes**.

Persister The very small sub-population of an **inoculum** of **microorganisms** which survives contact with an **anti-microbial** substance in concentrations lethal to the remainder of the inoculum, and yet retains all the characteristics of the susceptible majority, including **MIC**.

Pertussis (Commonly known as 'whooping cough'). An **acute** respiratory **infection** caused by *Bordetella pertussis*, and almost exclusively affecting children. Characteristically there is a paroxysmal cough followed by an inspiratory 'whoop'. The paroxysmal stage may persist for many weeks or months. Several toxins are produced by the organism, including one which is thought to be responsible for the paroxysmal cough. There is no effective specific treatment although **erythromycin** renders patients non-**infectious**, and can also be given prophylactically to contacts.

Peterfi See **Double embedding**.

Petri dish A shallow dish with a loose-fitting cover, into which molten **agar**-based **culture media** can be poured and allowed to solidify to produce a sterile flat surface for the growth of **bacteria**. The dishes vary in size and are usually circular, although square and sub-divided variants are available. Originally made of glass, most are now made of polystyrene and are intended to be disposable.

Perl's Prussian blue A coloured pigment − potassium ferric ferrocyanide − formed between **haemosiderin** and potassium ferrocyanide. A classical microscopical staining method.

Peyer's patches Areas of lymphatic tissue attached to the small intestine.

PF3 See **Platelet Factor 3**.

PF4 See **Platelet Factor 4**.

pH See **Hydrogen ion concentration**.

Phage type A classification of the strains of a species of **bacteria** by their differential susceptibility to a range of **bacteriophages**. Such patterns of susceptibility (phage types) are usually stable and can be used for the study of **epidemiology**.

Phagocyte A cell which ingests bacteria or other particles.

Phagocytin A **bactericidal** protein found in the **lysosomes** of **phagocytes**.

Phagocytosis The process of ingestion by a **phagocyte**.

Phagolysosome A structure found in the **cytoplasm** of phagocytes following phagocytosis. It is the fusion product of a **lysosome** and a **phagosome**.

Phagosome A structure formed in the **cytoplasm** of a phagocyte following phagocytosis. The injected material is enclosed in a portion of the phagocyte cell **membrane**. The phagosome then fuses with a **lysosome** to form a **phagolysosome**.

Pharmacokinetics The study of the behaviour of drugs in the human or animal body, including rates of absorption, binding to tissues and **plasma** constituents, degradation or inactivation, penetration into various body compartments and excretion. Such studies enable a prediction to be made of the plasma or tissue level after a given dose, and therefore allow avoidance of toxicity, assurance of optimum effect, and calculation of dose and frequency of administration.

Pharmacology   The study of the action of drugs on the human or animal body. In the case of **anti-microbial** substances this mainly concerns unwanted or unexpected side-effects and toxicity.

Pharyngitis   Inflammation of the pharynx, usually caused by a **virus** or by *Streptococcus pyogenes*. It is a very common symptom of upper respiratory tract infections.

Phase contrast   In microscopy, a principle which exploits slight structural differences in **refractive index**, which induce phase changes in otherwise non-absorptive objects. These changes are converted into changes in amplitude, which are sensed by the eye as differences in light intensity, resulting in images of high contrast.

Phenistix⊕   A paper test strip which has an absorbent area at one end impregnated with ferric ammonium sulphate, a buffer and a magnesium salt. The presence of phenylpyruvic acid is shown by a green/blue colour.

Phenolic disinfectant   A phenol-based **disinfectant** of a type widely used in bacteriology. They are poorly effective against **viruses**, however, non-**enveloped** types in particular surviving them well.

Phenotype   The apparent characteristics (in serology, **blood group**) of an individual, without indication of all the individual **genes** responsible for the characteristic. See also **Genotype**.

Phenylalanine   See **Phenylketonuria**.

Phenylketonuria   An inherited disorder of amino acid metabolism in which there is a lack of phenylalanine hydroxylase. This results in phenylketonuria, in which phenylpyruvic acid and other compounds are excreted in the urine.

Phenyl methane dye   An important group of **dyes** derived from phenyl substituted methane. Formed via a **carbinol**, they are most commonly amino or hydroxy derivatives of triphenyl methane and include such dyes as malachite green and basic fuchsin.

Philadelphia chromosome   An abnormal **chromosome** found in about 80% of patients with **chronic myeloid leukaemia**, and resulting from deletion of the long arms of a G22 chromosome.

Phlebitis   Inflammation of a vein, which may be due to chemical or physical damage, as in the intravenous administration of drugs, or to **infection**. A potentially serious consequence is thrombosis of the affected vessel.

PHLS   Public Health Laboratory Service (in England and Wales).

Phosphodiesterase   An **enzyme** which in **platelets** regulates cyclic adenosine monophosphate (cAMP) levels by converting cAMP to 5'AMP. Drugs which inhibit phosphodiesterase cause cAMP to accumulate in the platelet and interfere with **platelet aggregation**.

Phosphotungstic acid   An electron-dense heavy metal compound frequently used for **negative staining** in **electron microscopy**.

Photometry   A system of measuring the amount of light transmitted through a solution.

Phototherapy   A form of treatment for **hyperbilirubinaemia** in the newborn − especially in **haemolytic disease of the newborn** − in which the infant is exposed to ultraviolet (290−320 nm) light or to visible light. As **bilirubin** circulating in the superficial blood vessels is exposed to light it combines with oxygen and is broken down into other, more readily excreted, products.

Phytagglutinin   See **Lectin** and **Phytohaemagglutinin**.

Phytohaemagglutinin   (PHA) A **lectin**, extracted from the seeds of *Phaseolus* spp, which **agglutinates** certain **erythrocytes** and acts as a **mitogen** on **T cells**.

Picogram   The **SI** unit corresponding to 10^{-12} g. In **haematology** it is the unit of measurement for **mean cell haemoglobin**.

Picornaviridae   A large family of non-**enveloped** viruses 25−30 nm in diameter. There are four genera: **enterovirus, rhinovirus,** aphthovirus and cardiovirus. The name is derived from the Greek *pico* (small) and **RNA**.

Pig-bel   An **acute** necrotising **enterocolitis** due to the beta-toxin of *Clostridium perfringens* type C. Typically it affects residents of Papua-New Guinea following infrequent pig feasts, when undercooked pig carcasses are eaten.

Pigeon fancier's lung   A **type III reaction** of hypersensitivity due to the inhalation of **antigens** derived from the blood, faeces or feathers of pigeons. See **Bird fancier's lung**.

Pigmentation   The deposition of pigment or coloured material.

Pilus   A tubular appendage of the bacterial cell, also known as **fimbriae**. They are mainly concerned with adhesion of one cell to another, and to some surfaces such as **epithelium**.

Pink disease   An artefact of tissue sections with a patchy failure of nuclear haematoxylin staining, and subsequent eosin staining of the same areas. Most noticeable in lymphoid tissue and epithelium.

Pinocytosis   The process by which **macrophages** ingest **proteins** and colloids too small to be ingested by **phagocytosis**.

Pin worm   *Enterobius vermicularis*. Also known as Seat worm. A very common **nematode** with world-wide distribution. Particularly associated with young children of primary school age, in whom it produces anal itching (pruritus).

Piperacillin   A semi-synthetic **penicillin** derivative, active against **Enterobacteriaceae, Pseudomonas, Bacteroides** and **cocci** which are positive by **Gram's stain**, including **enterococci** but not **penicillinase**-producing **staphylococci**.

Piperazine   An anti-**helminth** drug which causes expulsion of live paralysed worms.

Pipette A glass or plastic tubular device for transferring and/or measuring small volumes of fluid. Pipettes may or may not be calibrated in terms of volume. See also **Pasteur pipette**.

Pirani gauge A simple thermocouple gauge for vacuum measurement, operating from atmospheric pressure to medium vacuum levels. See also **Penning gauge**.

Pituitary gland An **endocrine** gland located at the base of the brain, which produces **hormones** which influence the function of other endocrine glands.

Pityriasis versicolor Syn. *Tinea versicolor*. A superficial fungus infection of the skin, commonly seen in young adults and presenting as hypopigmentation on dark-skinned individuals. The causative organism is *Malassezia furfur*.

PIVKA See **Proteins Induced by Vitamin K Absence or Antagonism**.

Pivmecillinam A pivaloyloxymethyl ester of **mecillinam** which is absorbed from the gastro-intestinal tract, unlike mecillinam, and is then converted to the active drug by hydrolysis.

PK See **Pyruvate Kinase**.

Placebo An inert **control** treatment, such as a dummy pill, often used when testing a new treatment so that subjects – and sometimes the person giving the treatment – do not know which treatment they are receiving. See **Control**.

Planapochromat A type of **apochromatic** objective lens, corrected for flatness of field.

Planococcus A **bacterium** which is a genus of the family **Micrococcaceae**, whose members exhibit **motility** by means of **flagella**. They are **catalase** positive **cocci** and strict **aerobes** which are positive by **Gram's stain** and live in sea water.

-plasia A suffix word indicating formation, growth or development (e.g. **hypoplasia**).

Plasma The fluid portion of circulating blood and of shed blood which has not been allowed to clot, and which therefore contains fibrinogen. In **whole blood** collected for **transfusion** the plasma is diluted with an **anticoagulant**/preservative solution (usually **Acid Citrate Dextrose** or **Citrate Phosphate Dextrose**) and is more properly termed 'citrated plasma'.

Plasma cell A mononuclear cell which is the end point of **differentiation** of the **B-lymphocyte** and which participates in the **immune response** through production of **antibody**.

Plasma derivatives See **Blood fractions**.

Plasma expander A solution of known viscosity used in **transfusion** to replace lost fluid volume. Plasma expanders should be retained in the circulation for reasonable periods of time but must eventually be completely excreted. The most common example is **Dextran**.

Plasma haemoglobin See **Haemoglobinaemia**.

Plasmapheresis **Apheresis** applied for the purpose of harvesting plasma from a **blood donor**.

Plasma protein fraction See **Plasma Protein Solution**.

Plasma protein solution A preparation of human **albumin** used in transfusion as a **plasma expander**.

Plasma thromboplastin antecedent See **Coagulation factors**.

Plasma volume The total volume of plasma in the body, which can be measured following injection of radio-labelled albumin. The normal adult values are approximately 49–59 ml/Kg body weight. See **Blood volume**.

Plasmid Extrachromosomal genetic material which is replicated along with the host **genome**. **Genes** borne on plasmids can code for resistance to **anti-microbial** substances, formation of a **capsule**, and transferability of the plasmid to other cells, as well as many other properties. They can be transduced by **bacteriophage** but are also lost spontaneously due to failure to replicate.

Plasmin In the blood, the **serine protease** enzyme formed from **plasminogen** as the major product of the fibrinolytic system. The major biological function of plasmin is to digest **fibrin**, forming **fibrin degradation products**.

Plasminogen The main inactive precursor **protein** of the fibrinolytic system in the blood. It may be converted to **plasmin** by a number of **plasminogen activators**. Circulating plasminogen normally has NH_2-terminal glutamic acid (glu-plasminogen), but an NH_2-terminal lysine type (lys-plasminogen) may form as a result of partial degradation of the glu-form.

Plasminogen activator A general term for any **protein** capable of converting **plasminogen** to **plasmin**. See also **Streptokinase**, **Tissue plasminogen activator** and **Urokinase**.

Plasmodium A genus in the class Sporozoa which also includes **Toxoplasma** and **Babesia**. Plasmodium is an obligate intracellular **parasite** which causes **malaria**. Four species, *P. falciparum*, *P. vivax*, *P. malariae* and *P. ovale* cause human disease. The sexual reproductive stage takes place in the mosquito and the asexual stage occurs in man. The **infectious** sporozoites are introduced when the mosquito bites, and multiply in the liver before emerging as merozoites to invade **erythrocytes**. Here they can be detected by **Giemsa stain**. Sexual reproduction begins by both male and female merozoites or gametocytes being ingested by another mosquito.

Platelet A small non-nucleated blood cell found in peripheral blood and numbering approximately 150 000 to 400 000 per mm^3. Platelets are part of the mechanism of **coagulation**, forming part of the haemostatic 'plug' at the site of skin puncture. Also known as thrombocytes.

Platelet activating factor An ether-lipid mediator of inflammation, produced by and active on both **platelets** and endothelial cells. It is capable of inducing **platelet aggregation** and **neutrophil chemotaxis** as well as a wide range of other pharmacological actions, and is being used increasingly as a **platelet aggregation** reagent in the laboratory.

Platelet adhesion The ability of **platelets** to adhere to a foreign surface, and which is the first stage of **haemostasis**. In the laboratory this may be assessed by measuring the platelet count of blood before and after passing through a column of glass beads, and calculating the percentage of platelets which have been retained.

Platelet aggregation The process by which **platelets** aggregate and adhere to each other during the formation of a haemostatic plug. In the laboratory, platelet aggregation can be assessed in **platelet-rich plasma** or whole blood, and is commonly used to assess platelet function. Popular aggregating agents are **adenosine diphosphate**, **collagen**, **epinephrine**, **thrombin**, **ristocetin**, **arachadonic acid** and **platelet activating factor**.

Platelet concentrate The concentrated **platelets** from one or more units of **whole blood** collected for **transfusion**. Platelet concentrates must be stored at 20−22°C with constant agitation and may remain viable for no more than 3 or 5 days (depending upon the formulation of the plastic container in which they are stored), even though intact platelets can still be counted. The **pH** of the preparation must not be allowed to fall below 6·0.

Platelet-derived growth factor A basic **protein**, found in **platelet** alpha-granules, which has a number of biological activities including inducing endothelial cell growth, fibroblast **chemotaxis**, and promoting activation of **macrophages**.

Platelet factor 3 A **platelet**-derived **coagulation factor** of phospholipid-like composition. It may be defined as the contribution of the blood platelets to coagulation factor interaction during activation of factor X and prothrombin in the **intrinsic blood coagulation** system.

Platelet factor 4 The name given to the **heparin**-neutralising activity of **platelets** due to a low molecular weight protein released during **platelet aggregation**.

Platelet lifespan The length of time the blood **platelet** remains in circulation: normally 8−10 days. The platelet survival time can be measured directly with radio-labelled **platelets**, or indirectly by measuring **malonyldialdehyde** production following aspirin ingestion.

Plateletpheresis **Apheresis** performed to harvest **platelets** from the donor.

Platelet poor blood **Whole blood** for **transfusion** from which the **platelets** have been removed to prepare a **platelet concentrate**. (Note. Whole blood stored for more than 48 h will also be deficient in viable platelets, but the term 'platelet poor' is not normally used for these donations.)

Platelet-poor plasma (PPP) Plasma obtained from blood which has been centrifuged at relatively high speed (>1000 x g for 20 min) to sediment all **platelets**. PPP is usually required for blood coagulation assays and as a blank in **platelet aggregation** studies by optical **aggregometry**.

Platelet-rich plasma (PRP) Plasma obtained from blood which has been centrifuged at relatively low speed (160 x g for 10 min) to sediment the **erythrocytes** while leaving the **platelets** in suspension. PRP is required for optical **platelet aggregation** tests as well as other tests of **platelet** function.

Platelet substitute A phospholipid preparation derived from chloroform-treated brain extracts, used as a substitute for **platelet factor 3** in some blood coagulation tests, for example in the **thromboplastin generation test**.

(beta) Pleated sheet An arrangement of poplypeptide chains which gives **amyloid** its characteristic properties when stained with Congo red.

Pleomorphism 1. Exhibiting general variation in form. 2. The assumption of various distinct forms by a single species or organism.

Plesiomonas A genus of rod-shaped **bacteria** in the family Vibrionaceae, which exhibit **motility**, are facultatively **anaerobic** and negative by **Gram's stain**, and which are found in water and in human **faeces**. They are occasionally suspected of causing **enteritis**.

Pleural effusion Collection of fluid in the pleural space. This may be due to circulatory or cardiac disease, pancreatitis, malignancy or **infection**. Infective causes are **pneumonia**, **tuberculosis** and actinomycosis, or fungal respiratory infections.

Pluripotential stem cell A type of cell which is difficult to identify morphologically, but which is believed to give rise to the several lines of differentiated blood cells – **erythrocytes**, **leucocytes** and **platelets** in blood and **bone marrow**.

Pneumocystis carinii A **protozoon** which forms both **cysts** and **trophozoites** and which produces an interstitial pneumonia, seen as endemic illness of premature and malnourished children and associated particularly with immunocompromised subjects and those receiving prolonged corticosteroid therapy. It also appears to be a fairly common cause of disease in animals. In humans the cysts are found in the alveoli, where they cause an **acute** alveolitis. Diagnosis is made radiologically and by finding cysts in lung **biopsies**, but the organism has also been cultured on **vero cells** and other cell lines. Demonstration of the organism is more successful in biopsy material than in sputum. Treatment involves the administration of pentamidine or co-trimoxazole. See also **Acquired immune deficiency syndrome**.

Pneumonia An **acute** lower respiratory tract **infection** involving **oedema** and infiltration of the alveoli with exudate, and sometimes haemorrhage. The affected area loses its elasticity and becomes X-ray opaque. One pulmonary lobe only may be affected, or the whole lung field can be involved. Primary atypical pneumonia, associated with *Mycoplasma pneumoniae* and *Chlamydia psittaci*, is shown by diffuse areas of damage in both lungs. Community-acquired pneumonia is usually due to *Streptococcus pneumoniae*, *Legionella pneumophila* or **influenza**, para-influenza and respiratory syncytial **viruses**, **Coxiella** and **Mycoplasma**. Hospital-acquired pneumonias are also caused by **pseudomonas**, **enterobacteriaceae** and *Staphylococcus aureus*. Pneumonia in the immuno-suppressed individual may be due to *Pneumocystis carinii*, **aspergillus**, **candida** and other **fungi**. Aspiration pneumonia in those with a swallowing defect such as the unconscious, the inebriated or those with neurological deficiencies is often due to mixtures of **anaerobes**.

Pneumonitis Strictly, inflammation of the lungs. It can occur alone but is more usually part of other lung diseases such as **pneumonia**.

Pneumovirus A genus of the **Paramyxoviridae**, characterised by lack of haem**agglutinin** and **neuraminidase**. The only member of the genus is **respiratory syncytial virus**.

PNH See **Paroxysmal Nocturnal Haemoglobinuria**.

Poikilocyte An **erythrocyte** of irregular (e.g. tear-drop or helmet-shaped) outline, commonly seen in the peripheral **blood films** of patients with **myelofibrosis** and **megaloblastic anaemia**.

Point sampling A simple method of establishing the proportional area occupied by a given component in a tissue section. The method relies on a number of random points falling on a particular area being directly proportional to the total size of that area. It is given by the formula $s/S = p/P$, where P = total points on total area S, and s = the particular area on which points p fall.

Poke In computing, an instruction used in **BASIC**, which enables the programmer to insert information in any location in **Random Access Memory**.

Pokeweed mitogen A collection of **mitogens** derived from *Phytolacca americano*. Depending on which fractions are used, **T cells** and **B cells** may be activated.

237

Polarising microscopy A form of microscopy which employs polarised light as the illuminant. Two sheets of material impregnated with organic dyes (polars) are placed, one below the condensing lens (the 'polariser') and one in the eyepiece (the 'analyser'). As the analyser is rotated through 360°C the light intensity changes from bright to nearly black twice during the rotation. If **birefringent** or **anisotropic** materials are introduced in the light path at the nearly-black position they will appear as bright images on a dark field.

Pole piece The soft iron part of an electromagnetic lens, where the strong axial field is generated.

Poliomyelitis Inflammation and **necrosis** of motor **neurones** in the spinal cord, and occasionally the medulla, resulting in irreversible paralysis of the muscles served. The disease is caused by **poliovirus** types 1–3, and (rarely) by **coxsackie** virus type A9. The disease has become rare in developed parts of the world due to the widespread use of killed and live **vaccine**.

Poliovirus Types 1–3 are members of the **enterovirus** genus of the **Picornaviridae**. They are commonly found in the gastro-enteric tract, where they cause little damage. A proportion of infections spill over from the gut into the blood, in which they may be transported to the central nervous system, causing **meningitis** or poliomyelitis. They are readily isolated from faeces in **primary cell** culture, producing a rapid **cytopathic effect**.

Polyacrylamide gel electrophoresis A system for separating charged macromolecules (usually **proteins**) by **electrophoresis**, in which acrylamide is used as a **substrate**. If sodium dodecyl sulphate is included in the system, proteins separate according to their molecular weights.

Polyagglutination **Agglutination** of red cells by a number of different sera, apparently non-specifically, but not by the serum of the cell donor.

Polychromasia The presence in **blood films** which have been **Romanowsky stained** of **erythrocytes** with a 'blue' tint rather than the normal eosinophilic appearance. Such cells are often larger than the surrounding red cells and represent **reticulocytes** in which the reticular material takes up both acid and basic stain components, resulting in the polychromatic appearance.

Polyclonal Derived from several cells. In serology, usually referring to an **antibody** produced as part of the **immune response**.

Polycythaemia Strictly defined as an increase in the numbers of all cellular elements of the peripheral blood (i.e. **erythrocytosis, leucocytosis** and **thrombocytosis**). The condition may be primary **(polycythaemia rubra vera)** or secondary to other conditions (e.g.

anoxia). In the latter group, the term polycythaemia has become synonymous with **erythrocytosis**, even though **leucocyte** and **platelet** levels are not usually increased.

Polycythaemia rubra vera A disorder characterised by **hyperplasia** of the **bone marrow** resulting in **erythrocytosis, leucocytosis** and **thrombocytosis**. It is a malignant condition and a member of the group of **myeloproliferative disorders**.

Polyenes A group of anti-fungal **anti-microbial** substances produced by **Streptomyces** species, and characterised by a macrolide ring and a cyclic lactone formation. The two most commonly used are **Nystatin** and **Amphotericin B**. They act by forming complexes with sterols in the fungal **cell membrane**, causing cytoplasmic leakage. Toxicity on parenteral administration of amphotericin includes thrombophlebitis and renal damage.

Polymicrobial A term used to describe **infections** where more than one putatively causative organism is present.

Polymixins A group of polypeptide **anti-microbial** substances produced by the **Bacillus** species, and active against rod-shaped **bacteria** which are facultative **anaerobes** and which are negative by **Gram's stain**, including **pseudomonas** but excluding **proteus**. Most Gram-positive bacteria are resistant. The site of action is the bacterial **cell membrane**. Polymixins are nephrotoxic and also cause vestibular damage and peripheral neuropathies. The group includes polymixin B and polymixin E (**colistin**).

Polymorphism Literally, many different shapes or forms. Used in genetics to refer to the occurrence of two or more **alleles** at the same locus, as in the **blood groups**.

Polymorphonuclear Having a **nucleus** which is deeply lobed so as to appear like a multiple nucleus.

Polynucleotide A polymer of **nucleotides**; long polymers are nucleic acids.

Polyomavirus A genus of the **Papovaviridae**, including the **SV40** virus of monkeys and the human **virus** JC, which is thought to be a cause of **progressive multi-focal leucoencephalopathy** in the **immunocompromised** host.

Polyp A growth protruding from the mucous membrane.

Polypeptide The generic term for compounds containing 6–30 amino acids linked together by peptide bonds.

Polystyrene latex test See **Latex particle test**.

Polyuria An increase in the daily volume of urine excreted. It occurs in many conditions including **diabetes** mellitus and diabetes insipidus.

Polyvalent anti-serum A **serum** containing **antibodies** directed against a wide variety of **antigens**. The term is sometimes used in a

239

more restricted manner to describe an **anti-serum** containing anti-bodies against antigens carried on a single genus of a **bacterium**.

Polyvalent vaccine A **vaccine** containing **antigens** from a number of **micro-organisms** of a single genus (e.g. TAB vaccine, active against the **bacteria** causing typhoid, para-typhoid A and para-typhoid B).

Pontiac fever A form of **Legionellosis**.

Population In statistical usage this can either be a true (often very large) collection of individuals, or a hypothetical collection of the results which would be obtained if an experiment or study was repeated under identical conditions an extremely large number of times. See also **Sample**.

Porin A type of **protein** found in the outer **membrane** of **bacterial** cells which are negative by **Gram's stain**. Porins create a discrete hydrophilic area which allows passage of hydrophilic substances into the cell − a mechanism which is important in the entry of **anti-microbial** substances into the organism. Altered porins, or reduction in their numbers, account for some cases of resistance to **anti-microbial** substances.

Porphobilinogen An intermediate in the pathway of haem syn-thesis, formed by the condensation of two mols of delta-amino-laevulinic acid.

Porphyria A rare group of inherited disorders characterised by over-production of **porphyrins** and/or porphyrin precursors, due to faulty regulation or blocking of haem synthesis. These condi-tions may be associated with photosensitivity and dermatitis, as well as neurological and endocrine disorders.

Porphyrin A cyclic compound formed by four pyrrole rings which are linked by methylene bridges. It consists of resonating, red-coloured molecules formed by irreversible oxidation of porphy-rinogens during haem synthesis. They are lost from the haem synthesis pathway and excreted in bile and urine.

Porphyrinuria See **Porphyria**.

Port In computing, a physical area for the connection of a com-munications line between the **central processing unit** and any of its **peripherals**.

Positive strand A strand of nucleic acid capable of **transcription** of information to **messenger RNA** or **translation** from **RNA** to **protein**.

Post chroming Treatment of tissue with 30 g/l potassium dichromate following normal **fixation**. Reputed to improve preservation.

Post coupling A method of demonstrating enzymes in tissues. The insoluble primary reaction product of enzyme/substrate interac-tion is coupled with a coloured or opaque marker at the site of activity.

Post fixation   A term applied to (i) the secondary **fixation** of **lipid-**rich tissue following processing through **clearing** agents; and (ii) the **fixation** of **freeze-dried** tissue using the vapour phase of the fixative.

Potency   Literally strength, power. Used in serology to refer to the degree of ability of an **antibody** to react with its specific **antigen**.

Poxviridae   A large family of ovoid or brick-shaped **viruses**, 250–300 by 300–350 nm in size, and large enough to be just visible by **light microscopy**. Two genera infect man, **orthopoxvirus** and para-**poxvirus**. The **genome** of their **DNA** is enclosed in a complex **protein** coat with no discernible symmetry.

PPF   See **Plasma Protein Solution**.

PPS   See **Plasma Protein Solution**.

Prausnitz-Kustner reaction   A skin test to detect **IgE**. Human serum containing IgE is injected intradermally, where it may bind to sub-epithelial **mast cells**. After 48 h, **antigen** is injected into the same site. A 'weal and flare' response indicates a specific reaction between antigen and mast cell-bound IgE. See **Passive cutaneous anaphylaxis** – a similar test used in experimental animals.

Pre-albumin   A **protein** with a molecular weight of 61 000. It binds T_3 (and, to a lesser extent, T_4) and on **electrophoresis** it is more mobile than **albumin**. See **Protein binding**.

Precipitation   The result of a compound becoming insoluble so that the solute is no longer soluble in the solvent.

Precipitin   An **antibody** which reacts with a soluble **antigen** to form visible **precipitation**.

Precision   The degree of reproducibility in a set of replicate results. It is usually expressed in terms of **standard deviation** or **coefficient of variation**.

Pre-kallikrein   The plasma precursor of **kallikrein**, one of the **co-agulation factors** involved in **contact activation**. Pre-kallikrein may be converted to kallikrein by activated factor XII.

Pre-leukaemia   Any condition associated with an abnormal **clone** of **bone marrow** cells which has a greater probability than normal of further abnormal maturation into a frankly leukaemic state. Several myelodysplastic conditions such as sideroblastic anaemia, **polycythaemia rubra vera** and **paroxysmal nocturnal haemoglobinuria** are thought to be pre-leukaemic.

Price-Jones curve   A now obsolete method of determining **mean cell diameter** by measuring images of red cells from stained **blood films** projected on to white paper. The measurements are then expressed as a grouped frequency distribution curve.

Primary cell culture   A **monolayer cell culture** derived directly from the disruption by **enzymes** of excised tissue or organs.

Primary immune response   The **immune response** of an individual

241

to the first exposure to an **antigen**. Usually, only low levels of **antibody** or **cell-mediated immune** response are seen. On subsequent exposure to the same antigen a heightened response is seen. This is called the secondary, memory, or **anamnestic response**.

Primary standard A very pure material that can be used to prepare a solution at varying concentrations to calibrate a system accurately.

Primigravida A woman pregnant for the first time.

Priming dose The first dose of an **antigen** administered to an individual. This will elicit the **primary immune response**, after which the individual is said to be 'primed' for, or sensitised to, the antigen.

Primipara A woman who has had one previous pregnancy. In her second pregnancy she is para 1 and gravida 2.

Prism A triangular glass, silica, quartz or rock salt structure through which polychromatic white light is passed. The refractive index of the material, being different to air, causes the light to be bent (refracted) according to its wavelength. A specific wavelength can then be transmitted from the prism to form the incident light beam in a **spectrophotometer**.

PRIST Abbreviation for **P**aper **R**adio**I**mmuno**S**orbent **T**est, used to measure **IgE** in **serum**. Test serum is allowed to react with paper discs coated with anti-IgE. Following washing of the discs, radio-labelled anti-IgE is added. The amount of radioactivity detected on the discs is proportional to the IgE level in the test serum.

'Private' antigen See **Family antigen**.

Privileged site A site in the body where **antigens** or grafts may be placed without stimulating an **immune response** (e.g. hamster cheek-pouch and the anterior chamber of the eye).

Probenecid Dipropyl sulphamoyl benzoic acid, a drug which partially inhibits renal tubular secretion of **beta lactam** types of **antimicrobial** substances, and thereby increases serum half-life. It also blocks renal excretion of **rifampicin**, although this is insufficiently reliable to be of practical use.

Processing 1. In **histopathology**, the passage of tissue through a series of reagents prior to **embedding** in a final medium for **microtomy**. Normally includes **fixation**, **dehydration**, **clearing** and **impregnation**. 2. In **transfusion science**, the separation of a unit of **whole blood** into various components for **transfusion**. See **Blood components** and **Blood fractions**. 3. In computing, the manipulation of input data by a **central processing unit** in order to derive other data from it.

Proctitis Inflammation of the rectum. It is found most often in prostitutes and male homosexuals, where it can be caused by **chlamydia** or *Neisseria gonorrhoeae*.

Proerythroblast The earliest recognisable **erythrocyte** precursor in the **bone marrow**. It is a relatively large cell, $14-19 \times 10^{-6}$ m in diameter, possessing a deep blue, agranular **cytoplasm** with no evidence of **haemoglobin** synthesis.

Progesterone A **hormone** produced by the *corpus luteum*.

Proglottid The mature segment of a tape worm, which is passed out in faeces. If infected faeces is shed indiscriminantly the proglottid disintegrates and the released eggs are eaten by an intermediate host. *Taenia solium* (pig) and *T. Saginata* (beef) are the most common examples, but other tape worms infective to man and their intermediate hosts are known to occur in many parts of the world. The definitive host (man) thus becomes infected by eating under-cooked meat.

Program In computing, the complete sequence of instructions and routines for the computer to carry out a given task. (Used as a verb, to write such a program.)

Progressive multi-focal leucoencephalopathy A rare and fatal central nervous system disease of the **immunocompromised** host, probably caused by a **polyomavirus**.

Progressive staining A method in which tissue sections are immersed in a **dye** bath and various structures are stained sequentially. The section is removed when the desired staining has been achieved. See also **Regressive staining**.

Prokaryote A type of single-celled **micro-organism** which lacks a nuclear **membrane**, has a single **chromosome**, does not undergo **mitosis**, and has no mitochondria or other cytoplasmic organelles. **Bacteria** belong to this group, while **fungi** are **eukaryotes**.

Prolactin A **hormone** secreted by the anterior pituitary gland. It stimulates the secretion of milk in mammary glands.

Promegakaryocyte A very large cell ($20-80 \times 10^{-6}$ m in diameter) with a large convoluted nucleus, present in the **bone marrow**. The cell is formed from the **megakaryoblast** and is the precursor of the **platelet**-forming **megakaryocyte**.

Promonocyte The precursor of the **monocyte**, $14-20 \times 10^{-6}$ m in diameter, with a large folded nucleus and basophilic **cytoplasm**. It is infrequently seen in **bone marrow** smears, but can be identified as the more immature of the two types of marrow cell capable of adhering to glass.

Promyelocyte The largest of the **granulocyte** precursor cells in the **bone marrow**, with abundant basophilic **cytoplasm** containing red (azurophilic) granules. The promyelocyte is formed from the **myeloblast** and subsequently develops into the **myelocyte**.

Pronormoblast See **Proerythroblast**.

Properdin A **protein** component of the **alternative pathway** of **complement** activation. Properdin stabilises C3bBb and extends the half-life of C3bBb as a convertase of complement component C3.

Prophase The first stage in **mitosis**, including all the processes up to the **metaphase**.

Prophylaxis Prevention of disease. In **immunology**, active prophylaxis uses **immunogens** such as live or killed **vaccines** to induce **active immunity**. Passive prophylaxis is achieved by inoculation of pre-formed **antibody** to provide short-term **passive immunity**. Chemical prophylaxis provides protection by the maintenance of active levels of **chemotherapeutic** agents such as **antibiotics**.

Propionibacterium Rod-shaped **bacteria** which do not exhibit **motility**, are non-branching, do not form **spores** and are **catalase** positive **anaerobes** which are positive by **Gram's stain**, and whose main product of **fermentation** is propionic acid. They are found on human skin and occasionally cause wound infections, particularly after neuro-surgery. They also sometimes colonise **prostheses**.

Propositus The member of a family in which a genetic pedigree has been studied and with whom the investigation was started.

Prostacyclin The popular name for one of the **prostaglandins** (prostaglandin I_2) synthesised by endothelial cells, but not by **platelets**. Prostacyclin is a potent stimulator of the **platelet** enzyme **adenylate cyclase**, thus elevating platelet **cAMP** concentration and inhibiting **platelet aggregation**.

Prostaglandins A family of biologically active compounds, with a wide range of pharmacological actions, formed from the metabolism of **arachadonic acid**. Almost all tissues are capable of prostaglandin production, although the major products vary between tissues. In **platelets**, prostaglandins are responsible for both pro-aggregatory and anti-aggregatory functions. See **Prostacyclin**.

Prostatitis Inflammation of the prostate gland, usually caused by rod-shaped **bacteria** which are facultative **anaerobes** and negative by **Gram's stain**. In **acute** prostatitis **anti-microbial** substances are able to penetrate the gland and effect a cure, but in **chronic** prostatitis relapse is common.

Prosthesis A replacement for an absent, removed or defective structure or function in the body. Surgically implanted prostheses (as opposed to, e.g., artificial limbs and dentures) include joint replacements, ascites shunts, urinary sphincters, cardiac pacemakers and valves, hydrocephalus shunts and peripheral and central vascular catheters. Implanted prostheses often become colonised or **infected** with **micro-organisms** such as **coagulase**-negative **staphylococci**.

Prosthetic valve endocarditis Colonisation of a valve **prosthesis**, and **infection** of the surrounding tissues. Early prosthetic valve endocarditis is contracted at implantation and is usually caused by **coagulase**-negative **staphylococci**, whereas late prosthetic valve endocarditis is often caused by *Streptococcus viridans* or by **enterococci**. Treatment often involves surgical removal of the prosthesis.

Protamine sulphate A basic **protein** which is clinically useful as an antidote for the anticoagulant effect of **heparin**. In the laboratory, protamine sulphate is used for the measurement of plasma heparin levels prior to reversal of the anticogulant effect, and forms the basis for a **paracoagulation test** for **fibrin monomers**.

ProtargolⓉ Ⓜ A combined reagent of silver and partially hydrolysed protein, used to demonstrate nerve fibres.

Protectin A specific haemagglutinin (but *not* an antibody) found in extracts of certain animal tissues. See also **Lectin**.

Protein An ubiquitous tissue component formed of amino acids linked by peptide bonds of variable sequences and chain lengths.

Protein A A protein isolated from the cell wall of *Staphylococcus aureus*, with a strong affinity for the Fc portion of **immunoglobulin** molecules. Used as a marker of **antigen/antibody** reactions. May be labelled with **FITC**, peroxidase, ferritin, etc.

Protein binding One of the mechanisms for transporting compounds in the **plasma**. For example, the binding of **anti-microbial** substances to **plasma** albumen and other proteins; a process which is often reversible and the therapeutic significance of which is unclear as it provides a reservoir of drug which is released as the free plasma drug levels fall, thus prolonging the plasma half-life of the drug. (However, bound drug fails to penetrate some body components.)

Protein C One of the **vitamin K**-dependent **coagulation factors** which, when activated by **thrombin**, exerts a powerful anticoagulant action by neutralising activated factors V and VIII.

Protein S A **vitamin K**-dependent **protein** which acts as a co-factor in the inactivation of activated factor V by activated **protein C**.

Proteins Induced by Vitamin K Absence or Antagonism (PIVKA) The precursor forms of the **vitamin K**-dependent **coagulation factors** II, VII, IX and X, which lack the gamma-carboxyglutamic acid residues normally added to these proteins during the post-synthetic process catalysed by vitamin K. PIVKA lack the ability to bind calcium ions and therefore cannot take part in normal blood coagulation.

Proteolytic enzyme A substance capable of digesting protein. A number of these are used in blood group serology.

Proteus Rod-shaped **bacteria** which exhibit **motility** and swarming, are facultative **anaerobes, catalase** positive, **oxidase** negative and negative by **Gram's stain.** With the exception of *P. mirabilis* they deaminate phenylalanine and produce indole. Citrate is utilised and urease is produced. The organisms are **commensals** of the intestine and cause urinary tract and wound **infections.**

Prothrombin See **Coagulation factors.**

Prothrombinase The name given to the complex formed from activated factor X, factor V, **platelet factor 3** and calcium ions which act as the physiological activator of **prothrombin** in the **intrinsic blood coagulation** system.

Prothrombin Consumption Index (PCI) A test of **intrinsic blood coagulation** based on the fact that **prothrombin** is almost completely consumed during clotting. An estimation of **prothrombin time** is made on the **serum** remaining 1 hour after whole blood has clotted in a glass tube, and compared with the clotting time of anticoagulated **plasma.** The PCI is calculated as:

$$\frac{\text{Plasma clotting time}}{\text{Serum clotting time}} \times 100\%$$

More accurate results are obtained by specific measurements of **prothrombin** before and after clotting has occurred.

Prothrombin time The time taken for plasma to clot after addition of brain **thromboplastin** and calcium chloride. The test is sensitive to deficiencies of **coagulation factors** II, V, VII and X and is widely used in the laboratory control of oral anticoagulant therapy.

Prothrombotic state A condition thought to exist, although often difficult to detect by laboratory tests, in which an individual is at increased risk of developing thrombosis. This may occur in an individual who is apparently well, or in association with other conditions which predispose to thrombosis (e.g. **antithrombin III** deficiency and **polycythaemia**).

Protoplasm A general term for the substance of a living cell.

Protoporphyrin A **porphyrin**, the iron complex of which constitutes haem which, together with protein, forms **haemoglobin.**

Protozoa Simple unicellular organisms, eukaryotic cells, the bodies of which are covered by a trilaminar unit **membrane.** Protozoans move by **flagella, cilia, pseudopodia** or undulating ridges. Central and peripheral zones of **cytoplasm** can frequently be distinguished as **endoplasm** and **ectoplasm.**

Protozoology The study of protozoa. Medical protozoology deals with the nucleated single cell-like micro-organisms which may be referred to as either unicellular or acellular, and which act as **parasites** in man.

Providencia Rod-shaped **bacteria** which exhibit **motility** and are **catalase** positive, **oxidase** negative, facultative **anaerobes** which are negative by **Gram's stain** and which deaminate phenylalinine but fail to hydrolyse urea. They are associated with urinary tract infections, particularly in those with indwelling urinary catheters.

Prozone phenomenon The phenomenon that occurs when an **antibody** fails to react with its specific **antigen** in high concentrations but begins to react at lower concentrations.

PRP See **Platelet-rich plasma**.

Prussian blue Potassium ferric ferrocyanide: a highly coloured reaction product of **haemosiderin** and potassium ferrocyanide.

Prussian blue staining A method for the cytochemical demonstration of iron in blood, **bone marrow** or tissue preparations. It is based on the reaction between **haemosiderin** and acidified potassium ferrocyanide (Perl's reaction). See **Prussian blue**.

PRV See **Polycythaemia Rubra Vera**.

Psammoma body A small round and concentrically arranged structure, often calcified, frequently present in ovarian and other papillary **tumours**.

Pseudocollagen A term to describe mature **fibrinoid**, which stains as collagen rather than fibrin.

Pseudokeratosis A reaction in the stratified **squamous epithelium** of the uterine cervix, characterised by the presence of several layers of small polygonal cells overlying the surface of the stratified squamous mucosa.

Pseudomelanosis pigment An **autofluorescent** pigment found in *lamina propria* of the colon, usually in **macrophages** and, particularly, in pseudomelanosis coli − a condition of unknown **aetiology**.

Pseudomembranous colitis An **acute** inflammation of the colon and caecum involving necrosis and sloughing of the mucosa with formation of a thick membranous fibrinous exudate. The most usual cause is *Clostridium difficile*, a common organism which overgrows when broad-spectrum **anti-microbial** substances are used. The organisms often produce **toxins** which are cytotoxic. While **clindamycin** was originally implicated, the condition is now known to be a complication of therapy with a variety of anti-microbial substances.

Pseudomonas Rod shaped **bacteria** which exhibit **motility**, are **catalase** positive, **oxidase** positive, negative by **Gram's stain** and are obligate **aerobes**. They are metabolically versatile and can use complex organic compounds as carbon sources. An example is the ability to utilise chloroxylenol and other **antiseptic** substances. They have a wide growth temperature range, some species being able to grow slowly at temperatures around freezing. Some species produce pigments, some of which are fluorescent. They are common in both everyday and hospital environments. *Ps. aeruginosa* and several other species cause serious sepsis in hospitalised patients if a portal of entry to the host is provided or if the immune system is severely compromised. They are often resistant to a wide range of **anti-microbial** substances and present serious therapeutic problems.

Pseudopodium An extension of the **cytoplasm**, used for movement or to gather food. Seen (e.g.) in living **trophozoites** of parasitic amoebae.

Psittacosis A **zoonosis** of birds which can affect humans. The causative agent, *Chlamydia psittaci*, is an obligate intracellular **bacterium** which enters the body by being inhaled along with dust from bird droppings or feathers. The lung is primarily involved but the infection is systemic. The incubation period is up to 2 or 3 weeks after exposure, and the symptoms are high fever, headache, myalgia and anorexia with a dry cough. The diagnosis is made by serological means. The **anti-microbial** substance of choice is **tetracycline**.

PT See **Prothrombin time**.

PTH See **Parathormone**.

'Public' antigen The converse of 'Private' or 'Family' **antigen**. **Blood group** antigens which are found in the blood of nearly all individuals. Also know as 'high incidence' antigens.

Purine A class of compounds of which the end point of **metabolism** in man is uric acid. In most mammals it is acted upon by uricase to form allantoin.

Pus A collection of both living and dead **neutrophils** and **macrophages**, plasma proteins, **bacteria** and debris resulting from an **infection**. It is seen most often as the constituent of an **abscess** and usually drains spontaneously if allowed to do so.

Putrefaction Breakdown of tissue after removal or death, and due to the action of micro-organisms.

P-value See **Significance level**.

Pyelonephritis An **infection** of the parenchyma of the kidney causing scarring, **abscess** formation, shrinkage and eventually loss of function. Recurrent urinary tract infection precedes pyelonephritis which itself often becomes **chronic**. The symptoms are fever, loin pain, malaise, dysuria and frequency of micturition, with bacteriuria. The causative organisms include **Enterobacteriaceae** and **enterococci**.

Pyknocyte A term used to describe an **erythrocyte** with an irregularly contracted outline and abnormally deep staining reaction, seen in some **haemolytic anaemias**.

Pyknosis A degenerative change in which the **nucleus** shrinks in size and **chromatin** condenses to a solid amorphous mass.

Pyloric stenosis Congenital or acquired narrowing of the gastric outlet – either at the pylorus or within the duodenum – causing an obstruction.

Pyoderma An **infection** of the skin, involving **pus** formation and usually due to *Streptococcus pyogenes*. Commonly known as impetigo.

Pyogenic Denotes an association with **pus** formation.

Pyrazinamide A synthetic **anti-microbial** substance produced from nicotinamide and active against *Mycobacterium tuberculosis*. The mode of action is unknown. Side effects (including hepatotoxicity) and the low activity of the drug have led to it being rarely used.

Pyrexia Persistently elevated body temperature. A **febrile** condition. A **fever**. See also **Pyrogen**.

Pyrimethamine A synthetic **anti-microbial** substance similar to **trimethoprim**, and active against **plasmodia**. It is used to treat quinine-resistant **malaria**.

Pyrogen A substance capable of inducing **fever**. Usually refers to a polysaccharide by-product of bacterial metabolism which, when introduced by a **parenteral** route into a living body, precipitates a **febrile** reaction. Dead organisms, or even lipopolysaccharide derived from them, cause fever if injected. Pyrogens are commonly found in tap water and both solutions intended for intravenous use and infusion apparatus must be prepared using only water distilled in a special baffled still designed so as to exclude pyrogenic water from the final distillate. Endogenous pyrogens are secreted by **neutrophils** and other cells and are a cause of fever associated with **infections**.

Pyruvate A salt or metabolite of pyruvic acid.

Pyruvate kinase (EC 2.7.1.40) An enzyme of the **Embden Meyerhof pathway** which catalyses the conversion of phosphenolpyruvate to pyruvate with the formation of **adenosine triphosphate**. It is found in red cells, heart, brain, liver and kidneys. Hereditary deficiency of pyruvate kinase is associated with chronic non-**spherocytic haemolytic anaemia**.

Pyuria The presence of **pus** in the urine, due to urinary tract **infection**. It is usually associated with the presence of large numbers of organisms, but this may not be the case when there has been prior **chemotherapy** with **anti-microbial** substances directed against *Mycobacterium tuberculosis*, or in the case of a non-infective cause. Conversely, pyuria may sometimes be absent in the presence of significant **bacteriuria**.

Q

Q fever A pyrexial illness which is caused by *Coxiella burnettii*. It is a **zoonosis** of cattle and sheep which also affects humans, with **lymphadenopathy**, malaise, primary atypical **pneumonia** (though this may be asymptomatic), and **hepatitis**; the illness may progress to **endocarditis**. The organism is transmitted among animals by ticks, and to humans by inhalation of aerosols from products of parturition. A rising, or high, **titre** of serum **antibody** is diagnostic and the treatment of choice is **tetracycline** or **chloramphenicol**. The disease was first named 'Query fever' in 1937, hence its present name.

Quality The extent of compliance, or goodness. In the laboratory, in terms of **accuracy** and **precision** it is associated with nearness to truth and the ability to reproduce a result within defined limits. See **External quality assessment**, **Internal quality control**, and **Quality assurance**.

Quality assessment See **External quality assessment**.

Quality assurance A total system of ensuring that appropriate investigations are performed accurately in the laboratory under appropriate conditions on properly collected and transported samples, and that within-laboratory errors are minimised. Quality assurance includes staff training and performance as well as **internal quality control** and **external quality assessment**.

Quality control See **Internal quality control**.

Quantification The measurement of morphological or reactive features of cells and tissues, including microscopic and macroscopic features of dimension, volume, number, mass, concentration, biochemical and section analysis.

Quaternary ammonium compounds A group of **antiseptic** substances which are cationic surfactants. They are active against **bacteria** which are positive by **Gram's stain**, although not usually **bactericidal**. They have no useful activity against Gram-negative rod-shaped organisms and their activity is inhibited by anionic detergents such as soap, and other organic materials. Benzalkonium chloride is an example of this group.

Quellung reaction The reaction of **antibodies** on the **capsule** of *Streptococcus pneumoniae*, causing it to swell and to increase its refractive index. After exposure to antibody and examination by **light microscopy** the diplococci appear surrounded by a clear zone. The reaction is type-specific and can be used for studies of **epidemiology**. Other capsulated organisms react in a similar way with specific anti-sera.

Quenching In **histopathology**, rapid freezing of small pieces of tissue at low temperature to avoid the formation of ice crystals, and diffusion of labile substances.

Quinolones Synthetic **anti-microbial** substances which act by inhibiting the **DNA** gyrase of **bacteria**. The group contains **nalidixic acid**, **enoxacin**, **norfloxacin**, **ciprofloxacin** and others. The newer compounds such as norfloxacin and ciprofloxacin have a wide spectrum of activity against **bacteria** which are both positive and negative by **Gram's stain**. Resistance, if it occurs, is due either to alteration of DNA gyrase or to exclusion of the compound from the cell. Side effects of quinolones include central nervous system disturbances.

Quinone S Non-protein substances which play an important role in electron transport within the cell, being readily oxidised or reduced.

R

Rabies A fatal disease of the central nervous system, with a greatly variable incubation period, and caused by the **rabies virus**. Man frequently acquires the **infection** from infected dogs or cats, which will almost certainly have been exhibiting bizarre behaviour at the time. Man develops severe fits, often induced by the offer of water (hydrophobia), dementia, coma and death. Only three individuals are known to have survived the onset of symptoms. A successful vaccine and a specific **immunoglobulin** for prophylaxis are now available.

Rabies virus A member of the **Lyssavirus** genus, causing **rabies** in man and a wide variety of animals. The main reservoir of **infection** is in carnivores such as foxes, skunks, racoons, jackals and vampire bats, in which the disease may have an incubation period of several months. The **virus** is spread to man and other animals by biting injury inflicted by an infected animal. The virus has been kept out of the United Kingdom and other islands by strict quarantine of imported animals. Laboratory diagnosis of **rabies** is often made post-mortem by detection of **negri bodies** in brain cells, using **immunofluorescence** or the methods of **histopathology**. The virus may be isolated from brain and saliva, although this task is usually undertaken with some reluctance.

Radial diffusion test A test for quantitating soluble **antigen**. Wells are cut into an **agar** gel incorporating specific **antibody**. Antigen is placed in the wells and allowed to diffuse radially into the gel. A circular zone of **precipitation** develops, the diameter of which is proportional to the concentration of the antigen.

Radial haemolysis test See **Single radial haemolysis**.

Radiation response The percentage of **benign** forms of **squamous cells** in vaginal smears displaying radiation effects after radiation therapy.

Radioactivity The property of spontaneous disintegration of the nucleus of an atom, resulting in emission of alpha or beta particles or gamma rays.

Radio allergosorbent test A method for measuring **allergen**-specific IgE in human **serum**. Test serum is exposed to dextran particles coated with allergen and radio-labelled anti-human IgE then added. Following washing of the particles their radioactivity is proportional to the amount of allergen-specific IgE in the test serum.

Radioimmunoassay An **antigen/antibody** reaction in which a **radioisotope** is attached to one of the reactants — usually the antibody — and the extent of the ensuing reaction is measured by counting the number of **radioactive** particles emitted by the antigen/antibody complex. The result may be expressed initially as 'counts per minute', and by comparison with a **control test** containing a known amount of the substance for **assay** this can be converted into the appropriate units of measurement for that substance.

Radio immunoelectrophoresis A modification of **immunoelectrophoresis** in which radio-labelled **antibody** is used. Arcs of **precipitation** can be detected by **auto-radiography**.

Radioimmunosorbent test A method for measuring the total amount of **IgE** in **serum**. Test serum is mixed with radio-labelled IgE and the mixture then exposed to dextran particles coated with anti-human IgE. The labelled and unlabelled IgE compete for the anti-human IgE, and following washing the radioactivity of the particles is inversely proportional to the IgE level in the test serum.

Radioisotope A **radioactive** form of an element, consisting of unstable forms of the atoms of the element emitting alpha, beta or gamma radiation. See **Radiation**.

Radiometry A method of detecting metabolism of **bacteria** — and, by implication, their presence, multiplication or continued survival — by their ability to release radio-labelled carbon dioxide from ^{14}C-labelled glucose into the **culture medium**. Other radio-labelled compounds can also be used. The system can be used for blood cultures and for **anti-microbial** susceptibility testing.

Raji cell assay A test used to detect **complement**-fixing **immune complexes** in **serum**. Test serum is exposed to Raji cells (a human **lymphoblast**oid cell line). Immune complexes containing complement components bind to the Raji cells. Following washing of the cells, radio-labelled rabbit anti-human **IgG** is added. The amount of **radioactivity** detected on the cells is proportional to the level of complement-fixing immune complexes in the test serum.

Rake In histology, the angle formed between the knife facet closest to the cut surface of a block of material, and a line drawn vertically at right angles to the block surface. See also **Slant**.

RAM See **Random Access Memory**.

Ramsden circle The point at which rays emerging from the eyepiece of a microscope come to a focus.

Ramsden eyepiece A microscope eyepiece which comprises two plano-convex lenses with the convex surfaces of the eye and field lenses mounted in opposition. Also known as a positive eyepiece.

Random access memory In computing, **memory** which can be both read and written into by the computer during normal operation.

Randomisation The allocation of treatments to individuals at random, in order to avoid statistical **bias**.

Range Statistically, the smallest and the largest observations in a series. Looking at these gives a rough measure of the spread of the **distribution** being studied. See **Standard deviation**.

Rank Statistically, this is the position of an observation when the observations are ordered from the smallest to the largest. Ranks are used when using **normal probability paper**, and in the **Wilcoxon signed rank test** and the **Mann-Whitney U-test**.

RAST Abbreviation for **Radio AllergoSorbent Test**.

Rat-bite fever An illness involving **pyrexia**, with a rash and arthralgia occurring a few days after a bite by a rat or other small rodent. The causative organisms, *Streptobacillus moniliformis* or *Spirillum minor*, form part of the normal pharyngeal flora of rodents and are also found in laboratory rats. The disease may be of short duration but it may also relapse several times over a period of months. *Streptobacillus moniliformis* can be isolated on ordinary **culture media** from blood or joint aspirates, and *Spirillum minor* can be seen by dark ground microscopy. Serological tests are also helpful. One in four patients gives a false positive test for syphilis. The drug of choice for treatment is **penicillin**, although **tetracycline** is also useful.

Raynaud's phenomenon A condition characterised by reduced blood flow in peripheral blood vessels, precipitated by emotional stress or − more commonly − exposure to cold. Typically this gives rise to cyanosis and whitening of the fingers and other extremities.

RCF See **Relative Centrifugal Force**.

RCPath The Royal College of Pathologists. Founded 1963.

Reaction of identity A **precipitation** reaction in a **gel diffusion test**, which demonstrates that two **antigen** solutions are identical. This is seen by the fact that the arcs of precipitation produced merge together to give a continuous, combined arc.

Reaction of non-identity A **precipitation** reaction in a **gel diffusion test** which demonstrates that two **antigen** solutions are not identical. This is seen by the fact that the arcs of precipitation produced do not merge together, but cross and continue independently. See **Reaction of identity**.

Reaction rate analyser An analyser which measures the speed or rate of a reaction as it proceeds rather than at the end point. It is particularly useful for measurements of **enzyme** activity.

Read only memory In computing, **memory** containing fixed data or instructions, which are permanently loaded as part of the manufacturing process. The memory can be read but cannot be altered by writing fresh data into it. See also **Erasable Programmable Read Only Memory**.

Reagin 1. An **antibody** (IgE) which becomes attached to **mast cell** surfaces. When specific **antigen** binds to the mast cell surface antibody the mast cells de-granulate and liberate vaso-active amines which cause **type I reactions** of **hypersensitivity**. 2. An obsolete term for the **complement**-fixing antibody detected in some serological tests for syphilis.

Reaginic antibody See **Reagin**.

Real image An optically formed image of an object.

Recalcification time The time taken for a clot to form following addition of calcium chloride to citrated **plasma**. The clotting time is prolonged in **coagulation factor** deficiencies of the **intrinsic system**, but has been replaced for clinical purposes by the **activated partial thromboplastin time**.

Receptor An area of a molecule or cell which can bind specifically to another molecule or cell.

Recessive gene A gene which manifests itself only in the **homozygous** state. The converse of a **dominant gene**.

Recirculating pool In **immunology**, a term used to describe the **T cells** and **B cells** which circulate around the body in the blood and lymph.

Recombinant A **genome** or organism produced by artificial genetic recombination. A recombinant substance is the product of 'genetic engineering'.

Red cell See **Erythrocyte**.

Red cell volume See **Blood volume**.

Reducing rinse In **histology**, a potassium metabisulphite/hydrochloric acid solution used to remove non-reacted **Schiff** reagent from tissue sections. Of doubtful value.

Reducing sugar A sugar which, on boiling with an alkaline copper reagent, reduces the cupric copper to cuprons. These sugars include glucose and lactose but other non-sugar compounds such as salicylate will also reduce the reagent.

Reduvid bug The vector of *Trypanosoma (schitzotryparum) cruzi*, known clinically as Chaga's disease or South American **trypanosomiasis**.

Refractive index The constant value for light travelling from air into an optically dense medium, according to the formula:

$$\frac{\text{sine of the angle of incidence}}{\text{sine of the angle of refraction}}$$

Regression Statistically, the use of one or more **variables** (explanatory variables) to explain or predict another variable. If one variable is thought to follow approximately a straight line relationship with a second variable, this is called simple linear regression. If several explanatory variables are used, then this is called multiple regression. See also **Scatter diagram**.

Regressive staining Exploitation of the different **avidity** of various tissue groups for different **dyes** by over-staining all tissue structures and then selectively removing the dye from unwanted tissue groups.

Reider cell A type of **lymphocyte** with a deeply clefted nucleus, and which may be observed in **chronic** lymphatic **leukaemia**.

Reiter's syndrome A disorder involving rash, arthritis, uveitis and mucous membrane lesions, occurring in association with urethritis or gastroenteritis. The disease lasts for several months and reoccurs over many years. There is a positive association with histocompatibility **antigen** HLA-B27. **Tetracycline** is also alleged to be helpful in treatment.

Relapsing fever A syndrome of headache, **fever**, arthralgia, myalgia, rash and often cough and meningism, caused by **infection** with **Borrelia** species. The organisms are introduced by the bites of ticks or lice. The symptoms disappear in a few days, only to reappear at intervals of 1 or 2 weeks. Death can occur due to shock or disseminated intravascular coagulation. Diagnosis is by demonstration of **spirochaetes** in blood films. The drugs of choice for treatment are **penicillin**, **tetracycline** or **chloramphenicol**.

Relative Centrifugal Force The relative weight of a particle being subjected to centrifugation compared with its normal weight. Centrifugal force is measured in terms of gravities. Relative centrifugal force (RCF) may be calculated from the formula $11 \cdot 18 \times 10^{-6} \times r \times N^2$), where r is the radius of the centrifuge (measured from the centre of the shaft to the base of the container) and N^2) is the number of revolutions per minute.

Reoviridae A family of RNA **viruses** without **envelopes**, 50–80 nm in diameter and with a double layer of **capsomeres** arranged in concentric spheres around the **nucleoprotein**. The **genome** is unique among animal **RNA** viruses in being double-stranded; it is also segmented. There are three genera, **Reovirus**, **Rotavirus** and Orbivirus.

Reovirus A genus of the **Reoviridae**, found in various species including man. The **RNA** has 10 segments. They are not known to cause any human disease.

Replica plating A method of transferring growth of a **micro-organism** from a whole **Petri dish** to several different **culture media** so that on non-inhibitory media an exact replica of the colonised distribution is obtained. A block of wood or metal with a flat face, and a diameter just less than that of the Petri dish, is covered with sterile velvet and used to sample the growth by lightly pressing the velvet onto it. The velvet is then lightly pressed onto further plates to produce replicate cultures. The method is used to study mutations in cultures.

Replicate Observations on different individuals or samples which receive the same statistical treatment. These should not be confused with duplicate readings, which are repeat observations on the same individual or sample.

Reptilase⊛ Commercially-available purified venom from the snake *Bothrops atrox*, which has a **thrombin**-like action and is used in blood coagulation studies. Unlike thrombin, however, Reptilase cleaves only **fibrinopeptide** A from **fibrinogen**, and is not affected by the presence of **heparin**.

Resazurin An indicator of **oxidation-reduction potential**, or Eh. The **dye** is colourless when reduced and blue when oxidised. It is used in **culture media** intended for the growth of **anaerobic** types of **bacteria**.

Resin 1. A type of product obtained from the sap of certain plants. 2. In microscopy, synthetic chemicals used for **embedding** specimens, e.g. for **transmission electron microscopy**.

Resistance In **bacteriology**, the lack of susceptibility of a **microorganism** to an **anti-microbial** substance at a stated concentration. If that concentration is within the range likely to be achieved during clinical use then therapeutic failure is to be expected. Resistance to anti-microbials is mediated by several factors including **plasmids**, **transposons**, **bacteriophage** and spontaneous **mutation**.

Resolving power The ability of a lens to distinguish fine detail.

Resonance The property of certain molecules which possess electrons excited to change bond position by the energy of light waves.

Respiratory syncytial virus The only member of the pneumovirus genus of the **Paramyxoviridae**. The **virus** differs from other members of the family in lacking both haem**agglutinin** and **neuraminidase**. It commonly infects children causing, if anything, a common cold-like illness. **Infection** during the first year of life may induce a severe life-threatening bronchiolitis, and it may be the cause of some cases of sudden infant death syndrome (cot deaths). Laboratory diagnosis has traditionally been by isolation of virus in **cell culture**, although use of labelled **monoclonal antibodies** in **immunofluorescence** tests on **exfoliated** cells from the nasopharynx is now the method of choice.

Resorption The biological removal or degradation of calcified tissue by specialised cells and their products.

Respiration 1. In common usage, breathing. 2. In **bacteriology**, a method of energy production in which adenosine triphosphate is formed during the transfer of electrons to an inorganic acceptor. In aerobic respiration the acceptor is oxygen, while in anaerobic respiration the inorganic acceptor is usually sulphate, nitrate or carbonate.

Restricted clone A population of cells derived from the proliferation of a small number of different cells. See **Monoclonal**.

Restriction endonuclease A bacterial **enzyme** that will cleave both strands of **DNA** in a genome at points identified by a specific short sequence of **nucleotides**, giving a characteristic pattern of fragmentation. The fragments are then separated by gel electrophoresis and the patterns compared.

Reticulate body The replicating form of the **Chlamydia** species of **micro-organism**.

Reticulin Delicate, frequently branching, connective tissue fibres supporting dense cellular organs such as liver and lymph node. Periodicity is identical to **collagen**, but reticulin contains more interfibrillar material.

Reticulocyte A young **erythrocyte**, slightly larger than a mature red cell, and which still contains some reticular material after expulsion of the nucleus in the late **normoblast** stage. The reticulocyte can be demonstrated supravitally with **brilliant cresyl blue** and may exhibit **polychromasia** in **blood films** which have been **Romanowsky stained**. In normal peripheral blood between 0·2% and 2·0% of the erythrocytes are reticulocytes.

Resolving power The ability of a lens system to separate two closely adjacent points. It depends upon the **numerical aperture** of the system and the wavelength of the illuminant.

Reticulo-endothelial system A collective term for the system of phagocytic cells which derive from a common precursor in the **bone marrow**, which have both **endothelial** and reticular attributes and which show a common **phagocytic** behaviour towards dyes. The mature **macrophage** is one example of a cell which is part of this system, which is concerned with the formation and destruction of blood cells and plays a defensive role in establishing immunity and in cases of inflammation. It is also known as the mononuclear phagocytic system.

Reticulum A small network, such as that of protoplasm in cells.

Retroviridae A family of **enveloped** cubical **RNA viruses** 100 nm in diameter, unique in the possession of a **reverse transcriptase**. Replication of all retroviruses involves integration of transcribed viral **DNA** into the cell **genome**. There are three sub-families, oncovirinae, lentivirinae and **spumavirinae**.

Reversed passive agglutination test A type of **inert particle agglutination test**.

Reverse transcriptase The popular term for **RNA**-dependent **DNA** polymerase, the unique enzyme of the **retroviridae** which mediates the **transcription** of a DNA copy of the viral RNA.

Reye's syndrome A severe, often fatal, fatty encephalopathy. It has occurred in association with infection sufficiently frequently for several **viruses** to have been proposed as the cause, but without clear proof to date.

R-factor A type of **plasmid** which encodes for **resistance** to **antimicrobial** substances.

Rhabdomyosarcoma A **malignant neoplasm** composed of striated muscle.

Rhabdoviridae A family of **enveloped** helical **RNA** viruses. The envelope is cell-derived with added viral **proteins**, and frequently bestows a bullet-shaped **morphology** on the whole **virus** particle. The **virions** are 70−90 nm wide by 300−350 nm long. Two genera infect man and economically important animals, **lyssavirus** and vesiculovirus.

Rh blood group The **blood group** which is second in clinical importance after the **ABO blood groups**. More than 60 different Rh types can be recognised although for clinical purposes blood for **transfusion** is defined only as Rh-positive or Rh-negative, depending upon the presence or absence of an **antigen** called D. Rh **antibodies** − especially anti-D − can cause severe haemolytic reactions following the transfusion of blood carrying the appropriate antigen, and in pregnancy **IgG** forms of anti-D can pass the placental barrier and cause **haemolytic disease of the newborn**.

Rheology The study of the flow behaviour of fluids. Haemorheology is, more specifically, the study of the flow properties of blood, including measurements of blood and plasma **viscosity** and red cell **deformability**.

Rhesus Literally, referring to the rhesus monkey, *Macaccus rhesus*, in which a **blood group antigen** believed to be the same as one found in 85% of white Americans was discovered. It is now known that the monkey antigen is not the same as the human antigen which was named Rhesus (or Rh) after it, although the name has become inseparably attached to the human antigen. See **Rh blood group**.

Rheumatoid arthritis A **chronic** inflammatory condition characterised by swollen joints, anaemia, lymph node enlargement and connective tissue disturbance. The disease may have an **autoimmune** basis.

Rheumatoid factor An **antibody** present in the **serum** of many individuals with **rheumatoid arthritis**. Rheumatoid factor combines with denatured **IgG** and can be detected by a **latex particle test**.

Rhinovirus A genus of the **Picornaviridae**, distinguished from others by their acid lability and **buoyant density**. There are over 100 **serotypes** affecting man, and many more in animals. Some types will grow in **monolayers** in **cell culture**, producing **cytopathic effect**. Others will only grow in organ cultures of human ciliated **epithelium**. Yet more have only been found in volunteer studies. Rhinoviruses are the commonest infectious agents occurring in winter months, causing much morbidity. Years of research have not yet produced any prophylactic agent.

Rhodococcus A **micro-organism** which is **coccus**-shaped and negative by **Gram's stain**. It is found in stagnant water and is a photoorganotroph which produces a red pigment in light and air.

Rhodotorula An asporogenous **yeast** which is widespread in nature and which very occasionally causes systemic **infection** in the **immunocompromised** host. It produces a yellow or red pigment on culture. Microscopically it has been confused with **cryptococcus**. It is asaccharolytic.

RIA See **Radioimmunoassay**.

Riboflavin Vitamin B_2, a fat soluble **vitamin** found in the liver, kidneys and muscles of the body as well as in eggs and some leafy vegetables.

Ribonucleic acid Nucleic acid found in all living cells. The major chemical constituent of the **nucleolus** and a polymer of ribo**nucleotides** which carries the code for **protein** production from **DNA** to ribosomes, and then initiates the actual production.

Richardson's method (for preservation of complement) A method requiring dilution of **complement**-rich **serum** (usually obtained from guinea pigs) in borate buffers prepared in saturated sodium chloride solution. This mixture is stable for up to 1 year at $+4°C$. Prior to use an initial dilution must be made in distilled water to restore the correct physiological osmotic pressure.

Rickettsia A class of rod-shaped − or sometimes coccoid − **bacteria** resembling those which are negative by **Gram's stain**, but which are obligate intracellular **parasites**. They possess both **RNA** and **DNA**, multiply by binary fission, and have bacterial **cell walls**. Only one of the group is a natural infection of man (*R. prowazekii*, the cause of **epidemic** typhus fever). All the group, with the exception of *Coxiella burnettii*, have as **vector** haemagogous arthropods such as lice, fleas, ticks and mites. They are **risk group 3 pathogens** which cause a variety of diseases including typhus (*R typhi*, *R. tsutsugamushi*, *R. proazekii*) and spotted fever (*R. rickettsii*, *R. conorii*); the related *Coxiella burnettii* causes **Q fever**. The main symptoms of rickettsial infection are fever, rash and headache, and diagnosis is by serological tests. *Chloramphenicol* and *tetracycline* are the drugs of choice for treatment.

Rifampicin A derivative of rifamycin, which is produced by the **Streptomyces** species of **micro-organisms**. The drug is active against most **bacteria** which are positive by **Gram's stain**, including *Mycobacterium tuberculosis*, as well as against **neisseria** and **haemophilus**. Activity against other Gram negative organisms is variable. **Chlamydia, rickettsia** and some **protozoa** are also susceptible. On oral or intravenous dosage the drug penetrates widely, including into the normal cerebrospinal fluid and into **neutrophils**. It acts by inhibiting RNA synthesis after binding to RNA polymerase. Side-effects are uncommon but may include abnormalities of liver function. Resistant mutants rapidly develop when the drug is used alone, and it is usually used in combination with **trimethoprim, vancomycin** or **isoniazid**.

Ringer's solution An aqueous solution of sodium chloride 9 g/l, potassium chloride 4·2 g/l, calcium chloride 4·8 g/l and sodium bicarbonate 2 g/l.

Ringing media Material applied to the outer edges of coverslips to seal wet or aqueous preparations. Nail polish and paraffin wax are common examples.

Ringworm A superficial **mycosis** due to **infection** with **fungi** of the **dermatophyte** group.

Risk group *n* **pathogen** Specifies **micro-organisms** of high risk to laboratory personnel, which fall into four groups. *Group 1* are not, in fact, readily **pathogenic**, being organisms that rarely cause disease in spite of regular contact. *Group 2* are those which may often cause disease in laboratory staff, but this (i) can be prevented by administration of a **vaccine**, (ii) can be treated with readily-available and non-toxic drugs, or (iii) may cause self-limiting disease with only moderate morbidity. They require to be handled with reasonable care and good aseptic technique. *Group 3* pathogens are those presenting a serious risk to laboratory personnel. They must be handled in a **class I exhaust protective cabinet** sited in a room away from the general work. (However, specimens containing **hepatitis B virus** or **human immunodeficiency virus** need not be processed in a cabinet provided that steps are taken to avoid needle stick injury and mucous membrane contamination.) *Group 4* pathogens are those presenting a risk of serious illness in laboratory personnel and the community at large. They must be handled in a **class III exhaust protective cabinet** sited in purpose-built accomodation.

RIST Abbreviation for **RadioImmunoSorbent Test**.

Ristocetin Originally used as an **antibiotic**, ristocetin is a potent **platelet aggregation** reagent. **Platelets** from individuals suffering from **von Willebrand's disease** do not aggregate in response to ristocetin.

261

Ristocetin cofactor That portion of the **coagulation factor** VIII molecule that is responsible for **platelet aggregation** to **ristocetin**, and which is deficient in patients with **von Willebrand's disease**.

RK13 cells Cells grown as a **monolayer** in **cell cultures** derived from a normal rabbit kidney. They are particularly useful for the isolation and identification of **rubella virus**.

RNA See **Ribonucleic acid**.

Robot A machine designed to function in place of a living agent.

Robotics The application of **robots** to specific tasks.

Rocket immunoelectrophoresis See **Laurell test**.

ROM See **Read Only Memory**.

Romanowsky, Dimitri Leonidowitsch (1861−1921) Russian physician who in 1891 was first to recommend a method of staining the malaria parasite with eosin and methylene blue. This became the basis of virtually all modern staining methods for blood films. See **Leishman's stain**, **Jenner's stain** and **Wright's stain**.

Romanowsky stains A range of **stains** designed for the staining of cells and **parasites** in **blood films**. The subtle discriminant properties of these stains depends on the presence of derivatives of the interaction between methylene blue and **eosin**. The presence of 'methylene blue azure' is particularly important and is responsible for the 'azurophilic' staining of **neutrophil** granules. **Giemsa's stain**, **Leishman's stain** and **Wright's stain** are examples of Romanowsky methods. **Jenner's stain** and May-Grunwald stain contain unripened methylene blue and therefore are not true Romanowsky stains; however, they are generally used in conjunction with **Giemsa's stain**, which is.

Room temperature A loosely-applied phrase for ambient temperature. Unless otherwise indicated, a range of 18−22°C is generally implied.

Rosette A term used to describe the flower-like appearance of several cells of one type adhering to the surface of a single cell of another type. For example, human **T cells**, mixed with sheep **erythrocytes**, become surrounded by the erythrocytes. The resulting complex has the appearance of a rosette.

Rotavirus A genus of the **Reoviridae**, and a common cause of human and animal **gastroenteritis**. The viral **genome** is segmented in 11 pieces. A number of **antigenic** variants and **electropherotypes** cause disease in man, usually in children and the elderly. Human rotaviruses do not grow readily in **cell culture**; laboratory diagnosis is by **electron microscopy** or **enzyme immunoassay** on clarified faecal samples.

Rothera's test A urine test for acetoacetic acid and acetone, using ammonium sulphate and sodium nitroprusside. When ammonia is layered on to the mixture a purple ring appears at the junction of the layers.

Rothia Rod-shaped **bacteria** which are **aerobes**, do not exhibit **motility** and which are **catalase** positive. They are found typically in dental plaque and carious teeth. They also occasionally cause endocarditis.

Rouleaux formation Aggregation of red cells in a high molecular weight environment, which may superficially resemble agglutination. Typically, when viewed microscopically the cells adhere together with their biconcave surfaces touching, in a formation which has been likened to a pile of coins.

Roundworm Popular name given to **nematode** worms.

Rubella A common childhood illness caused by **rubella virus**, presenting with erythematous rash, cervical **lymphadenopathy**, and mild **pyrexia**. It is of no real concern unless the infection occurs in the first trimester of pregnancy, when severe fetal damage may occur. Rubella syndrome is the term applied to the condition in children born with the more severe symptoms of intrauterine rubella infection such as heart disease, cataracts, deafness and microcephaly.

Rubella virus The only member of the Rubivirus genus of the **Togaviridae**. It is the cause of **rubella** and of severe intrauterine damage when acquired in the first trimester of pregnancy. A wide variety of laboratory tests have been devised for the diagnosis of rubella-like illness early in pregnancy, including **haemagglutination inibition tests**, **single radial haemolysis** and **MACRIA**.

Rubin's technique A method of **elution** of **antibodies** from the surface of red cells by agitation in di-ethyl ether.

Runt A small immature individual. This state can be produced in mice by the injection of **allogenic** lymphocytes into immunologically immature individuals and is an example of **graft-versus-host reaction**.

Russell body A **hyaline inclusion body** sometimes seen in the **cytoplasm** of **myeloma cells**.

Russell viper venom The venom obtained from the Russell viper, and which is capable of activating **coagulation factor** X in the absence of other coagulation factors. The time taken for the **plasma** to clot after addition of the venom and calcium chloride is known as the RVV or Stypven™ clotting time, and is commonly used to distinguish between deficiencies of coagulation factors VII and X in patients with a prolonged **prothrombin time**.

RVV See **Russell viper venom**.

S

Sabin Feldman dye test   A test used to detect the presence of serum **antibodies** of *Toxoplasma gondii*, in which the domestic cat plays a major role as the host. *T. gondii* is found in a high proportion of children with mental disorders.

Sabouraud agar   A **culture medium** for the growth of **fungi**. It has a high concentration of either glucose or maltose, and a low **pH**. Anti-bacterial agents can be added to confer greater selectivity.

SAG-M   See **Optimal additive solution**.

Salicylsulphonic acid   An anionic precipitant which neutralises **protein** cations and thus precipitates the protein. Used in 250 g/l solution as a test for the presence of protein in (e.g.) urine.

Saline   1. Literally, a solution of salts in water. 2. In medical laboratory practice, specifically a solution of sodium chloride of a precise concentration. See **LISS** and **Normal saline** (also known as **NISS**).

Salivaria   The group of **trypanosomes** disseminated by the tsetse fly in its saliva during feeding. See **Trypanosomiasis**.

Salmonella   Rod-shaped **bacteria** which constitute a genus in the **Enterobacteriaceae**. They are usually facultative **anaerobes** which exhibit **motility**, are **catalase** positive, **oxidase** negative and negative by **Gram's stain**. Many serologically distinct species exist. *Salm. typhi* and *Salm. paratyphi* are the causes of typhoid fever and the remaining species are responsible for enteritis or food poisoning, the difference being mainly in the propensity of the organism to invade the blood stream from the gut in the case of typhoid fever. Salmonella species will grow on ordinary **culture media**, but selective media such as deoxycholate citrate **agar** are usually used to suppress the normal intestinal flora.

Salpingitis   Inflammation of the fallopian tubes, usually due to infection with *Neisseria gonorrhoeae*, *Bacterioides fragilis*, *Chlamydia trachomatis* and other organisms. The **antibiotic** of choice for treatment is **tetracycline**, though some cases might need surgical drainage.

Salt link   Union between reactive chemical groups of opposite electrostatic charge. See **Coulombic forces** and **Electrostatic bonding**.

Salzman method   A technique for assessing **platelet adhesion** in which venous blood is withdrawn, under constant vacuum, through a column of glass beads. After a fixed period of time a second blood sample is obtained without passage through glass beads, and **platelet** counts are performed on both samples. The percentage platelet adhesiveness may then be calculated, the normal range being 25−60%.

Sample In statistical usage, part of the **population** which is examined in order to make inferences about the population. Individual members of the sample are usually chosen from the population at random.

Sandfly fever An acute infectious disease characterised by fever, severe headache, orbital pain, etc. Caused by a specific **virus**, inoculated when female sandflies take a blood meal. Occurs commonly in summer around the Mediterranean basin.

Sandwich technique A fluorescent **antibody** technique used to detect antibody in tissue sections. **Antigen** is applied, followed by antibody (labelled with a fluorescent substance) specific for the antigen. The section is then examined by **fluorescence microscopy**. Fluorescing areas indicate antibody present in the original tissue.

Saponification Treatment of tissue sections with alcoholic potassium hydroxide to restore reactivity blocked by **acetylation** or **methylation**, or to render acetylated hydroxyl groups **PAS** reactive.

Sarcoma A **malignant tumour** derived from embryonic connective tissue. These tumours include ones made of immature cells – including **undifferentiated** spindle cells or round cells – and those made up of differentiated cells of such a nature that the tumour may be so designated (e.g. fibrosarcoma, osteosarcoma, etc.).

Saturated fatty acid Fatty acid in which all the free bonds are saturated with hydrogen (i.e. they contain no double bonds).

Saturated lipids See **Saturated fatty acid**.

Scabies A skin disease caused by the scabies mite, *Sarcoptes scabiei*. See **Mite**.

Scalded skin syndrome Also known as **Lyell's disease** or Ritter's disease. It is caused by superficial infection with a strain of *Staphylococcus aureus* which produces exfoliative **toxin**.

Scanning coil Electromagnetic coils used to scan the electron beam over the surface of the specimen in the **scanning electron microscope**.

Scanning electron microscope An electron microscope which scans specimens with a beam of electrons to reveal very fine surface detail. See **Microscopy, electron** and **Transmission electron microscope**.

Scarlet fever An accompaniment of streptococcal **pharyngitis** in which a diffuse red rash appears over the trunk and limbs, due to production of erythrogenic **toxin** by the infecting strain. In most cases the rash subsides in about a week, to be followed by desquamation.

Scatter diagram A statistical diagram in which the value of one **variable** is plotted against a second variable for each individual in the **sample**. This is used to see if there is any relationship between two variables, and should be examined before **regression** analysis is performed.

Schiff reagent Basic fuchsin (or, more accurately, **pararosaniline**) decolourised by sulphurous acid. Used to detect dialdehydes, with which it combines to form a coloured reaction product. See **PAS**.

Schilling count A **differential leucocyte count** modified from the **Arneth count** and widened to classify the **neutrophils** into **myelocytes**, **metamyelocytes**, 'stab cells' and mature, fully segmented neutrophils.

Schilling test A method for assessing **vitamin B12** absorption following oral administration of radio-labelled vitamin B12 and measurement of total radioactivity in a 24 h urine sample.

Schistocyte A red cell containing fragments which may occur in the peripheral blood as a result of mechanical damage within the circulation. Such cells are particularly characteristic of **microangiopathic haemolytic anaemia**.

Schistosoma Digenetic trematodes: human schistosomes or blood **flukes**. The genus *Schistosoma* contains three species (*S. haematobium*, *S. mansoni* and *S. japonicum*), which are important as agents of disease in man. These **parasites** inhabit the mesenteric-portal blood vessels.

Schistosomiasis The name given to a group of diseases caused by trematodes of the genus *Schistosoma*. See **Fluke**.

Schizont A cell undergoing schizogony, a form of asexual reproduction in which multiple **mitosis** occurs; e.g. the **parasites** of malaria produce schizonts which, when mature, release **merozoites** that in turn appear in red blood cells as small ring forms of the parasite. See **Malaria**.

Schumm's test A test for detecting the presence of **methaemalbumin** following addition of yellow ammonium sulphide to **plasma**. Methaemalbumin is converted to ammonium haemochromogen, which gives an intense absorption band on **spectroscopy** at 558 nm.

SCOTEC Scottish Technical Education Council. From 1973 to 1985 the body responsible in Scotland for technical education and training. Replaced in 1985 by **SCOTVEC**.

Scotochromogen A species of **mycobacterium** which produces a pigment only when grown in the dark. An example is *M. scrofulaceum*.

Scott's tap water substitute A mildly alkaline solution of potassium bicarbonate and magnesium sulphate, used for **blueing** of **haematoxylin**-stained tissue sections.

SCOTVEC Scottish Vocational and Educational Council. Since 1985 the body responsible in Scotland for technical education and training.

Secondary cell culture A **monolayer cell culture** derived from a single **passage** of a **primary cell culture**.

Secondary electron Electrons generated from the surface of specimens, struck by the illuminating beam of electrons in a **scanning electron microscope**.

Secondary fixation Sequential application of two fixatives, the first rendering the tissue more resistant to the undesirable effects of the second.

Secondary infection Infection occurring during, or as a result of, a surgical procedure or a course of **anti-microbial** substances to treat a primary infection. An example is candidiasis following a course of broad-spectrum **anti-microbial** substances to treat septicaemia.

Secondary standard A **standard** which has been calibrated against a primary source and to which a value, concentration or activity has been assigned. It is often in the form of a **serum** which is **lyophilised** for long-term storage.

Second-set rejection A term used to describe the heightened **immune response** to a tissue graft seen when a previous similar graft has been rejected. Second-set rejection is more rapid than **first-set rejection**.

Secretin A **hormone** secreted by the duodenum and which stimulates the pancreas to secrete a fluid rich in bicarbonate but low in enzyme content.

Secretion 1. The cellular process involved in production of a specific substance or **hormone** by an organ or gland. 2. Any substance produced by the act of secretion.

Secretor An individual who secretes blood group specific substances in his saliva in a water-soluble form. The state is genetically determined by a dominant gene called *Se*.

Secretory IgA A dimeric form of **IgA** which is present in secretions.

Secretory piece A polypeptide chain associated with dimeric **IgA**. Secretory piece is produced in secretory tissue and may be concerned with the secretion of IgA and/or the protection of IgA against hydrolysis by enzymes in secretory fluids.

Sector In computing, a division of a **track** on a **floppy disc**.

Sedimentation rate See **Erythrocyte sedimentation rate**.

Selective medium A **culture medium** containing an inhibiting substance which is intended to prevent, or considerably diminish, the growth of unwanted organisms, while allowing the growth of those being sought. Selective agents include **anti-microbial** substances, dyes and bile salts.

Selectivity (in staining) See **Specificity**.

Self antigen Any **antigen** expressed on an individual's own normal tissues.

267

Self recognition A term used to describe the capacity of an individual's **immune** system to recognise **self antigens**.

Self tolerance The capacity of the **immune** system of an individual to recognise, but not respond to (tolerate), **self antigens**. This is thought to be acquired during fetal life and/or the neonatal period.

SEM See **Scanning electron microscope**.

Semi-apochromat A type of objective lens intermediate in correction between an **achromat** and an **apochromat**.

Semi-continuous cell line A cell line which can be **passaged** a finite number of times *in vitro*. Laboratory existence is often extended by careful storage of low passage cells.

Sendai virus A mouse **paramyxovirus** serologically identical to para**influenza** type 1 **virus**, and often used to prepare **antigen** for laboratory tests instead of the human strain.

Sensitisation 1. The administration of a **primary dose** of **antigen** to an individual. On subsequent administration of antigen a more pronounced **immune response** is seen in the sensitised individual. 2. The coating of cells (e.g. **erythrocytes**) with specific **antibody**, either *in vitro* or *in vivo*.

Sensitivity (in staining) The ability of a **dye** or staining method to detect tissue substrates in low concentration.

Sensitised cells Red cells to which specific **antibody** molecules have become attached, but which are not **agglutinated**.

Sephadex℠ A substance used for **molecular exclusion chromatography**. It consists of particles of cross-linked dextran which swell to form a semi-solid gel when soaked in **buffer** solutions.

Sepsis A state of **infection**, ranging from wound sepsis which may be trivial or severe, to generalised sepsis with **septicaemia** and metastatic **abscesses**.

Septicaemia An infective state with multiplying **micro-organisms** present in the blood, and associated generalised toxic features such as **fever** and hypotension. A primary focus is often present and secondary foci often develop in the form of metastatic **abscesses**, **meningitis** or **endocarditis**.

Septic shock A collapsed state with **fever**, hypotension and consumption of coagulation factors and **platelets**, mediated by **endotoxin**, or sometimes by other toxic products of **micro-organisms**. Endotoxin activates factors which lead to hypotension, fibrinolysis and coagulation, as well as causing inflammation by activating the **complement** cascade. **Anti-microbial** substances, though important, are not the only factor in the management of this serious condition.

Sequential Multiple Analyser Computer An automatic multi-channel **continuous flow analyser** in which the same repertoire of multiple tests is performed on all samples presented to the analyser. The analytical and data handling processes are controlled by a computer, which is an integral part of the analyser.

Sequestered antigen An **antigen** which is hidden from, or protected from contact with, an individual's **immune** system.

SequestreneⓂ See **Ethylene di-amino tetra-acetic acid**.

Serial In computing, a system in which electrical patterns of **bits** travel in sequence along a wire. See also **Parallel**.

Serial sections In **histology**, the procedure of retaining every section as it is cut from a block of tissue. The sections may be retained loose or mounted on slides. The coarser methods of semi-serial, deeper or cut-down sections are used to ensure that representative levels of the tissue blocks are examined, thus ensuring that small foci of pathology are not missed.

Serine protease Any enzyme which has a serine residue as its active site. Many of the activated **coagulation factors** are serine proteases and therefore can be inhibited by **antithrombin III**.

Seroconversion Describes the difference in levels of **antibody** in **serum** collected in **acute** disease, compared with those found in **convalescent serum**.

Serology The study of serum factors. In particular, the aspect of **immunology** concerned with *in vitro* **antigen/antibody** reactions. For example, serological tests may be used to assist diagnosis or monitoring of an infective process. Such tests rest on the principle that a particular infective agent will give rise to one or more antibodies which will be to some degree specific for that agent, and that their demonstration in abnormally high quantities will therefore imply infection with it. Time must be allowed for such antibodies to be produced, and preferably the results should be compared to a baseline relating to a sample taken during the **acute** phase of the illness before antibody production had increased. Conversely, antisera may be used to identify organisms isolated on culture, or to detect them in biopsy material. Serological tests are also used to determine **blood groups** and **tissue types**.

Serosa A **serous** membrane such as the serous or peritoneal coat of the intestine.

Serotonin See **5-Hydroxytryptamine**.

Serotype 1. In **immunology**, a **blood group** or **tissue type**. 2. In **bacteriology**, a strain of a **micro-organism** which bears **antigens** which can be detected and identified using specific **antibodies**, so that the antigens can be listed as a codified profile. This allows similar strains of organisms to be distinguished for prognostic purposes or for study of their **epidemiology**.

Serratia Rod-shaped **bacteria** which are members of the family

Enterobacteriaceae and which exhibit **motility**, are facultative **anaerobes** and are **catalase** positive, **oxidase** negative, and negative by **Gram's stain**. Usually (but not always) they produce pink or red pigments on culture, and deoxy-ribonuclease is produced. The organisms are found in soil, water and sewage as well as the human intestinal flora. They cause **opportunistic infections** in debilitated or **immunocompromised** patients. Because of their ability to develop resistance to a wide range of **anti-microbial** substances, treatment of such infections is difficult.

Serum The fluid portion of blood which has been allowed to clot, and which therefore does not contain fibrinogen.

Serum iron The total amount of iron carried in the **serum**, and which is bound to **transferrin**. See also **Iron-binding capacity** and **Iron turnover**.

Serum sickness A **type III reaction** of **hypersensitivity** to the injection of **antigens** contained in an **immune** serum. The reaction may occur several days after the administration of the serum and is thus distinct from an **anaphylactic shock** reaction.

Severe combined immunodeficiency (SCID) A **congenital** state of **immunodeficiency** in which both the **T cells** and the **B cells** fail to function normally. The condition is usually recognised in the first few weeks of life.

Sex chromosome A **chromosome** associated with the determination of sex. In mammals they constitute an unequal pair called X and Y.

Sexually transmitted disease An **infection**, the main or only means of transmission of which is by sexual activity, including vaginal or anal intercourse as well as other activities such as fellatio and cunilingus. The features range from the asymptomatic through mild irritation to pelvic inflammatory disease and immune complex sequelae. The causative organisms include *Neisseria gonorrhoeae*, *Chlamydia trachomatis* and the causative organisms of **non-specific urethritis**, as well as **viruses** such as **Herpes simplex**, **Human Immunodeficiency Virus** (HIV) and **Hepatitis B**. The classical example of **Syphilis** is no longer common in developed western countries.

Sezary syndrome A disease characterised by erythroderma and keratosis. The total **leucocyte** count is increased due to the presence of large numbers of Sezary cells, which are of **T cell** origin and show clefted nuclei when examined by **electron microscopy**. Similar cells infiltrate the skin and their presence is diagnostic for the condition.

Shear rate The relative speed of movement between adjacent layers of fluid when that fluid flows in a streamlined fashion. The unit of shear rate is velocity (distance per unit time) divided by distance, which becomes inverse seconds (s^{-1}). See also **Viscosity**.

Shear stress The amount of tangential force per unit area applied to a fluid to produce shearing. The unit of measurement is the Pascal (Pa) or millipascal (mPa). See also **Shear rate** and **Viscosity**.

Shell sort In computing, a **program** which sorts numerically identified data into ascending order, one item being considered at a time and each new item being inserted into the appropriate position relative to the previously sorted items. In the method introduced by Donald L. Shell in 1959 the sorting is done in diminishing increments. For example, if 16 records are to be sorted a 'pass' is made over them in eight groups of two each, which are sorted separately; a second pass is made over the records in four groups of four each; a third pass sorts the records in two groups of eight; and a final pass sorts all sixteen records separately. The increments of 8, 4, 2, 1 are not immutable and other series may be more useful in particular circumstances; it is only necessary that the last increment equals 1. The method has the advantages of being simple to program, it uses minimum space in **random access memory**, and is reasonably rapid in operation. See also **Bubble sort**.

SHHD Scottish Home and Health Department. In Scotland, the government department responsible for health care services.

Shift to the left A term applied to the appearance, in peripheral **blood films**, of **neutrophils** with fewer than the normal number of nuclear lobes.

Shift to the right A term applied to the appearance, in peripheral **blood films**, of **neutrophils** with a greater than normal number of nuclear lobes. Also known as **hypersegmentation**.

Shigella Rod-shaped **bacteria** which are members of the family **Enterobacteriaceae** and which do not exhibit **motility**, are facultative **anaerobes**, usually **catalase** positive and **oxidase** negative, and are negative by **Gram's stain**. The species can be distinguished biochemically and on the basis of **serotypes**. Shigella species are important causes of dysentry in the community.

Shingles The painful recrudescence of herpes varicella/zoster infection, presenting as a cluster of **vesicular** lesions along the line of a spinal or cranial nerve. It is common in the elderly. The disease may disseminate in the **immunocompromised** host, and requires rapid diagnosis and treatment.

S.I. *Systeme international d'Unités.* An internationally accepted system of nomenclature for weights and measures, which has been approved by the World Health Assembly and widely adopted in the medical sciences. The system comprises three types of units: base units, derived units and supplementary units − although the

271

latter are of no relevance in the medical sciences. The base units are: for length, the metre (m); for mass, the kilogram (kg); for time, the second (s); for electric current, the ampere (A); for thermodynamic temperature, the kelvin (K); for luminous intensity, the candela (cd); and for amount of substance, the mole (mol). The derived units are of two kinds. The main kind is derived by multiplying a base unit by itself, or by combining two or more base units by simple multiplication or division. Thus the derived unit for area is the cubic metre (m^3), and that for substance concentration is mole per cubic metre (mol/m^3). Some derived units have special names, however, and those most relevant to the medical laboratory are: for pressure, the pascal (Pa); for energy or quantity of heat, the joule (J); for temperature, the degree Celsius (°C); and for activity of a radionuclide, the becquerel (Bq). Decimal multiples and sub-multiples of SI units are indicated by a series of 16 prefixes (e.g. kilo (k) represents a factor of 10^3; milli (m) represents a factor of 10^{-3}; femto (f) represents a factor of 10^{-15}). Eight very widely used non-SI units have been retained for general use with the SI. They are: for time, the minute (min), hour (h) and day (d); for plane angle the degree (°), minute (') and second ("); for volume, the litre (l) − which is defined in SI terms as 1 dm^3; and for mass, the tonne (t), which in SI terms equals 1000 kg.

Sialic acid Naturally-occuring N-acetylated neuraminic acids, comprising the carboxylated **glycoproteins** of **serum, blood group substances** and **mucins** of the alimentary tract.

Sialidase See **Neuraminidase**.

Sialomucin A **glycoprotein** originating primarily in the **epithelium** and found in salivary glands and other parts of the alimentary system.

Sibling A brother or sister.

Sickle cell The crescent, or 'sickle'-shaped, **erythrocytes** that result from the de-oxygenation of red cells containing **haemoglobin** S. Such cells may be observed in the peripheral **blood films** of patients with **sickle cell anaemia**.

Sickle cell anaemia A form of **haemoglobinopathy** found in individuals who are **homozygous** for the **sickle cell** gene. This results in the replacement of normal adult **haemoglobin** with the abnormal haemoglobin S. Under conditions of relative anoxia, normally encountered in the micro-circulation, sickle cells may be formed. Although initially a reversible phenomenon, irreversible sickling eventually occurs with consequent **haemolytic anaemia**.

Sideroblast A **normoblast** with **Prussian blue**-positive granules in the **cytoplasm**. In normal individuals about half the normoblasts in the **bone marrow** may possess small iron-containing granules.

The so-called 'ringed sideroblast' contains a full or partial ring of larger siderotic granules around the nucleus and is only seen in pathological conditions (e.g. sideroblastic anaemia).

Siderocyte An **erythrocyte** containing iron granules demonstrable by the **Prussian blue** staining technique, and which has persisted from the **sideroblast** stage.

Siderophore A protein with a high affinity for iron. Siderophores are produced by certain **bacteria** in order to bind and transport iron, which is an essential mineral for most organisms. *Yersinia enterocolitica* is able to cause septicaemia in patients with a long history of **blood transfusion**, and therefore potentially of iron overload, and siderophores are considered to be an important factor in the pathogenesis of septicaemia.

Significance level Most statistical **hypothesis tests** involve calculating the value of a function of the data, and then comparing it with tabulated values. The **significance level** is the probability of observing such a value, or a more extreme one, if the hypothesis being tested is true. The smaller the significance level, the more certain it can be that the hypothesis being tested is not true.

Sign test A simple statistical **non-parametric test** used when two observations are taken on the same or related individuals (e.g. the level of a substance in the blood of an individual before and after an operation) in order to see if there has been a change in that **variable**. See **Wilcoxon signed rank test**.

Silent gene A **gene** which produces no detectable product.

Simian herpes virus See **B virus**.

Simpson's rule In **histology**, a method for calculating the total volume of an irregular solid by dividing it into slices of equal thickness and measuring the area of each cut surface.

Simultaneous coupling In **histochemistry**, an enzyme demonstration method in which a reagent present in the incubation medium combines with the enzyme reaction product to form an insoluble, coloured final reaction product.

Single radial diffusion test A **radial diffusion test** in which one reactant is allowed to diffuse radially into an **agar** gel containing the other reactant.

Single radial haemolysis A technique in which **antigen**-labelled **erythrocytes**, mixed with **complement** and molten **agar**, is poured into Petri dishes. **Heat inactivated** serum containing specific **antibody**, when introduced into wells cut into the set agar, will induce the development of zones of **haemolysis** around the well. The size of the zone of haemolysis correlates well with the amount of antibody present. The test is widely used for screening ante-natal samples of blood for **immunity** to **rubella**.

Sinus 1. An anatomical cavity in a bony structure such as the skull, communicating with the atmosphere by way of the upper respiratory tract. The sinuses of the facial region can become congested and infected with **anaerobic bacteria** and other **micro-organisms** (such as *Haemophilus influenzae* or *Streptococcus pneumoniae*), to cause **sinusitis**. 2. A cavernous structure in the vascular system, such as the sagittal sinus in the dura. Septic thrombosis as a result of draining of a facial infection can cause severe life-threatening disease. 3. A track draining **pus** or exudate from a site of **infection** to the outside, or to a hollow viscus. Draining sinuses are seen in staphylococcal **osteomyelitis** and as a feature of actinomycosis.

Sinusitis Inflammation or **infection** of a **sinus** (1) forming part of the upper respiratory tract. The features are headache, local pain and pressure, erythema of the overlying skin, and nasal congestion, often with a post-nasal drip. The commonest **micro-organisms** involved are *Streptococcus pneumoniae*, *Haemophilus influenzae*, **anaerobes** and **rhinoviruses**. An important predisposing factor is air pollution, and particularly tobacco smoke. Complications include brain **abscesses** by direct extension from the sinus.

SIRC cells Cells grown in a **monolayer** in **cell culture** and derived from the cornea of a normal rabbit. **Rubella virus** induces a clear and rapid **cytopathic effect** in these cells.

Sisomycin An **aminoglycoside** type of **anti-microbial** substance produced by **Streptomyces** species, with a spectrum of activity almost identical to that of **gentamicin**. It is not widely used.

Sixteen bit computer A computer which handles data in **words** of sixteen bits at a time. Such a computer is faster in operation than an **eight bit computer**.

Sjorgen's syndrome A condition characterised by inflammation of the salivary and lacrimal glands and usually the conjunctiva (sicca complex). The disease is associated with an **auto-immmune** form of **arthritis**, usually **rheumatoid arthritis**.

Skewness In **statistics**, an alternative term for asymmetry in a **distribution**.

Slant In **microtomy**, the angle between the outer surface of the knife and the surface of the block. This angle is unchanged by variations in the **facet**. See **Rake**.

Sleeping sickness A common name given to African **Trypanosomiasis**. As the infection progresses, so the sufferer becomes more and more lethargic and eventually appears to be constantly asleep.

Slime layer A layer of glycoprotein external to the **cell wall** of **bacteria**, with a loose structure consisting largely of water. Slime layers are found commonly in bacteria of no medical significance in aquatic environments, and are also found under certain conditions in some medically important organisms such as *Pseudomonas* *aeruginosa* and *Staphylococcus epidermidis*. In some cases they undoubtedly contribute to pathogenicity, although their exact functions are unclear.

Slow-reacting substance A A vaso-active amine released from **mast cells** during **type I reactions** of **hypersensitivity**. Its pharmacological activity is similar to that of **histamine**, but it acts more slowly and is not inhibited by anti-histamines. The 'A' stands for **anaphylaxis**.

Slow virus 1. A term applied generally to **virus** infections that take a number of years to induce overt disease. 2. Strictly, the unusual agents causing **spongiform encephalopathy** in man, sheep and mink.

SMACⓉᴹ See **Sequential Multiple Analyser Computer**.

Small pool plasma (Obsolete) **Dried plasma** for **transfusion** prepared from a pool of no more than 10 donations of **whole blood**, in order to limit the spread of **viral hepatitis B**. A volume of 400 ml was **lyophilised** in a bottle and for use was reconstituted by the addition of 400 ml of **pyrogen**-free **distilled water**.

Smallpox The **haemorrhagic fever** with typical **vesicular** rash caused by **Variola** major and Variola minor **viruses**. Once a serious world-wide problem, the disease has been eradicated by the use of a **vaccine** and by aggressive public health measures. See also **Jenner, Edward**.

Smear cell A term usually applied to degenerate **lymphocytes** which appear to have burst and smeared during the preparation of a **blood film**. They are particularly common in **chronic** lymphatic **leukaemia**.

Snap freeze See **Quenching**.

SNBTS Scottish National Blood Transfusion Service.

Somatic Pertaining to the body of a cell.

Somatic mutation In **immunology** the term is used to describe a theory for the **generation of diversity** of **B cells** and **T cells**. The theory suggests that the genes within these cells, coding for surface **immunoglobulin** or T cell **receptors**, mutate during the differentiation of the cells. See **Germ line theory**.

Southern blotting A technique for transferring fragments of **DNA** from the gel in a **polyacrylamide gel electrophoresis** to a nitrocellulose filter paper sheet, followed by exposure to a **radioactive** complementary nucleic acid, and identification of their position by **autoradiography**. A similar technique, referred to as Northern blotting, is used to identify **RNA**. Compare with the technique of **Western blotting**.

Specific gravity The density of a substance compared to that of water. (Also known as relative density.)

Specificity 1. In **Immunology** and determination of **blood groups**,

275

Spectrin

the characteristic of an **antibody** which causes it to react only with one particular **antigen**. 2. In staining, the ability of a **dye** or staining method to discriminate between tissue components.

Spectrin A long fibre-like **protein** assembled into pairs of interwoven chains, which forms the main structural component of the **erythrocyte** membrane.

Spectrophotometer An instrument which is capable of splitting an incident light beam into the parts of the spectrum so that light of a narrow wavelength range can be transmitted selectively. The amount of this light absorbed by a solution is then measured.

Spectroscope An instrument for developing and analysing the spectrum of a substance.

Spectroscopy The study and use of the absorption and emission of light radiation by matter.

Sperm (Spermatazoon) The male gamete (sex cell).

Spherical aberration The failure of rays passing through the periphery of a lens to come to a common focus with those passing through the centre, so producing images with hazy outlines.

Spherocyte A small, densely-staining **erythrocyte** which has lost its central concavity and therefore appears without an area of central pallor in stained **blood films**. Such cells have increased **osmotic fragility**.

Spherocytosis The term used to describe the presence of **spherocytes** in the peripheral **blood film**. The condition may be **congenital** (hereditary spherocytosis) or secondary to other conditions (e.g. **auto-immune haemolytic anaemia** or burns).

Sphingomyelin See **Lecithin/Sphingomyelin ratio**.

Spiramycin A **macrolide** type of **anti-microbial** substance with a spectrum of activity similar to that of **erythromycin**. The drug persists in the tissues for longer than erythromycin.

Spirillum Rod-shaped **bacteria** which exhibit **motility**, are **oxidase** positive and are **aerobic** or **microaerophilic**. They are members of the family Spirillaceae and vary considerably in length. *Spirillum minor* causes **rat-bite fever**.

Spirochaete A general term describing **micro-organisms** which are members of the family Spirochaetaceae, which consists of the genera Spirochaeta, Cristispira, **Treponema**, **Borrelia** and **Leptospira**. They are highly coiled **motile bacteria**, many of which are pathogenic to man, including the causative organism of syphilis (see *Treponema pallidum*).

Spongiform encephalopathy A progressive and fatal disease of the central nervous system caused by the **Kuru** and **Creutzfeldt-Jakob disease** agents.

Spore A resting stage in the metabolism of certain **bacteria** – notably **Bacillus** and **Clostridium** species – in which the organisms

276

are resistant to heat, dessication and starvation. Most sporing organisms have soil as their natural habitat. The spores are usually formed within the body of the cell (**endospores**) and, with some exceptions, possess a thick wall. Calcium dipicolinate is present in high concentrations. Each spore germinates to produce one vegetative cell.

Sporotrichosis A subcutaneous granulomatous **infection** also involving local lymphatic vessels, and caused by the dimorphic **fungus** *Sporothrix schenkii*. Infection commonly follows trivial trauma from thorns or wood splinters. While **amphotericin** B or **miconazole** are indicated in disseminated cases arising in the **immuno-compromised** host, the cutaneous form is usually treated with oral potassium iodide.

Sporozoite The stage of the malaria **parasite** which the infected female mosquito inoculates when taking a blood meal.

Spumavirinae A sub-family of the **Retroviridae**, including the **foamy viruses** of monkeys. They are not known to cause any human disease. In laboratory practise they are important causes of poor sensitivity of primate **cell cultures** used for **virus** isolation.

Sputter coater An apparatus used to apply a very thin conductive coating of metal onto the surface of specimens prior to examination in the **scanning electron microscope**.

Sputum Mucus derived from the lower respiratory tract, and normally removed by the ciliated epithelium or by coughing. In **infective** states such as **bronchitis** or **pneumonia** the sputum is thickened and contains **pus**, plugs of **fibrin** and **erythrocytes**.

Squamocolumnar junction The variable location transition zone border between the stratified **squamous epithelial** lining of the ectocervix and the granular columnar epithelium of the endocervix.

Squamous cell A flat, scale-like cell of the **epithelium**. Four types are recognised: (i) Basal – a small rounded **cyanophilic** cell with a centrally placed **vesicular nucleus** derived from the basal layer; (ii) Parabasal – a small round or oval cyanophilic cell with dense **cytoplasm** and a vesicular nucleus; (iii) Intermediate – a polygonal cell with a cyanophilic cytoplasm and a vesicular nucleus; (iv) Superficial – a large polygonal cell with a **pyknotic** nucleus and cytoplasm which may be either **eosinophilic** or cyanophilic.

ssDNA Single stranded **deoxyribonucleic acid**.

Stab cell A term used to describe a **neutrophil** in which the nucleus has not yet become fully segmented, but which is more mature than the **metamyelocyte**.

Stable factor See **Coagulation factors**.

Stage micrometer A microscope slide with an etched scale, usually divided in units of 0·01 and 0·1 mm. Used in conjunction with an **eyepiece graticule** in **micrometry**.

Stain A compound that will impart colour to tissue and be resistant to simple washing. It is common (but not universal) practice to use the term 'stain' for a **dye** in solution.

Standard A material which is used to calibrate a system, and with which unknowns are compared. See **Primary standard** and **Secondary standard**.

Standard deviation In statistical usage, the most widely used measure of the variability of a quantity in a **population**. It is equal to the square root of the **variance** and is **estimated** by the square root of the **variance** of the **sample**.

Standard error A statistical measure of the accuracy of an **estimated** quantity. The **standard error** of the **mean** of a **sample** equals the **standard deviation** of the **population** divided by the square root of the sample size.

Staphylococcal clumping test A method of detecting **fibrin degradation products** (FDP), based on the fact that certain strains of **staphylococci** are **agglutinated** by serum containing FDP.

Staphylococcus Spherical **bacteria** which do not exhibit **motility**, are **catalase** positive and **oxidase negative**, and are facultative **anaerobes** which are positive by **Gram's stain**. They are members of the family **Micrococcaceae**, along with the genera **Micrococcus** and Planococcus, and 24 species are known to exist. Staphylococci are traditionally divided into those which form **coagulase** and those which do not. Several schemes exist for their classification and identification. *Staphylococcus aureus* causes **abscesses, osteomyelitis, pyoderma, pneumonia, endocarditis** and **septicaemia**, as well as a variety of toxic manifestations such as **toxic shock syndrome**. Coagulase negative species – predominantly *Staph. epidermidis* – cause such lesions only in the **immuno-compromised** host. However, they are the causative organisms of most infections associated with implants such as central venous catheters and hydrocephalus shunts. Staphylococci constitute a major proportion of the normal flora of the skin and mucous membranes. They are usually susceptible to **flucloxacillin** and **aminoglycosides**, and often to **erythromycin** and **fusidic acid**. The only drug to which no strains have yet been reported as resistant *in vitro* is **vancomycin**.

Statistics The mathematical science dealing with the collection, analysis and interpretation of data.

Steatorrhoea The presence of excess fat in the faeces.

Stenosis A narrowing or stricture of a duct.

Stercobilinogen A colourless breakdown product of bilirubin which is oxidised to stercobilin in the gut. Stercobilin contributes to the brown colour of faeces. Some stercobilinogen is excreted in the urine as urobilinogen.

Stercoraria   The group of **trypanosomes** disseminated by the reduvid bug in its faeces, during feeding. See **Trypanosomiasis**.

Stereo microscope   A microscope which provides a three-dimensional image. Usually employing a large split-field objective lens and beam-splitting prisms to provide separate images to each eye. Used principally in the medical laboratory for dissection and for plate culture work.

Steric hindrance   A term used to describe a situation in which two molecules which are able to combine are prevented from doing so, because the shape or presence of other molecules hinders interaction between the combining sites on the two reactants (e.g. interaction between **antigen** and **antibody**).

Sterile   1. Free of living organisms such as bacteria, etc. 2. Unable to produce offspring. See **Sterilisation**.

Sterilisation   1. The killing or removal of all viable **micro-organisms**. Various means exist, each with a different degree of efficiency and reliability, and their use depends to a great extent on the material to be sterilised. Wet heat at temperatures above the boiling point of water – as produced at increased pressure in an **autoclave** – is most efficient and reliable and is to be recommended where possible. Dry heat in the form of incineration is also efficient, but obviously destroys the article to be sterilised, and is only suitable for the disposal of waste. Dry heat at lower temperatures is satisfactory if exposure time is prolonged, and thus is not suitable for many materials although it is very efficient for non-porous materials such as glassware or metal instruments. Chemicals are generally relatively unreliable and inefficient but some, such as glutaraldehyde, have to be used for certain heat-and/or moisture-sensitive objects such as some surgical devices (e.g. fibre-optic scopes) and laboratory equipment (e.g. centrifuges). Fluids are best sterilised by autoclaving, but those which are heat-sensitive can usually be filtered using a filter which will remove **bacteria** and **fungi**, although not **viruses**. See also **Autoclave**, **Disinfectant**, and **Sterile**. 2. The act of rendering an individual incapable of procreation. This may be by means of surgery or the use of drugs. See also **Sterility**.

Sterility   1. The complete absence of viable **micro-organisms**. 2. The inability of a living organism to procreate.

Steroid   A compound which has the basic steroid **nucleus** consisting of saturated phenonthrene cyclic rings with an additional five-membered ring attached.

Sternberg-Reed cell A giant mesenchymal cell with multiple **nuclei** and large **nucleoli**. A characteristic **histological** feature of Hodgkin's disease.

Stillbirth The non-living product of pregnancy, in the human delivered after 28 weeks gestation.

Stimulation The action that results when a compound initiates a response from another compound or organ.

Stomatocyte An **erythrocyte** which in **blood films** which have been **Romanowsky stained** shows a slit-shaped unstained central area in contrast to the circular area of central pallor seen in normal red cells.

Stray light In microscopy, radiant energy in an incident beam which is outside the spectral band pass selected by the monochromator, and which reaches the detector. It is often caused by imperfections in the monochromator.

Streptavidin A **protein** with four high affinity sites for **biotin**; isolated from *Streptomyces avidinii*.

Streptobacillus Rod-shaped **bacteria** which do not exhibit **motility**, are **catalase** and **oxidase** negative facultative **anaerobes** which are negative by **Gram's stain**, and which usually appear in chain or filament formation. They can be isolated on **culture media** enriched with 20% serum. *S. moniliformis* causes **rat-bite fever** and is a **commensal** of the oral cavity of the rat. The drug of choice for treatment is **penicillin**.

Streptococcus Spherical **bacteria** of the family Streptococcaceae which usually do not exhibit **motility**, are **catalase** and **oxidase** negative facultative **anaerobes** which are positive by **Gram's stain**, and which occur in pairs or in a chain formation. Many can be allocated serologically to one of the **Lancefield groups** according to the **cell wall** carbohydrate. *Strep. pyogenes*, the cause of tonsillitis, wound infection and scarlet fever belongs to Group A; *Strep. agalactiae*, a cause of neonatal **sepsis**, belongs to Group B; **enterococci** belong to Group D − and some strains in this group exhibit motility. *Strep. pyogenes* is susceptible to **penicillin** but Group D strains generally are not. Group A strains can be further **serotyped** according to the presence of **antigens** known as M, T and R.

Streptococcus viridans See **Viridans streptococcus**.

Streptokinase A **plasminogen activator** purified from culture filtrates of haemolytic **streptococci**, and which may be administered intravenously as a thrombolytic agent.

Streptolysin A **haemolysin** produced by the **Streptococcus** species of **bacteria**, and especially by those of **Lancefield group** A. Two main types of streptolysin are produced, known as O and S. Streptolysin O is beta-haemolytic and is reversibly inactivated by oxygen. Streptolysin S is produced only in the presence of serum and is oxygen-stable. Streptolysin O is **antigenic**, and **antibody** to it in the serum can be measured for diagnostic and monitoring purposes.

Streptomyces Rod-shaped **bacteria** found in soil and which are filamentous and positive by **Gram's stain**. They produce a number of **anti-microbial** substances, some of which (for example, **streptomycin** and **chloramphenicol**) are clinically useful and are used industrially for the production of potent **antibiotics**. Together with the genus *Nocardia* they are known principally as the cause of serious disease in man and animals.

Streptomycin An **aminoglycoside** type of **anti-microbial** substance produced by the **Streptomyces** species of **micro-organisms**. It is active against a wide range of **bacteria** both positive and negative with **Gram's stain**, including *Mycobacterium tuberculosis*. It acts by binding to the 30s sub-unit of bacterial ribosomes, thus inhibiting protein synthesis. Like other aminoglycosides it is ototoxic and nephrotoxic.

Striated border A specialisation of the free surface of a cell, consisting of rod-like structures which greatly increase the surface area. Noted particularly on the intestinal **epithelium**.

String In computing, a set of characters arranged in sequence and treated by the computer as a single item.

Stripping film Photographic emulsion which may be removed from its backing and floated over tissue sections to reveal sites of **radioactivity**. Used in **autoradiography**.

Stroma 1.The supporting tissue or matrix of a cell or organ. 2. The remaining portion of the **membrane** of a red blood cell after **haemolysis**.

Strop A flexible or rigid length of leather (horsehide) or treated canvas, used to polish a knife edge for **microtomy**.

Stuart (Stuart-Prower) factor See **Coagulation factors**.

Student's test See **t-test**.

Stypven timeᵀᴹ See **Russell viper venom**.

Sub-acute sclerosing pan-encephalitis A progressive and fatal complication of **measles** infection which manifests itself some years after the original disease. Diagnosis is made by the presence of high levels of antibody to **measles virus** in the **serum** and cerebrospinal fluid.

Subset A term used to describe cells with different functions and/ or characteristics within a general cell type. The term is most usually used to describe variations in T cells (e.g. T **helper cells** and T **suppressor cells**).

Substrate 1. A substance or liquid on (or in) which a micro-organism or a tissue **cell culture** grows. 2. A substance which may be transformed into a product or products by the action of an enzyme.

Substrate film A method for the detection of active enzymes (mainly hydrolases) by bringing a thin film of substrate into immediate contact with tissue sections, and subsequently demonstrating the presence or absence of **substrate** in the original film.

Substrate plasma A plasma used in **one-stage clotting assays** which provides all factors necessary for clot formation except the factor under test. In **two-stage clotting assays** a **substrate** plasma may be a normal plasma, containing all **coagulation factors**, which acts as an indicator of the clotting reaction in the first stages of the assay.

Suckling mice These animals are particularly sensitive to laboratory infection with some **viruses**. Choice of this system for the isolation of **Coxsackie** viruses requires that the mice be less than 48 h old, as older animals are not susceptible.

Sucrase The enzyme which is responsible for splitting of sucrose prior to its absorption in the jejunum as glucose.

Sucrose lysis test A test for the diagnosis of **paroxysmal nocturnal haemoglobinuria** (PNH), and based on the fact that red cells adsorb **complement** components from serum at low ionic strength. Because of their abnormal sensitivity to complement, PNH **erythrocytes** undergo haemolysis whereas normal cells do not.

Sudan black stain A cytochemical method to stain the granules of **leucocytes**, many of which contain lipids. The staining pattern closely parallels that of the **peroxidase reaction**.

Sulphaemoglobin A poorly-characterised derivative of **haemoglobin** which can be produced by the action of various **oxidant drugs**. It may be distinguished from **methaemoglobin** by **spectroscopy** and cannot be re-converted to normal **oxyhaemoglobin**.

Sulphite time See **Reducing time**.

Sulphomucin Sulphate containing **glycoprotein** and **sialic acid**, and found in the human colon. Not to be confused with sulphated **acid mucopolysaccharide**.

Sulphonamides A large group of synthetic drugs with **anti-microbial** and other activities. Depending on their structure, sulphonamides may be short-acting (rapidly absorbed and rapidly excreted), medium-acting (rapidly absorbed but slowly excreted) or long-acting (rapidly absorbed but very slowly excreted). In addition, another group is poorly absorbed. These properties allow the choice of an appropriate compound based on frequency of dosage needed as well as site of **infection**. The drugs act by blocking competitively the synthesis of dihydrofolic acid, and therefore purine synthesis. They have a wide potential spectrum of activity against **aerobes** and **anaerobes**, and organisms which are both positive and negative by **Gram's stain**, as well as *Chlamydia trachomatis* and **protozoa**, etc. *Treponema pallidum* is resistant. Unfortunately, wide usage has resulted in development of resistance in most of these organisms. Toxic side effects include rashes, and occasionally agranulocytosis.

Sulphosalicylic acid   See **Salicylsulphonic acid**.

Superinfection   A **secondary infection** arising as a result of suppression of normal **bacterial** flora and overgrowth of resistant organisms during therapy with **anti-microbial** substances. *Candida albicans*, *Pseudomonas   aeruginosa* and *Clostridium difficile* are common causes.

Suppression   The action that results when a compound antagonises, poisons or slows down the response or activity of another compound or organ.

Suppressor cell   (T_s cell). Any lymphoid cell capable of modulating the activity of **T cells** and **B cells**. The term is most usually applied to a **subset** of T cells called T-suppressor cells.

Supravital staining   The staining of cells after removal from the body, but without **fixation**, so that their biochemical functions are preserved. In **haematology**, examples of supravital staining are the demonstration of **reticulocytes** with **brilliant cresyl blue**, and the observation of **leucocyte** mobility after staining with Janus green and neutral red.

Surface decalcification   A method of removing calcium salts from the surface of tissue **embedded** in **paraffin wax** ready for **microtomy**. Usually entailing immersing the surface of the block in 50% hydrochloric acid.

Surface membrane immunoglobulin   (SmIg). **IgD** or monomeric **IgM** found on the surface of **B cells**, where it serves as an antigen **receptor**.

Susceptibility   The inhibition or killing of a culture of **micro-organisms** by a stated concentration of an **anti-microbial** substance, under standard cultural conditions. Such tests provide predictive data from which a choice of an appropriate anti-microbial can be made.

Svedberg unit   A unit of measurement used for the determination of sedimentation coefficients of molecules subjected to **ultracentrifugation**. For examples of the use of the unit see **7S Antibody** and **19S Antibody**.

SV40 virus   A **polyoma** virus of monkeys (SV = Simian Virus). Some people become infected after receiving a **vaccine** prepared from killed **poliovirus**, the polyomavirus having survived the inactivation process. There is no evidence to date of disease resulting from the infection.

Sweat test A test used for the diagnosis of cystic fibrosis. Sodium and chloride concentrations are measured in sweat, which is collected onto a pre-weighed gauze or filter paper.

Swimmers' itch Caused by attachment to the skin, when bathing in streams and ponds, of **cercaria** of **Schistosoma**. See also **Fluke**.

Swimming pool granuloma An ulcerated granulomatous lesion occurring at the site of a trivial injury during swimming or the cleaning of swimming pools or aquaria, and due to infection with *Mycobacterium marinum*.

Synacthen A synthetic ACTH-like product which is used to test the ability of the adrenal cortex to secrete glucocorticoids. After the injection or infusion of synacthen the adrenal cortex response is assessed by measuring blood cortisol.

Syncytium A multi-nucleate cell or aggregate of cells in which the **nuclei** are irregularly arranged and individual boundaries of **cytoplasm** are not visible by light microscopy. They are derived either by arrested cell division or by fusion of adjacent cells. **Virus**-induced syncytia can be very large, containing hundreds of nuclei.

Syndrome A group of symptoms which are present at the same time and are characteristic or diagnostic of a particular disease.

Synergistic gangrene A group of similar syndromes due to **infection** with **streptococci**, **anaerobes**, **staphylococci** and coliform **bacteria** following trauma or surgery. Certain types are very rapidly progressive and require immediate treatment. Most cases require extensive excision of **infected** or necrotic tissue along with high doses of appropriate **anti-microbial** substances such as **penicillin** and **metronidazole**.

Synergy The combined activity of two or more causes or agents, such as drugs or **anti-microbial** substances, which amounts to more than the effects of the individual components simply added together. Such activity often occurs only with certain proportions of some causes or agents, and may be lost or reversed at others.

Syngamy Sexual reproduction. The union of **gametes**. In **protozoology**, as opposed to reproduction by binary fission.

Syngeneic A term which means genetically identical. It is most usually used to describe tissue grafts within an **inbred strain** of experimental animal.

Synthesis 1. Literally, the process of forming, or building up. 2. A series of chemical reactions or metabolic processes leading to the formation of a specific end product.

Synovial fluid A transparent viscid alkaline fluid secreted by the synovial **membrane** and contained in joint cavities, bursae and tendon sheaths.

Syphilis A **sexually transmitted disease** caused by *Treponema pallidum*. A few weeks after exposure a painless lesion or chancre appears which heals spontaneously after a few weeks. About 6 weeks later the secondary stage appears with rash, mouth ulcers, fever, malaise, arthralgia, meningism and sometimes nephritis. This stage may relapse after a latent period of varying duration, but often years long. The tertiary stage then appears with gummas and cardiovascular and neurological involvement. The symptoms of each stage are varied and complex and are not shown by all patients. Treatment with **penicillin** in large doses is usually curative, except in cases of neurosyphilis where success is less certain. Diagnosis of syphilis is by serological tests.

Systematic error In **statistics**, a constant error in a method or result. All results are affected and it may have the effect of shifting the position of results relative to their true value. It will occur (for example) if a standard has been prepared incorrectly or has deteriorated.

Systemic lupus erythematosus (SLE) An **auto-immune** disease characterised by widespread degeneration of many tissues including connective tissue, joints, skin and kidneys. The **serum** of the patient contains **anti-nuclear factor**, and **LE cells** may be demonstrated in the blood.

T

T₃ See **Tri-iodothyronine**
T₄ See **Thyroxine**.
Tadpole cell An elongated club-shaped cell with one broad and one narrow end.
Taipan snake venom The venom of the Taipan snake (*Oxyuranus scutellatus*), which is capable of converting **prothrombin** to **thrombin** in the absence of any other **coagulation factors**.
Takatsy technique A method of producing multiple dilutions, using wire loops to transfer known volumes from well to well in a plastic **agglutination** reaction plate.
T antigen 1. Tumour **antigen** appearing in cells transformed by **adenoviruses** or **polyoma**viruses. They may be the only remaining trace of the transforming **virus**. 2. A **blood group** antigen found on the red cells of all normal adults.
Tape worm The name describes particularly two species, *Taenia solium* and *T. saginata*, generally distributed world wide. Man becomes infected by eating under-cooked meat. See **Proglottid**.
Target cell A form of **leptocyte**, the abnormally thin **erythrocyte** commonly seen in cases of **thalassaemia**. In **blood films** which have been **Romanowsky stain**ed the **haemoglobin** appears at the outer rim and at the centre of the cell, separated by an unstained area, giving the 'target' appearance.
Tartrate lability The condition of an acid phosphatase which is prostatic in origin and is inhibited by tartrate.
TBG See **Thyroxine binding globulin**.
T cell See **T lymphocyte**.
T cell-B cell cooperation The process by which T-**helper cells** interact with **B cells** for the production of **IgG**.
t-distribution Statistically, a bell-shaped **distribution**, symmetrical about zero. Like **normal distribution** but with a larger probability of extreme values. See **t-test**.
TEC Technician Education Council. From 1973 to 1983 the body responsible in England, Wales and Northern Ireland for technician education and training. Replaced in 1983 by **BTEC**.
Teichoic acid Chain-like polymers of polyalcohol phosphates linked to **peptidoglycan** in the **cell wall** of **bacteria** which are positive by **Gram's stain**. They do not appear to be structurally important and their biological function is unclear. Two main types are found − polyribitol and polyglycerol. They are antigenic and can function as **antigens** in diagnostic tests, such as those for *Staphylococcus aureus* infection, though they are not commonly used.

Teichoplanin A glycopeptide **anti-microbial** substance of the **vancomycin** type, produced by Actinoplanes species. Like vancomycin, it acts by inhibiting **cell wall** synthesis. Teichoplanin appears to have greater activity against **enterococci** than does vancomycin, but less activity against **coagulase** negative staphylococci. However, it is probably not **bactericidal** for enterococci, and unlike vancomycin it can be given intramuscularly as well as intravenously, and it has a longer half-life. The implications of *in vitro* studies for clinical results are not yet clear.

Telophase The last of the four stages of **mitosis**, in which the daughter **chromosomes** resolve themselves into a **reticulum** and the daughter **nuclei** are formed. The **cytoplasm** divides to form two complete daughter cells.

TEM See **Transmission electron microscope**.

Template bleeding time See **Bleeding time**.

Template theory An **instructive theory** for **antibody** production which suggests that **antigen** is taken into a **lymphocyte** and used as a template for the production of antibody with a combining site which exactly fits the antigen. This theory is now largely disregarded by modern biologists as being scientifically doubtful.

Terpene resin In **histology**, a useful substitute **mountant** for Canada balsam.

Testosterone An androgenic steroid **hormone** secreted by the testis. It is responsible for the development and maintainance of male sex characteristics such as the genitals, and also of secondary sex characteristics such as growth of beard, deepening of voice at puberty, and bone and body structure. A high local concentration of testosterone is essential for spermatogenesis.

Test strip A solid support medium, usually paper or plastic, which is impregnated with reagents to be used for a test. It may be dipped into the fluid to be analysed or may have the fluid to be tested dropped or smeared on it.

Tetanus A serious neuromuscular syndrome resulting from the action of the **toxin** of *Clostridium tetani*. **Infection** with the organism often follows relatively trivial injury such as a nail puncture wound or a deep scratch from a plant thorn. The greatest risk is trauma which produces a deep, though not necessarily extensive, wound which contains foreign material such as soil, road grit or wood splinters. This provides ideal **anaerobic** conditions for germination of the spores of *Clostridium tetani*, and the relatively mild local infection which results gives rise to a usually generalised intoxication. The **toxin** acts both at the neuromuscular junction and in the spinal cord synapses, and produces characteristic muscular spasms. In developing countries, neonatal tetanus can occur due to the use of animal dung as an umbilical dressing. Tetanus can be prevented by immunisation with the **toxoid**. Treatment is complex and involves surgical debridement of the original site of the trauma, administration of **penicillin**, curarisation and ventilation for prolonged periods.

Tetracyclines A large group of **anti-microbial** substances with very similar chemical structure. They have a wide spectrum of activity, including acting against **bacteria** which are positive by **Gram's stain**, as well as Gram negative organisms with the exception of **Serratia, Proteus** and **Pseudomonas**. They are active against **Mycoplasma, Rickettsia** and **Chlamydia**. The drugs act by binding to the 30s sub-units of bacterial ribosomes, thus inhibiting protein synthesis. Unfortunately, wide usage has led to emergence of resistance in many organisms. The most important side-effects of tetracyclines are secondary infection due to overgrowth of **candida** and deposition in bones and teeth.

Tetrazolium salt In **histochemistry**, a useful marker of enzyme activity, accepting hydrogen atoms (from dehydrogenases and diaphorases) and being reduced thereby to insoluble coloured **formazan**.

Terasaki plate A type of small multi-welled plastic plate used for **agglutination** reactions in immunological tests.

TGT See **Thromboplastin generation test**.

Thalassaemia A group of inherited disorders of **haemoglobin** synthesis, characterised by absent or diminished synthesis of one of the globin chains of haemoglobin.

T$_H$ cell See **Helper cell**.

Thecoma A fibroid **tumour** of the ovary, containing yellow areas of lipoid material derived from theca cells and regarded by some as a form of **granulosa cell tumour**.

Therapeutic index The relationship between toxicity and efficacy of an **anti-microbial** substance. It can be indicated by dividing the dose of a particular anti-microbial which produces toxic effects by the dose which is required for effective treatment (or, in practice, that which gives acceptable blood levels). Anti-microbials such as **aminoglycosides** have a low index because the blood levels associated with toxicity are not much higher than those required for effective therapy.

Thermal amplitude The range of temperature over which an **antibody** will react with its specific **antigen**, or within which a **micro-organism** can be grown in culture.

Thermal optimum The temperature at which an **antibody** will react optimally with its specific **antigen**.

Thermo-electric tissue drier A device for **dehydration** of tissue at low temperature, exploiting the **Peltier effect** and allowing direct infiltration by **paraffin wax** without the use of an ante-medium.

Thin layer chromatography A **chromatography** separation technique in which a solid adsorbent phase is spread on thin plates or films and a liquid phase − often a mixture of solvents − is used as a mobile phase.

Thiobarbituric acid assay A colorimetric test for the measurement of **sialic acid** and **malonyldaldehyde**.

Thioglycollate Sodium thioglycollate, a reducing agent often used in **bacteriology** in fluid and semi-solid **culture media** for relatively non-fastidious **anaerobes**.

Thixotrophy The property of a fluid which flows freely if recently stirred, but which reverts to a gel-like state on standing.

Thoracic duct drainage A method for withdrawing **lymphocytes** through a catheter inserted into the thoracic duct.

Thrombasthenia A **congenital** bleeding disorder characterised by a greatly prolonged **bleeding time** with a normal **platelet** count, but complete absence of **platelet aggregation** in response to **ADP**, **collagen** or **arachadonic acid**. The condition is due to a specific platelet membrane **glycoprotein**, and is also known as Glanzmann's disease.

Thrombasthenin The term once used to describe the **platelet** contractile **protein** responsible for platelet shape, change and contraction, before it was recognised as actomysin.

Thrombin A powerful **serine protease** enzyme derived from the inactive protein **prothrombin** by both **intrinsic blood coagulation** and **extrinsic blood coagulation** pathways. The main function of **thrombin** is to convert **fibrinogen** to **fibrin**, but it also activates **coagulation factors** V, VIII, XIII and **protein C**, as well as being a potent inducer of **platelet aggregation**.

Thrombin clotting time The time taken for citrated **plasma** to clot following addition of **thrombin**. The test is sensitive to **fibrinogen** concentration as well as to the presence of **heparin**, **fibrin degradation products** and **dysfibrinogenaemia**.

Thrombocyte See **Platelet**.

Thrombocythaemia A disorder characterised by the presence of extremely high **platelet** counts ($>800 \times 10^{12}$/l), together with increased numbers of **megakaryocytes** in the **bone marrow**. This malignant disease, also known as Essential Thrombocythaemia, is a member of the **myeloproliferative disorder** group. See also **Thrombocytosis**.

Thrombocytopenia A reduction in the peripheral blood **platelet** count below the lower normal limit of 150×10^9/l.

Thrombocytosis An increase in the peripheral blood **platelet** count above the upper normal adult limit of $450 \times 10^9/l$, usually secondary to an underlying disease state. See **Thrombocythaemia**.

Thromboelastograph An instrument devised to record the clotting time of a plasma sample, together with several physical properties of the clot during its formation and dissolution. It is now rarely used in clinical practice.

Thromboembolism The blocking of a small blood vessel by a blood clot which has been transported through the circulatory system by the blood stream, and which originated in a different, larger blood vessel. The result may be partial or complete destruction of an organ, or part of an organ, supplied by the occluded vessel.

(beta) Thromboglobulin A protein found in the alpha granules of blood **platelets**, which has anti-**heparin** activity, and when detected in plasma represents evidence of recent platelet activation.

Thrombolytic therapy The administration of a drug in an attempt to dissolve a thrombus (blood clot) which has formed inside a blood vessel. See also **Brinase**, **Streptokinase**, **Urokinase** and **Tissue plasminogen activator**.

Thrombomodulin A **protein** found on the surface of **endothelial** cells, which accelerates the activation of **protein C** by **thrombin**.

Thrombophilia A term sometimes used to describe a condition in which there is an abnormal tendency for **thrombosis**, as (e.g.) in individuals with congenital **antithrombin III** deficiency. See **Prothrombotic state**.

Thromboplastin An extract of human or animal brain tissue which accelerates the activation of **coagulation factor** X by factor VII in the **extrinsic blood coagulation system** ('extrinsic thromboplastin'). Thromboplastin is most widely used in the estimation of **prothrombin time**. See also **International reference preparation** and **International sensitivity index**. Thromboplastin is also a term sometimes used to describe the factor X-activating principle generated by activated factor IX, factor VIII and **platelet factor 3** in the **intrinsic blood coagulation** pathway ('intrinsic thromboplastin').

Thromboplastin generation test A test for **coagulation factor** deficiencies of the **intrinsic blood coagulation** system in which mixtures of normal **plasma** and of patient's adsorbed plasma, serum and **platelet substitute** are tested for their ability to clot a normal **substrate plasma**. In this way suspected **coagulation factor** deficiencies may be localised to the patient's plasma (factor V or VIII deficiency), serum (factor IX or X deficiency) or both plasma and serum (factor XI and XII deficiency).

Thrombopoietin A hormone, the presence of which is suggested by experimental evidence to stimulate and control the rate of **platelet** production by the **bone marrow**.

Thrombosis The formation of a blood clot (thrombus) within the vessels of the circulatory system. It is caused by *in vivo* activation of the blood coagulation system, either by a defect in the haemostatic mechanism, as a result of a blood vessel disease, or due to abnormalities in blood flow. The relative contributions of the **platelets, coagulation factors** and other blood cells depend on the site of **thrombosis**.

Thrombospondin A **protein** found in the alpha granules of the blood **platelets**, and which may be involved in **platelet adhesion** to **fibronectin** and **collagen**, and **thrombin**-induced **platelet aggregation**.

Thrombotest™ A commercially-available method for screening the **extrinsic blood coagulation system** and for the laboratory control of oral anticoagulant therapy. The reagent consists of bovine brain **thromboplastin** and modified bovine plasma, and is sensitive to deficiencies of **coagulation factors** II, VII and X. Unlike **Normotest**™, the test is sensitive to the presence of **PIVKA**.

Thromboxanes End products of **prostaglandin** synthesis during **arachadonic acid** metabolism. In **platelets** this pathway leads to the formation of **thromboxane** A_2, a potent inducer of **platelet aggregation**. This is rapidly hydrolysed (30 s) into the more stable and inert thromboxane B_2.

Thromboxane synthetase The **enzyme** which catalyses the conversion, in **platelets**, of the **prostaglandin** intermediates PGG_2 and PGH_2 to **thromboxane** A_2.

Thrush A colloquial name for candida **infection** of the skin and mucous membranes. It is considered by many to be harmless, yet it is often painful and interferes with feeding when it occurs in infants.

Thymectomy The surgical removal of the **thymus**. Neonatal thymectomy of mice leads to a lack of **cell-mediated immunity** and **antibody** response to some **antigens**.

Thymic hypoplasia A congenital abnormality of the immunological functions of the **thymus**. The main effect of this is the failure of **cell-mediated immunity** to develop in the affected individual.

Thymidine kinase An **enzyme** which mediates phosphorylation of thymidine to thymidilic acid. Some **viruses** either carry their own, or induce cells to make a virus-specific enzyme.

Thymosin A **hormone** produced by the **thymus**, which commits stem cells from the **bone marrow** to become **T cells**.

Thymus A lymphoid organ which lies retro-sternally and is responsible for the development of **T cells**.

Thyroid A gland situated in the neck. It secretes a number of **hormones** that are responsible for modulating the rate of metabolism of body cells including growth, mental alertness, etc.

Thyroid stimulating hormone A **hormone** which is secreted by the anterior lobe of the pituitary, and whose target is the **thyroid** gland. It causes the release of T_3 and T_4.

Thyrotrophin See **Thyroid stimulating hormone**.

Thyrotrophin releasing hormone A **hormone** which is secreted by the hypothalmus and which allows the direct stimulation of the anterior pituitary to secrete **thyroid stimulating hormone**.

Thyroxine A compound produced by the follicular cells of the **thyroid**. It acts in a way which increases the rate of **metabolism** of (e.g.) **protein**, carbohydrate and fat. Each molecule contains four atoms of iodine (hence T_4).

Thyroxine binding globulin The globulin which binds 99% of **tri-iodothyronine** (T_3) and 60%−70% of **thyroxine** (T_4). It controls the amount of free **hormone** available and migrates on **electrophoresis** in the alpha-1 and alpha-2 regions.

TIBC See **Total iron-binding capacity**.

Ticarcillin A semi-synthetic **beta lactam** type of **anti-microbial** substance. It has the same spectrum of activity as **carbenicillin**, except for a much higher activity against **pseudomonas**.

Tick Cosmopolitan, wingless eight-legged hard-shelled creatures which are important **vectors** of diseases. They are blood sucking and look like large forms of **mite**, and disseminate many **viruses** to man and animals.

Tinea A superficial **mycosis** affecting the keratinised layer of the skin, and sometimes including the hair and nails. Otherwise known as **ringworm**, it is caused by **fungi** of the **dermatophyte** group.

Tinea imbricata A specific clinical skin condition produced by the fungus *Trichophyton concentricum*, producing scaly lesions in parallel lines. Common in the south Pacific and far east.

Tissue factor The factor present in several body tissues − primarily brain, lung and placenta − which accelerates the activation of **coagulation factor** X by factor VII. The term is synonymous with tissue ('extrinsic') **thromboplastin**.

Tissue plasminogen activator (t-PA). An enzyme which can be isolated from blood, vessel walls and the **culture medium** of some cells (e.g. melanoma), which converts **plasminogen** to **plasmin**. Unlike **urokinase**, t-PA requires the presence of **fibrin** for efficient activation of **plasminogen** and thus may be useful in **thrombolytic therapy**.

Tissue typing The processes by which **histocompatibility antigens** are identified.

Titre 1. The highest dilution of a solution, expressed as a fraction, at which the agent in solution shows detectable activity in a given test system. Titres are usually derived by serially diluting a solution of the active agent by doubling or tenfold steps, and adding the detection system. 2. The reciprocal of the greatest dilution of an **antibody** which will still react in a detectable manner with its specific **antigen**.

TLC See **Thin layer chromatography**.

T lymphocyte See **Lymphocyte**.

Tobramycin An **aminoglycoside** type of **anti-microbial** substance similar to **gentamycin** and produced by **Streptomyces** species. It has a higher activity against **pseudomonas** and is considered to be less toxic than **gentamycin**.

Togaviridae A family of **enveloped** cubical **RNA** viruses 70–120 nm in diameter, with three genera: **alpha virus**, pestivirus and rubivirus. All except the latter are arthropod-borne.

Tolbutamide A compound that stimulates the pancreas to secrete **insulin**. It is used in a test to differentiate insulinomas from other causes of hypoglycaemia.

Tolerance 1. In **bacteriology**, the exhibition of a ratio of **minimum bactericidal concentration** (MBC) to **minimum inhibitory concentration** (MIC) of at least 32. In other words, the concentration of an **anti-microbial** substance needed to kill an organism is much greater than that needed to prevent its growth. Tolerance is not mediated by anti-microbial-inactivating or neutralising enzymes, but is probably due to lack of autolysing enzymes. The effect can be minimised by prolonged incubation. 2. In **immunology**, the capacity of the **immune** system of an individual to be non-reactive to specific **antigens**. Such tolerance may be induced. See also **High dose tolerance** and **Low dose tolerance**.

Tomography Any method of producing an image of a section through a body. This is usually achieved either by use of X-rays or by **nuclear magnetic resonance imaging**.

TORCH screen Acronym for a screening test for **antibodies** to *TOxoplasma gondii*, Rubella, Cytomegalovirus and Herpes simplex. The expression is often used on laboratory request forms accompanying **neonatal** blood samples.

Torulopsis A **yeast** similar to **Cryptococcus**, except that it is saccharolytic and does not produce intracellular starch. *T. glabrata*, the only species associated with human disease, causes a spectrum of disease similar to that of **Candida**, though it occurs less often.

Total iron-binding capacity See **Iron binding capacity**.

Tourniquet test A test for abnormal capillary fragility following the application of a sphygmomanometer cuff above the elbow. A positive result is indicated by the appearance of petechiae on the forearm and is most commonly the result of **thrombocytopenia**.

Toxic epidermal necrolysis A condition mainly affecting adults, and caused by drug hypersensitivity. Also known as **Lyell's disease**, it differs from **scalded skin syndrome** or Ritter's disease, as the latter is caused by a specific exfoliative **toxin** produced by *Staphylococcus aureus*.

Toxicology   1. The study of the poisonous effects of substances on human and animal tissues. 2. The study of poisons and their effects on human and animal tissues.

Toxic shock syndrome   A condition mainly affecting menstruating women, and characterised by **fever**, hypotension, rash, myalgia and thrombocytopenia, and often with diarrhoea, renal insufficiency and disturbance of consciousness. It is due to a **toxin** produced by strains of *Staphylococcus aureus* colonising the vagina, and is possibly aided by the use of tampons. Males and non-menstruating females occasionally develop the syndrome, when it is associated with toxigenic strains of *Staphylococcus aureus* in the skin or other tissues.

Toxin   A substance produced by a **micro-organism**, which has a deleterious effect on cells or tissues of a host, and which can produce this effect experimentally in the absence of the living micro-organisms. **Endotoxin** is a **lipo-polysaccharide** found in the **cell wall** of organisms which are negative by **Gram's stain**, and is released usually only on cell lysis. Exotoxins are proteins released from the organisms during life, during sporulation or germination, or at death. Some are known by their site of action, such as neurotoxin or enterotoxin. Many consist of two sub-units, and the production of some is mediated by **bacteriophage**.

Toxoid   A protein **toxin** which has been treated with formalin to render it non-toxic while retaining its antigenicity.

Toxoplasma   A **micro-organism** of the order **Coccidia**. *Toxoplasma gondii* is an intracellular **parasite** which commonly infects animals and humans, often producing mild or sub-clinical **infection**. The organism persists as tissue cysts throughout the life of the host, and may be re-activated if **immunity** becomes compromised. In the immuno-incompetent, infection usually results in lymphadenopathy with no symptoms, or with **fever** and sore throat, resembling infectious mononucleosis. In the immunodeficient, a severe, and usually fatal, illness results. Infection during pregnancy can result in **congenital** toxoplasmosis, with a high incidence of retinitis and hydrocephalus.

t-PA   See **Tissue plasminogen activator**.

TPHA test   *Treponema pallidum* haemagglutination test. A sensitive test for the presence of **antibodies** to the causative organism of syphilis.

TPI test   The *Treponema pallidum* immobilisation test, for diagnosis of **syphilis**. The test, which depends on the ability of **antibody** to immobilise *T. pallidum* in the presence of **complement**, is now rarely used.

Trachoma A **chronic** inflammatory eye disease caused by repeated **infection** with *Chlamydia trachomatis*. The disease is present in dry areas of the world, and in areas of poor hygiene; both of these features serve to exacerbate re-infection. It may be the commonest preventable blinding disease in the world.

Track In computing, the portion of a moving storage medium (such as a **floppy disc**) which is accessible to a given position of the read/write head (e.g. in a **disk drive**).

Tranexamic acid A water-soluble synthetic **amino acid** which acts as an **inhibitor** of **plasminogen** activation and may be used therapeutically as a fibrinolytic **inhibitor**.

Transaminase One of a group of enzymes involved in the transfer of an amino group from an alpha-amino to an alpha-oxo acid.

Transcobalamin A type of protein responsible for the binding and transport of **vitamin B12** in the peripheral blood. Most of the serum vitamin B12 is bound to transcobalamin I, but some is also carried by transcobalamin II.

Transcription The process of transfer of information from one nucleic acid molecule to another. Double-stranded **DNA** is transcribed to form **messenger RNA**. Single stranded nucleic acids transcribe their information to a **complementary strand**.

Transducer A device which converts information or energy from one form to another, especially physical effects (such as light or temperature) into an electrical signal.

Transduction In **bacteriology**, the transfer of genetic material from a donor to a recipient cell by a **bacteriophage**. A small amount of **DNA** is incorporated into the bacteriophage during its development in the donor. Various characteristics such as toxigenicity and resistance to **anti-microbial** substances can be transferred in this way.

Transfer factor A substance isolated from disrupted **leucocytes**, which is used to transfer **delayed hypersensitivity** to a particular **antigen** from one individual to another, the reaction becoming apparent from 1 to 7 days after administration of the transfer factor. The chemical composition is unknown.

Transferrin An iron-binding protein found in body fluids, and particularly in breast milk. It is a plasma *beta*-**globulin** which is responsible for the transport of iron in the blood to and from **iron stores** and **bone marrow**. Transferrin is synthesised in the liver and each molecule is capable of carrying two atoms of iron. By depriving **micro-organisms** of essential iron, transferrin is thought to increase resistance to **infection**.

Transformation Various assumptions are made when using statistical methods. For example, in **analysis of variance** it is assumed that the within-group **variances** are equal, whereas in **regression**

the variability about the true relationship is assumed to be constant over all values of the explanatory variable(s). If data do not obey the relevant assumptions then **transformations** can sometimes be made on the data to obtain a transformed data set where they do hold. Commonly used transformations are the square root and the logarithm.

Transfusion   The infusion of blood or blood products directly into the circulation of a recipient.

Transfusion medicine   The practise of the clinical aspects of **transfusion**. See also **Apheresis, Blood bank, Blood donor, Blood components, Blood fraction, Blood products** and **Transfusion science**.

Transfusion science   The practise of the laboratory aspects of **transfusion** and of **transplantation**. See also **Blood bank, Blood group, Blood components, Blood fraction, Blood products, Tissue typing** and **Transfusion medicine**.

Transitional epithelium   The **epithelium** lining the renal pelvis, ureters, bladder and urethra. It may demonstrate columnar or squamous features, depending on the degree of contraction of the bladder.

Translation   The process of manufacture of a **protein** from the information encoded on **messenger RNA**.

Transmission electron microscope   A microscope which produces highly magnified images by the use of electromagnetic lenses and a beam of electrons passing through a very thin specimen. See **Microscopy, electron** and **Scanning electron microscope**.

Transmitted light   Light passing from a source, through an optical train to the eye of the observer. The commonly employed mode of illumination in light microscopy.

Transplantation   The surgical procedure of removing tissue from one individual and transferring it to another. See **Autograft, Heterograft, Homograft, Transfusion** and **Transplantation antigen**.

Transplantation antigen   A tissue **antigen** which is capable of stimulating the rejection of a transplant to an individual who lacks the antigen. See **Histocompatibility antigen** and **Transplantation**.

Transport medium   A solution of reagents designed to protect a clinical sample in transit from the patient to the laboratory; in particular, the cotton wool swab commonly used for the collection of specimens for the isolation of **pathogens**.

***Trans* position**   In genetics, the location of two **alleles** on different **chromosomes** of a **homologous** pair.

Transposon   Segments of **DNA** which are able to translocate to foreign DNA and become integrated into it. They are known to transfer from host DNA to plasmid DNA and then be transduced with it to the recipient cell. Some transposons carry genes for resistance to **anti-microbial** substances.

Transudate Any substance which has passed through a **membrane** or been extruded from a tissue. Characterised by high fluidity and low protein content.

Trasylol⊕ See **Aprotinin**.

Traveller's diarrhoea A condition characterised by abdominal pain, watery **diarrhoea**, and sometimes nausea and vomiting. It occurs in association with foreign travel. Most cases are caused by enterotoxigenic *Escherichia coli* which have been ingested with food and drink, but some cases may be caused by (e.g.) **Giardia**.

Trench mouth Acute necrotising ulcerative **gingivitis**, with a characteristic foul odour. There may also be **fever** and malaise. The cause is **infection** by *Borrelia vincentii*. Treatment is local debridement and application of **antiseptics**, and often administration of **penicillin** and **metronidazole**.

Trephine An instrument used to take **biopsies** of bone. Similar to a wide-bore needle, with a serrated cutting edge. The term is also commonly applied to the biopsy so obtained.

Treponema A genus of **micro-organisms** of the family Spirochaetaceae. They are spiral rod-shaped organisms which exhibit **motility** and are strict **anaerobes**; they are associated with the mucous membranes of man and animals. *T. pallidum* causes **syphilis**, *T. pertenue* causes **yaws** and *T. carateum* causes pinta, a cutaneous contagious disease seen in south America. The organisms cannot be cultivated *in vitro*.

Treponema pallidum A **spirochaete**; the causative organism of syphilis. See **Treponema**.

Triangulation number The number of triangles occurring on each face of a **virus** with **icosahedral** symmetry.

Trichomonas A genus of flagellate **protozoa** of the superclass Mastigophora. *T. vaginalis* causes **vaginitis** while other species are sometimes found on other mucous membranes. The organisms can be detected by microscopy or on culture. The treatment of choice is **metronidazole**. See **Trichomoniasis**.

Trichomoniasis A clinical disease, usually referring to infections with *Trichomonas vaginalis*, causing a severe **vaginitis** in females. Two other species of Trichomonads are not uncommonly found, *Trichomonas hominis* seen in faeces and *Trichomonas tenax* of the mouth. See **Trichomonas**.

Trichophyton A genus of **fungi** of the **dermatophyte** group, which causes a superficial **mycosis** known as **ringworm**, or **tinea**, in man and animals.

Trichrome A term applied to **stains** for **connective tissue**, which dye nuclei with one colour and other elements (e.g. muscle, **collagen**, **fibrin**) in two contrasting colours.

Trichuris A nematode, or roundworm, which is a common cause of human intestinal infestation. The eggs are excreted in the faeces and mature in the soil. When ingested they hatch in the small intestine before migrating to the colon. **Infection** is usually asymptomatic.

Tri-iodothyronine (T$_3$) A compound produced by the follicular cells of the thyroid. It acts in a way which increases the rate of **metabolism** of (e.g.) **protein**, carbohydrate and fat. Each molecule contains three atoms of iodine in each molecule (hence T$_3$). Metabolically it is more active than T$_4$.

Trimethoprim A synthetic **anti-microbial** substance with a wide range of activity including many Gram positive and Gram negative rod-shaped organisms, but not Gram positive **aerobic** and **anaerobic** bacilli nor **Pseudomonas**. **Plasmodium** species are susceptible. The drug acts by inhibiting dihydrofolate reductase, thus preventing **purine** synthesis. It shows **synergy** with **sulphonamides**, but only in certain proportions.

Trimming In **histology**, the process of removing superficial wax from the surface of a tissue block and of exposing the complete face of the tissue prior to sectioning.

Triple vaccine A **mixed vaccine** containing **antigens** from three unrelated **bacteria**. The vaccine contains diphtheria **toxoid, pertussis** vaccine and **tetanus** toxoid, and is designed to provide **active immunity** against **diphtheria**, whooping cough and tetanus, simultaneously.

Tris Common abbreviation for the buffer salt Tris (hydroxymethyl) aminomethane.

Trisomy The presence of an additional (third) **chromosome** of one type in an otherwise **diploid** cell.

Tritiate To label with the **radioisotope** of hydrogen called **tritium** (^{3}H).

Tritium A **radioisotope** of hydrogen (^{3}H). A *beta*-emitter with low kinetic energy, making it an ideal agent for **autoradiography**. Used especially to label thymidine, which is firmly bound in **DNA**.

Trophozoite A vegetative or growing stage in **protozoa**.

Trough level That concentration of **anti-microbial** substance remaining in a body fluid or tissue immediately before the next dose is given. See **Peak level**.

True value The actual and accurate quantity of a substance, as determined by the best available reference method.

Trypan blue A **dye** used to distinguish between viable and non-viable cells when counting a suspension in a **haemocytometer**. Viable cells remain unstained while non-viable cells stain deep blue.

Trypanosomiasis Infection with **trypanosomes** which are haemo-flagellates. Disseminated either by tsetse flies (African trypano-somiasis − **sleeping sickness**) or American trypanosomiasis (Chaga's disease), which is disseminated by reduvid bugs.

Trypsin A proteolytic enzyme sometimes used in serological reactions. Obtained from the pancreatic secretions of vertebrates.

Tryptomastigote The morphological form of the **trypanosome** of **sleeping sickness** (African trypanosomiasis), seen in peripheral blood.

TSH See **Thyroid stimulating hormone**

t-test In **statistics**, a **hypothesis** test using the **t-distribution**. The **independent** groups **t-test** is used to compare the **means** of two independent **populations**, each of **normal distribution**, whereas the matched pairs t-test is used where the individual observations come in pairs (i.e. each sample to be **assayed** is divided into two). The two treatments to be compared are allocated so that each pair has one receiving one treatment and the other receiving the second treatment, and the observations are normally distributed.

Tuberculin A sterile fluid containing the growth products of, or extracts from, *Mycobacterium tuberculosis*. It is used as an **antigen** in the **Mantoux test** for delayed **hypersensitivity** to this organism.

Tuberculosis An **infection** with *Mycobacterium tuberculosis*, which tends to be **chronic** and give rise to granulomatous lesions. The infection may involve lungs, kidneys, bone, skin, bowel, central nervous system and other tissues. Factors predisposing to infection − which nowadays is mainly spread by inhalation of droplets − are poor nutritional status, overcrowding and genetic suscepti-bility. Diagnosis is by demonstration of acid-fast **bacilli** in smears of sputum stained by Ziehl-Neelsen's method, and by growth on a **culture medium** such as Lowenstein-Jensen **agar**. Latex tests for demonstration of **antigen** in cerebrospinal fluid have been used experimentally. Treatment of tuberculosis is usually prolonged. Drugs used, always in combinations, include **isoniazid**, **rifampicin**, **streptomycin**, **ethambutol**, **ethionamide** and others.

Tumour 1. A new growth of tissue. See **Neoplasm**. 2. A swelling − often a sign of inflammation.

Tumour marker A tissue component identified as being present on malignant, or absent from normal cells. Examples include **hormone receptors**, **antigens**, **enzymes** and fetal metabolites. May also be detected in body fluids.

Tumour-specific antigen An **antigen** expressed by a tumour cell, but absent from normal adult tissues.

Turnkey system In computing, a **program** which enables a predetermined **file** to be displayed automatically when a **disc** containing both that file and the turnkey program is used to **boot** the system.

Two-stage clotting assay A method for the determination of individual **coagulation factors**, based on the ability of a test plasma to correct a **thromboplastin generation test** (or other two-stage clotting procedure) performed using reagents grossly deficient in the factor under test.

Type and screen A procedure in which potential candidates for **transfusion** of blood products containing red cells have their **ABO blood group** and **Rh blood group** determined and their **serum** screened for the presence of atypical **antibodies**. Subsequent **compatibility tests** prior to transfusion may be simplified and shortened if the blood groups are already known and no unexpected antibodies have been detected. This avoids the need for stocks of a scarce resource being held in reserve, and so being unavailable for other patients, while awaiting a decision on actual transfusion.

Type I reaction (of hypersensitivity) A term used to describe a **hypersensitivity** state in which **antigen** (allergen) binds to specific pre-formed **antibody (IgE)** attached to **mast cell** surfaces. This leads to degranulation of the mast cells and the liberation of vasoactive substances. Asthma and hay-fever are examples of this type of reaction. See **Immediate hypersensitivity**.

Type II reaction (of hypersensitivity) A term used to describe a **hypersensitivity** state in which specific **antibody** binds to **antigens** on cell surfaces, leading to **complement** activation and cell lysis, or phagocytosis of the cell, or attack on the cell by **killer cells**. **Autoimmune haemolytic anaemia** is an example of this type of reaction.

Type III reaction (of hypersensitivity) A term used to describe a **hypersensitivity** state in which humoral **antibody** binds to soluble **antigen**, forming complexes which deposit on the vascular walls. These complexes cause inflammation, which may activate **complement** via the **alternative pathway**, aggregate **platelets** and attract **neutrophils**. **Arthus reaction** is an example.

Type IV reaction (of hypersensitivity) A term used to describe a **hypersensitivity** state in which **T cells** are stimulated by **macrophage**-bound **antigen**. The T cells liberate **lymphokines** and a **lymphocyte**-macrophage **granuloma** is formed. The **tuberculin** test **(Mantoux test)** for susceptibility to **tuberculosis** is an example of this type of reaction.

Typhoid A febrile illness caused by *Salmonella typhi* and *Salm. paratyphi*, and characterised by headache, anorexia, chills, **diarrhoea** or constipation, and the appearance of 'rose spots' – although not all cases exhibit these features and some have addi-

tional ones such as cough, muscle pains and neurological disturbances. The only known reservoir is man. The organism is ingested
with food or drink (including piped water), these sources usually
being contaminated from carriers, either by direct contact or by
faulty sewerage. After about 2 weeks, during which the organisms
multiply in the large intestine, symptoms of **bacteraemia** and
toxaemia appear. In untreated cases the disease is prolonged and
liable to give rise to **abscesses** and bowel perforation. The treatment of choice is **chloramphenicol**. Diagnosis is assisted by serological tests such as the **Widal test**, but this is less reliable than
culture of blood, urine and stools.

Typhus A **febrile** illness caused by *Rickettsia prowazekii* and characterised by headache, chills and muscle pains. The pattern of
fever is different from that of **typhoid**, being constant. Symptoms
appear about 1 week after a bite by an infected body louse, and a
macular rash soon appears. If untreated the illness lasts for about
2 weeks before spontaneous recovery, though this is very slow to
complete. Diagnosis is serological, using the **Weil-Felix reaction**,
which detects **antibody** by **agglutination** of **Proteus** OX19. Treatment of choice is **chloramphenicol** or **tetracycline**.

Tyrosine A naturally occurring amino acid which is an essential
component of the diet of persons with **phenylketonuria**, in whom
its synthesis is deficient.

Tyrosine pigments **Melanin** is the major acknowledged pigment,
derived from the aromatic amino acid **tyrosine**; although **enterochromaffin** and **adrenal chromaffin** are also sometimes included in
this group.

U

Ulex europaeus The common gorse, extracts from seeds of which are used as **lectins** with a **blood group** specificity of anti-H.

Ultracentrifuge A **centrifuge** capable of turning rotors at speeds in excess of 20 000 rpm, and up to 100 000 rpm. It is heavily armoured to protect the environment should a rotor failure occur, and is used for concentrating very small particles such as **proteins**, cell **organelles** and **viruses**, and for various forms of **density gradient centrifugation**.

Ultracryotomy In **histology**, the preparation of very thin sections at low (sub-zero) temperatures for **electron microscopy**. Performed using an **ultramicrotome** with the features of a **cryostat**.

Ultrafiltration A pressurised membrane filtration system which allows the removal, or characterisation by molecular size, of macromolecules such as **proteins**.

Ultramicrotome A special **microtome** for preparing very thin sections necessary for **transmission electron microscopy**.

Ultrasonic Sound waves beyond human hearing. In **histopathology** the energy of ultrasonic waves has been used in attempts to expedite **fixation**, **processing**, **decalcification**, and **staining**.

Ultra-thin section Slices of material cut very thinly − normally less than 100 nm − for examination in the **transmission electron microscope**.

Ultraviolet irradiation The use of short wavelength (<250 nm) **ultra-violet light** to kill **micro-organisms**. Vegetative forms of **bacteria** which are either positive or negative by **Gram's stain**, and **fungi**, are susceptible, but bacterial **spores** and **viruses** are relatively resistant. In addition, the radiation has low energy and does not **disinfect** surfaces such as microbiological **safety cabinets** and operating theatres; however, it has been used in attempts to disinfect water supplies and room air. Severe corneal damage and skin burns result if proper protection is not used.

Ultraviolet light That part of the electro-magnetic spectrum which is of short wavelength (below 380 nm), lying close to the blue/violet part of the visible spectrum. It is employed in **fluorescence microscopy**, the commonly used source being a mercury vapour lamp. See also **Ultraviolet irradiation**.

Undecalcified section A section cut from tissue containing calcium salts, usually bone. Used particularly in the diagnosis of osteomalacia, where **decalcification** would mask the diagnostic features.

Undulant fever A term used to describe **brucellosis**, because of the rising and falling pattern of **pyrexias** seen particularly in infection by *Br. mellitensis*.

Undulating membrane The fold between the **flagellum** and the body surface of flagellated **protozoa**.

Unna-Pappenheim stain A method for the demonstration of **ribonucleic acid** (RNA) in **bone marrow** or peripheral **blood films**, based on the staining reaction with methyl green and pyronin.

Unsaturated lipid Chains of **fatty acids**, containing double bonds (ethylene groups), a feature which is exploited to differentiate **saturated** and unsaturated lipids using (e.g.) the performic acid **Schiff** reaction.

Uraemia The retention of constituents and breakdown products of metabolism in the blood due to the failure of the kidneys to excrete these in the urine.

Uranyl acetate A heavy metal compound used as a **negative stain** in **electron microscopy**.

Ureaplasma A **micro-organism** previously known as 'Mycoplasma T-strains', and having an absolute requirement for urea. It is **anaerobic** and lacks a **cell wall**, being a member of the class **Mollicutes**. *Ureaplasma urealyticum* is a species of Ureaplasma found in the male and female urogenital tracts; its role in disease is unclear, although many attempts have been made to prove a causal association with non-gonococcal **urethritis**. An organism having similar growth characteristics is also found in the upper respiratory tract.

Urease An enzyme which hydrolyses urea to carbon dioxide and ammonia. It is produced by many **micro-organisms** including **Proteus**, some **staphylococci** and *Campylobacter pylori*, which does so extremely rapidly.

Urethritis Inflammation of the urethra, which may be due to **infection** with *Neisseria gonorrhoeae*, *Chlamydia trachomatis*, *Ureaplasma urealyticum*, and occasionally *Trichomonas vaginalis*. *Gardnerella vaginalis* and **anaerobes** are also implicated.

Urinary tract infection An **infection** of the urinary bladder (cystitis), the urethra (**urethritis**), or upper urinary tracts and kidneys ([B[**pyelonephritis**]). Important predisposing factors are breach of the integrity of the system or impedance of the free flow of urine with efficient bladder emptying. Usually the causative organisms are **aerobes** derived from the large bowel. *Staphylococcus saprophyticus* causes cystitis in young women, while in catheterised patients other organisms such as **Pseudomonas** and **Candida** are often implicated. When the predisposing factor is not corrected, infection often relapses or recurs. In the community, lower urinary tract infection can often be treated successfully by one large dose of an **anti-microbial** substance such as **amoxycillin**.

Urobilin See **Urobilinogen**.

Urobilinogen

Urobilinogen The urobilinogens (**urobilin** and urobilinogen) are formed from **bilirubin** by bacterial enzymes in the intestine, and form a red-violet colour with Ehrlich's aldehyde reagent. These compounds are easily metabolised to form urobilins, which cannot be demonstrated with Ehrlich's reagent but combine with zinc to form fluorescent green compounds (Schlesinger's reaction).

Urobilistix™ A commercial **test strip** in which *p*-dimethylamino-benzaldehyde in an acid **buffer** has been impregnated into one end. This is dipped into a sample of urine to detect the presence of excess **urobilinogen** or **porphobilinogen** in the urine.

Urokinase A **plasminogen activator** isolated from urine or kidney cell cultures, which differs from **tissue plasminogen activator** in that it does not require the presence of **fibrin** for efficient activation of **plasminogen**.

Uroporphyrinogen An intermediate product formed when porphobilinogen deaminase acts upon **porphobilinogen**. **Coproporphyrinogens** are then formed after the action of uroporphyrinogen isomerase.

V

Vaccine A product which contains **antigens** derived from whole or fractionated, live or dead **micro-organisms**, and which can be introduced into the body in order to provoke active **immunity** which should provide protection against subsequent **infection** by the organisms (and sometimes related organisms), but without causing the naturally attendant disease. Vaccines often consist either of an attenuated strain of the **virulent** organism which causes a given disease, or a similar avirulent strain or species which has antigenic similarities. An example of a fractionated vaccine is the multivalent pneumococcal capsule vaccine, and **BCG** is an example of an attenuated vaccine (*Mycobacterium bovis*) which also provokes protection against the related organism (*Myco. tuberculosis*). Note: strictly speaking a **toxoid** is not a vaccine.

Vaccinia virus A member of the **orthopoxvirus** genus of the **Poxviridae**, and closely related to **variola** virus. It was used as a **vaccine** for the control − and final eradication − of **smallpox**. Infection with the virus usually resulted in a localised **vesicular** lesion at the site of inoculation. Patients with **eczema**, and those with defective **immunity**, could develop serious − and sometimes fatal − complications. The virus is readily isolated in fertile hen eggs and a variety of **cell cultures**. See also **Jenner, Edward**.

Vacuole A small space or cavity formed in the protoplasm of a cell.

Vacuum embedding In **histology**, infiltration of tissue, especially with wax, during **processing** under reduced pressure, thus facilitating replacement of volatile fluids in particular.

Vaginitis Inflammation of the vagina, which can be due to **infection** with *Candida albicans*, *Trichomonas vaginalis*, *Gardnerella vaginalis* and occasionally *Streptococcus pyogenes*, especially in children. In most cases treatment with **metronidazole**, possibly together with an anti-fungal **anti-microbial** agent, is effective.

Valency 1. In chemistry, an obsolete concept referring to the combining power of an element. It was formerly defined as the number of atoms of hydrogen with which one atom of the element will combine. The concept has now been replaced by that of an oxidation number indicating the theoretical number of electrons gained or lost in converting the atom to the elemental form. 2. In **immunology**, a term used to describe the number of combining sites possessed by an **immunoglobulin** or a large **antigen**. **IgG**, **IgD**, **IgE** and monomeric **IgA** each have a valency of 2 (i.e. they each have two combining sites), but pentameric **IgM** has a theoretical valency of 10. Most large antigens are multivalent.

Vancomycin A glycopolypeptide **anti-microbial** substance similar to **teichoplanin**, and produced by **Streptomyces** species. Most **bacteria** positive by **Gram's stain** (including **enterococci** and **Clostridium** species) are susceptible, but Gram negative bacteria are resistant. Vancomycin acts by inhibiting transfer of murein subunits, and also has an effect on the cytoplasmic **membrane** of the organism. If serum levels are allowed to become excessive the drug is toxic to the eighth cranial nerve and to the kidneys. If it is administered intravenously too rapidly, a histamine-like reaction results. However, the drug is safe and effective with proper use, and can safely be given directly into the cerebral ventricular system.

Van der Waal's forces Intermolecular forces which act as polar attractions between dipoles (i.e. molecules possessing both positive and negative charges). Important in certain **dye**/tissue reactions, and especially in **metachromasia**.

Vapour fixation A method of tissue **fixation** using the vapour or gaseous phase of the fixative (e.g. heated paraformaldehyde). Reputed to give improved preservation and localisation of certain tissue constituents, such as glycogen.

Variable A statistical term for any quantity that can be observed or measured, and which is not always the same.

Variance In statistical terms, the measure of the spread of a **distribution**. It is usually **estimated** by summing the squared differences of observations from the **mean** of the **sample**, and dividing by one less than the sample size.

Varicella Commonly known as chicken pox, a relatively mild **vesicular** rash of childhood caused by herpes **varicella/zoster** virus. Characteristically, **vesicles** at various stages of development are found mainly on the head and trunk. The disease is more severe in adults, and may be life-threatening in the **immunocompromised** host.

Varicella/zoster virus A member of the **Herpetoviridae**, and the cause of varicella (chicken pox). The **virus** becomes **latent** after the primary **infection**, and may recrudesce to cause **shingles**. Infection or recrudescence in the **immunocompromised** host can be serious and life threatening. The virus may be isolated in **epithelial** and **fibroblast** human **cell cultures**, with slow development of a typical **cytopathic effect**.

Variola A **virus** of the **orthopoxvirus** genus of the **Poxviridae**, and the cause of **smallpox**. It has been eradicated as a naturally-occurring **pathogen**, and is held in strict security by a small number of laboratories only.

Vascular Pertaining to blood vessels.

Vasopressin See **Anti-diuretic hormone**.

VDRL Abbreviation for the Venereal Diseases Research Laboratory test for syphilis, which tests the ability of the patient's heated serum to floculate an **antigen** consisting of cholesterol, lecithin and **cardiolipin**.

Vector A vehicle for the spread of **infectious** agents. A carrier of disease or infection, examples in **parasitology** being mosquitoes, flies, **ticks**, **mites**, etc.

Veillonella A species of **bacterium** which appears as diplococci and which does not exhibit **motility**, is **anaerobic**, **catalase** and **oxidase** negative, negative by **Gram's stain**, and which requires carbon dioxide for growth. They are normal inhabitants of the oral cavity and may play a role in periodontal disease.

Venereal disease A sexually transmitted disease.

Ventriculitis Inflammation of the lining of the cerebral ventricles, usually due to **infection**. If this is due to **coagulase** negative **staphylococci** or **enterococci** the inflammatory response may be minimal, whereas if *Escherichia coli* is the cause there will be very high protein levels and grossly elevated **neutrophil** counts.

Vero cells A continuous line of **monkey kidney cells** derived from a normal monkey kidney. They are used in the isolation of **rubella virus** to enhance the number of **infectious** particles prior to inoculation into **RK 13 cells**. They will also support the growth of **herpes simplex**, and some **enteroviruses** and **adenoviridae**. See **Verotoxin**.

Verotoxin A **toxin** which is effective against **vero cells**. The cell line is used to test for bacterial **adhesion** due to **fimbriae**, and for verotoxin production. The toxin, produced by certain strains of *Escherichia coli* (and possibly other organisms), acts as an **enterotoxin**, giving rise to bloody **diarrhoea**, and it is also implicated in the **haemolytic-uraemic syndrome**.

Vertical transmission The spread of an **infectious** agent from parent to offspring via the ovum or the sperm, or *in utero*.

Very-low density lipoprotein Lipoprotein fractions which consist of about 55% triglyceride, 8% **protein** and 18% phospholipids. They migrate in the pre-*beta* **globulin** area on **electrophoresis**.

Vesicle A small blister. A lesion presenting as a localised swelling of the skin, covered by a thin layer of **epidermis** and filled with clear fluid.

Vesicular Usually applied to the description of a **nucleus** with a uniform and open delicate network of **chromatin**, as opposed to a heavily stained shrunken **pyknotic** nucleus.

V-factor Nicotinamide adenine nucleotide, a substance required for growth by *Haemophilus influenzae*. Other **micro-organisms** −

notably *Staphylococcus aureus* – produce the substance in excess, and in mixed cultures of the two organisms colonies of *H. influenzae* are large around the staphylococcal colonies.

Viable count Quantitation of the living **bacteria** in a culture or sample, using cultural methods involving serial dilution and counting of the resulting colonies. It is assumed (inaccurately) that each colony arises from a single colony-forming unit which roughly equates to a single bacterial cell. (Note: densitometric methods measure all the bacteria present and do not distinguish between living and dead cells.)

Vi antigen In **bacteriology**, a polysaccharide capsular **antigen** formed under certain conditions by *Salmonella typhi* and some other enteric organisms. It is related to **virulence** in that it has some protective action against **phagocytosis**. It prevents **agglutination** of the organism by O-antisera, but this can be restored by heating the bacteria.

Vibrating microtome An instrument used to prepare sections of unfixed tissue at temperatures above freezing. The blade vibrates as the tissue passes across the edge. It is the preferred method for demonstrating certain enzymes.

Vibrio Curved rod-shaped **bacteria** which exhibit **motility**, are facultative **anaerobes, catalase** and **oxidase** positive, negative by **Gram's stain**, and found in aquatic environments. Some, such as *Vib. cholerae* and *Vib. parahaemolyticus*, cause human disease; **cholera** is due to an **enterotoxin** produced by *Vib. cholerae*. The organism is ingested with contaminated water or washed vegetables. *Vib. parahaemolyticus* is halophilic (i.e. it has an exceptionally high requirement for sodium chloride) and is found in prawns and other sea food. It produces an enterotoxin but its effect is much milder than that of cholera. Other vibrios (such as *Vib. vulnificus*) occasionally cause human disease, including traumatic wound infections. The organisms will grow on **culture media** designed for enteric organisms, with added sodium chloride where appropriate.

Vicia graminea A south American leguminous plant, extracts of the seeds of which behave as an anti-N **lectin** used in determination of **blood groups**.

Vincent's angina Acute ulcerative **pharyngitis** caused by *Borrelia vincentii*. The treatment of choice is **penicillin**. Diagnosis is made by looking for the **spirochaetes** microscopically.

Viraemia The presence of **infectious** virus particles in the peripheral circulation.

Viral hepatitis See **Hepatitis A, Hepatitis A virus, Hepatitis B, Hepatitis B 'e' antigen, Hepatitis B surface antigen, Hepatitis B virus** and **Hepatitis non-A, non-B**.

Viridans streptococcus   A **streptococcus** which, when grown on horse blood **agar**, produces greening or *beta*-haemolysis around the colonies. Species falling into this group are *Strep. milleri*, *Strep. sanguis*, *Strep. mitior* and *Strep. mutans*. They form part of the normal flora of the oral cavity and the large intestine, and also cause **endocarditis** and **abscesses**. (NB *Strep. pneumoniae* also produces greening on horse blood agar).

Virion   A **virus** particle.

Viroid   1. A term applied to hypothetical **infectious** agents supposed to be the cause of viral mutation. 2. Small lengths of nucleic acid found in plants which are only capable of replication due to the presence of appropriate pathways in the cell. It has been suggested that they could be present in some animal cells.

Virology   The study of the nature of **viruses**. In the medical laboratory the term is particularly applied to the study of their **epidemiology** and **pathogenesis**, and to the means for their detection.

Virolysis   Irreversible structural damage to a **virus**.

Viropexis   Absorption of a **virus** particle into a cell; known in most other circumstances as **pinocytosis**.

Virostatic   An agent which prevents replication of **viruses** without inactivating them. Removal of the agent enables replication to continue.

Virtual image   An image formed by the apparent divergence of rays from a point, rather than their actual divergence.

Virulence   The capacity of a **micro-organism** to cause disease. This is dependent upon its ability to evade host defences and to elicit symptoms and signs of host damage. Evasion of host defences alone does not constitute virulence, as illustrated by 'avirulent' strains of *Corynebacterium diphtheriae* which cause local **infection** but fail to produce the toxic features of **diphtheria**.

Virus   An **infectious** agent consisting of a nucleic acid **genome** of either **RNA** or **DNA**, enclosed in a protective **protein** coat. They are dependent on the pathways of living cells for replication, having no metabolic enzymes.

Viscoelastic   The property of some fluids which, on application of a force, gives rise to a curvilinear rise of **shear stress**, followed by a similar-shaped fall on completion of shearing. In blood this is due to initial elastic deformation of **erythrocytes**, followed by release of elastic energy on completion of shearing.

Viscometer   An instrument for measuring the **viscosity** of fluids. In **haematology** the most common type is the **capillary viscometer**, which measures the time taken for passage of a specific volume of a test fluid along a capillary tube, and is used for measurement of plasma viscosity.

Viscosity   The resistance of a fluid to flow, which may be defined as the **shear stress** divided by the **shear rate**. The **SI** unit of viscosity is therefore the pascal second (Pa s). Plasma viscosity is largely determined by the plasma **protein** concentration, but whole blood viscosity is more complex and is determined by a combination of **packed cell volume**, plasma **viscosity** and **erythrocyte deformability**.

Visible light Radiation between wavelengths of 400 and 700 nm, emitted by tungsten lamps. The blue end of the visible spectrum is at 400 nm and the red end at 700 nm.

Vital staining A method of colouring living cells or tissue. Originally dependent upon **phagocytosis** of **dye** by cells. More recently, a method applied particularly to staining nerve endings in muscle.

Vitamin A general term for several unrelated water- or fat-soluble organic substances necessary for normal bodily metabolism. They are found in trace amounts in various foodstuffs and are designated by letters and numbers; for example, see **Vitamin B12** and **Vitamin K**.

Vitamin B12 A **vitamin** obtained from animal foodstuffs including milk, eggs and meat, which is absorbed from the ileum following its attachment to **intrinsic factor**. **Vitamin B12** is transported in **plasma** bound to the **transcobalamins** and acts as an essential cofactor in the conversions of homocysteine to methionine and methylmalonic acid to succinic acid. Deficiency of vitamin B12 is associated with **megaloblastic anaemia**.

Vitamin K A **vitamin** which, in nature, exists in two forms: vitamin K_1, found in various vegetable oils and leafy plants, and vitamin K_2, a group of compounds which are synthesised by various **bacteria**, including the common gut flora. Both forms are fat-soluble and are only absorbed in the presence of bile salts.

Vitamin K-dependent clotting factors Those **coagulation factors** which depend on **vitamin K** for their synthesis (factors II, VII, IX, X, **protein C** and **protein S**). **Coagulation factors** produced in the absence of vitamin K lack the ability to bind calcium ions essential for normal biological activity. See also **Proteins induced by vitamin K absence or antagonism**.

Voges-Proskauer test A test for acetylmethylcarbinol or acetoin in **micro-organisms**. The substance is a neutral product of glucose metabolism and is found in **Klebsiella**, **Serratia**, **Enterobacter** and other organisms, but not *Escherichia coli*, which produces acid end-products. Various cultural factors such as pO2 and **pH** are important.

Volatile memory In computing, **memory** which is lost when the power supply to the computer is interrupted.

Volume The space occupied by material. The volume of solid material is less affected by pressure whereas the volume occupied by a gas depends largely upon pressure and temperature.

Volutin granules Aggregates of polyphosphate produced in cells of certain **micro-organisms** in response to starvation and consequent impedence of nucleic acid synthesis. They are characteristic of *Corynebacterium diphtheriae* when grown on moist Loeffler's **culture medium** and stained with Albert's or Neisser's stain.

Von Magnus phenomenon Inoculation of large numbers of **virus** particles into a system, resulting in the production of a greatly increased number of **defective interfering viruses**.

Von Willebrand's disease A **congenital** bleeding disorder characterised by a prolonged **bleeding time**, defective **platelet aggregation** in response to **ristocetin**, and a mild to moderate deficiency of **coagulation factor** VIII. See also **Ristocetin cofactor**.

V region (domain) The N-terminal regions of **heavy chains** and **light chains** of **immunoglobulin** (IgG) molecules. The 'V' stands for variable, as these regions of **IgG** chains vary in terms of the amino acid sequence from one immunoglobulin to another. See **Constant region**.

V$_H$ region (domain) The variable region of a **heavy chain** of an **immunoglobulin** molecule. See **V region**.

V$_L$ region (domain) The variable region of a **light chain** of an **immunoglobulin** molecule. See **V region**.

W

Waldenstrom's macroglobulinaemia See **Macroglobulinaemia**.

Wand See **Light pen**.

'Warm' antibody An **antibody** with a thermal optimum of around 37°C.

Warm stage An electrically heated thin microscope stage piece, designed to carry a microscope slide preparation so that it can be examined while being maintained at an even temperature.

Washed cells Red cells freed from excess **serum** or **plasma** by repeated centrifuging through a large volume of a suitable diluent (usually **normal saline**).

Wasserman, August von (1866–1925) German bacteriologist and immunologist who developed the first serological test for syphilis – the **Wasserman reaction** (WR).

Wasserman reaction An obsolescent serological test for syphilis, which detects fixation of **complement** by the non-**treponemal antigen** cardiolipin.

Water-in-oil emulsion A dispersion of water droplets containing **antigen** in mineral oil. The emulsion is stabilised by the addition of an emulsifying agent. Water-in-oil emulsions are used as **adjuvants**.

Water soluble wax Solid polyethylene glycols used in **histopathology** to infiltrate and **embed** tissues, with the advantage of avoiding **dehydration** and **clearing**, and consequent shrinkage. It is difficult to handle and store tissues and sections so prepared.

Wavelength In **wave optics**, the distance measured in nanometres between the troughs conceived as part of the trough/crest formation.

Wave optics The concept that light travels in wave formation rather than in the rectilinear form assumed in **geometric optics**.

W 138 cell A well-characterised type of a **semi-continuous cell line** of fibroblasts, derived from a human embryo lung. They are sensitive to a variety of fastidious **viruses**, including many **serotypes** of **rhinovirus**. Careful storage has lead to their continuing availability many years after their establishment.

Wear and tear pigment A descriptive term applied to **lipofuscin**, to illustrate an association with tissue age, trauma, etc.

Wehnelt cylinder The metal cap which surrounds the **filament** of an **electron gun**.

Weigart, Carl (1854–1904) German pathologist (a cousin of Paul **Ehrlich**) who developed many bacterial and tissue stains and staining techniques, including the use of Weigart's iron **haematoxylin**, still in widespread use today.

Weil-Felix reaction A diagnostic test for the presence of a **Rickettsial** infection, utilising the fact that some Rickettsia share **antigens** with some **serotypes** of **Proteus**. The test involves **agglutination** of a strain of *Proteus vulgaris* (Proteus OX 19) by serum from patients with **typhus**, and depends on the cross-reactivity of somatic **antigens** in the OX 19 strain and *Rickettsia prowazekii*. The pattern of **agglutination** shown by the various Proteus types indicates the particular Rickettsia that may be causing disease. A similar test, using a strain of *Pr. mirabilis* (Proteus OXK) is used to diagnose scrub typhus due to *Rickettsia tsutsugamushi*.

Weil's disease See **Leptospirosis**.

Western blotting In **immunology**, a technique for identifying protein **antigens** (or **antibodies**) by transfer from the gel in **polyacrylamide gel electrophoresis** to a nitrocellulose sheet, upon which the proteins bind as a 'blot' in an identical pattern to that in the gel. This is followed by exposure to a specific antibody (or antigen) labelled with a marker such as a **radioisotope**, an enzyme or a fluorescent dye. In **virology** the technique has been used especially for confirmation of positive screening tests for the presence of antibodies to the **human immunodeficiency virus** (HIV). Compare with the technique of **Southern blotting**.

Wheat germ agglutinin A **lectin** extracted from *Tritium vulgaris*, and which **agglutinates** certain **erythrocytes**.

Whipple's disease A **chronic** systemic **infection** characterised by **diarrhoea**, malabsorption, low grade **pyrexia, lymphadenopathy** and arthralgia. If untreated, the disease progresses over 10–20 years. **Bacteria** have been demonstrated microscopically in tissues but none have been isolated on culture. The treatment of choice is **penicillin** and **gentamicin**, followed by **tetracycline** for up to a year.

WHO World Health Organisation.

Whole blood The blood collected from a **blood donor** for **transfusion**, taken into an **anticoagulant/**preservative solution and otherwise unmodified and not separated into **blood components**.

Whole blood clot lysis time Clotted whole blood is **incubated** at 37°C and the time taken for lysis of the clot is recorded. It is a simple, non-specific and relatively insensitive test for the overall blood fibrinolytic activity, affected by levels of **plasminogen activators, plasminogen, plasmin, fibrinogen** and fibrinolytic **inhibitors**.

Whole blood clotting time The time taken for native (i.e. non-anticoagulated) blood to clot in a glass tube. The normal range is 5–10 min. It is a grossly insensitive test of the **intrinsic blood coagulation** factors but is sometimes used in the laboratory control of **heparin** therapy.

313

Whooping cough See **Pertussis**.

Widal test In **bacteriology**, a test for an **agglutinating** type of **antibody** in the patient's serum to somatic O and flagellar H **antigens** prepared from *Salmonella typhi* and other locally **endemic** species. A test for **Vi antigen** should be included. The usefulness of the test in diagnosis of **typhoid** is disputed. When the individual has been vaccinated against typhoid the diagnostic value of the **titre** of O **antibody** is more reliable than that of antibody to H antigen.

Wide field eyepiece A microscope eyepiece lens designed to increase the field of view by approximately 40%.

Wiener, Alexander S. (1907–1976) American immunologist and blood group serologist who was jointly responsible with Karl **Landsteiner** for discovery of the **Rh blood groups**.

Wilcoxon signed rank test A statistical **non-parametric test** for comparing the **medians** of two **populations** where observations come in pairs, as for the matched pairs **t-test**.

'Wild white' virus A member of the **orthopoxvirus** genus of the **Poxviridae**, found in monkeys and closely resembling **Variola** virus.

Wilm's tumour Embryonal carcino**sarcoma** of the kidney.

Winchester See **Hard disc**.

Winter vomiting An **acute** form of **gastroenteritis**, usually of children, caused by **Norwalk virus** and related **viruses**.

Wiskott-Aldrich syndrome A rare gentically-determined X-linked **immunodeficiency** state characterised by progressively defective **cell-mediated immunity**, production of **antibody**, and bleeding due to **thrombocytopenia**.

Wobbler A focusing aid which produces cyclical electrical deflections of the illumination beam in the **transmission electron microscope**.

Woolsorter's disease Pulmonary **anthrax** caused by inhalation of **spores** of *Bacillus anthracis* from infected hides or wool.

Word In computing, the minimum number of **bits** which the **central processing unit** handles at one moment. It is usually 8, 16 or 32 bits long. (See **Eight bit computer** and **Sixteen bit computer**).

Wound infection Inflammation and **pus** formation in a wound. The causes will differ depending on whether the wound is surgically or traumatically acquired. Most surgical wound infections are due to members of the normal bacterial flora at or adjacent to the site of incision, or from any hollow viscus which was opened. Similarly, most traumatic wounds are infected at the time of infliction by impaction of debris. However, clean wounds can become infected later due to contamination before healing has taken place.

Wright, Almoth (1861–1947) English **pathologist** who developed many basic techniques in **serology**, and who introduced micromethods into **bacteriology**. He did much pioneering work on anti-**typhoid** inoculation and **vaccine** therapy.

Wright's stain See **Romanowsky stains**.

Write In computing, the process of transferring data from the computer's internal **memory** to **Random Access Memory** or to an external storage device such as a **floppy disc**.

Wu and Hoak test A test for the detection and measurement of circulating **platelet** aggregates. Blood is drawn into two syringes, one containing **EDTA** (which disperses **ADP**-induced platelet aggregates) and the other containing EDTA and **formalin** (which fixes platelet aggregates). The ratio of free (i.e. non-aggregated) platelets is a measure of the number of circulating aggregates.

X

Xanthine An intermediate metabolite of **purine**, and the immediate precursor of uric acid.

Xanthomatosis The deposition of yellowish lipid material in the **reticulo-endothelial** cells, skin and other organs.

Xanthrochromic The yellow pigment which is present in cerebrospinal fluid (CSF) following the release of **haemoglobin** into the CSF from **erythrocytes** as a result of subarachnoid or cerebral haemorrhage.

X-chromosome inactivation See **Lyon hypothesis**.

Xenic Growth in culture of multiples of unidentified **microorganisms**.

Xenodiagnosis Diagnosis of disease by infecting an animal. Specifically, a method of detection of certain **parasites**, such as **trypanosomes**, by allowing uninfected insect **vectors** to ingest suspect blood from an animal host. After a delay to allow multiplication, the vectors are examined *post-mortem*.

Xenogeneic Synonym for **Heterogeneic**.

Xenograft Synonym for **Heterograft**.

Xenon lamp A high pressure lamp emitting a spectrum similar to daylight, and of high intensity. Used particularly in projection microscopes, it has a marked tendency to bleach stained tissue sections.

X-factor Haemin, derived from **haemoglobin**, is required for growth of *Haemophilus influenzae* and several other species of **microorganisms**. Discs containing haemin or X-factor, along with those containing **V-factor**, are used in the identification of haemophilus species.

X-ray microanalysis A technique in **electron microscopy** for elemental identification and measurement by electron microscopy. The electron beam causes a characteristic electron shift in the atoms of the specimen, which in turn emit X-rays of characteristic wavelengths.

Xylose A pentose which is not metabolised but is absorbed in the gut and excreted in the urine. It may be given orally to test for intestinal malabsorption. See **Xylose absorption test**.

Xylose absorption test A test in which a dose of sugar (xylose) is given to test the ability of the small intestine to absorb compounds. Xylose is not metabolised and can be measured in blood or urine.

Y

Yaws A contagious non-venereal disease of the skin and bones caused by *Treponema pertenue*, found in tropical locations. Diagnosis, as in **syphilis**, is by microscopical demonstration of treponemes in exudate or by serological tests such as the **VDRL**. Treatment with a single large dose of **penicillin** is usually curative.

Y axis See **Ordinate**.

Yeasts Single-celled **fungi** whose predominant form is the **blastospore**. Some, such as *Cryptococcus neoformans*, do not produce any other structure (though a sexual stage exists), while *Candida albicans* produces pseudohyphae and **chlamydospores** under certain conditions. Other yeasts are sporogenous, but these are of no medical importance.

Yellow fever A **haemorrhagic fever** of man and primates caused by yellow fever **virus** − a member of the **Flaviviridae**. It is confined to those areas of the world where man, monkeys and the mosquito **vectors** co-exist. European colonisation of Africa, South America and the West Indies was severely affected by this virus.

Yersinia Rod-shaped **bacteria** which are facultative **anaerobes**, **catalase** positive, **oxidase** negative and negative by **Gram's stain**: they are non-capsulated members of the family **Enterobacteriaceae**. *Y. pestis*, the causative organism of plague, does not exhibit **motility** while *Y. enterocolitica* and *Y. pseudotuberculosis* are non-motile at 37°C but motile at 22°C. They grow on McConkey's medium to produce non-lactose fermenting colonies.

Yield stress The minimum force or **shear stress** that must be applied to a fluid before flow begins.

Z

Zein agar A **culture medium** containing zein, which is a protein derived from maize. The substance is superior to corn meal in its stimulation of the production of **chlamydospores** by *Candida albicans*.

Zero order kinetics A state when the rate of enzyme action is dependent on the enzyme concentration only. The concentration of **substrate** is in excess and other conditions, such as time and temperature, are constant.

Ziehl-Neelsen stain A staining method for acid-fast **bacilli**, used mainly to demonstrate **Mycobacterium** species in films and tissues. The fixed material is stained with hot carbol fuchsin followed by decolorisation with a mixture of ethanol and hydrochloric or sulphuric acid, and counter-staining with malachite green or methylene blue. *Myco. tuberculosis* appears as beaded red rod-shaped organisms in a green or blue background. For those 10% of males who are red-green colour blind, a blue-green filter will show the organisms as black rod shapes against a light background when malachite green is used.

Zoonosis An **infection** of animals transmitted occasionally to man, with man-to-man spread being rare. Such infections may be mild in the natural host and severe in man. Examples are **brucellosis** and infection with **Babesia** species.

Zygomycosis An **infection** with **fungi** of the class Zygomycetes (mainly Mucor, Rhizopus and Absidia). The fungi appear in **biopsy** material as broad-branched hyphae with no cross walls. They grow as moulds on ordinary **culture media**. Rhino cerebral zygomycosis occurs mainly in those with **diabetes**, and runs a rapid course. The fungus invades the nasal mucosa and underlying tissues, growing into the sinuses and orbit and extending rapidly into the brain, with **necrosis**, thrombosis and haemorrhage. **Amphotericin B** and surgical debridement are sometimes successful treatment if begun early in the infection.

Zymodeme A population of organisms differing from similar populations in the electrophoretic mobility of certain specified enzymes. Used in **parasitology** to differentiate and identify similar populations of worms, amoebae, **trypanosomes**, etc.

Zymogen A term used to describe an inactive enzyme precursor which becomes an active enzyme when activated by another specific enzyme (e.g. **coagulation factors** II, IX, X, XI, XII, XIII and **plasminogen**).

Zymosan A polysaccharide from the cell wall of yeast, which activates the **alternative pathway** of **complement**.